Recent Results in Cancer Research 71

Fortschritte der Krebsforschung
Progrès dans les recherches sur le cancer

Endocrine Treatment of Breast Cancer

A New Approach

Edited by
B. Henningsen, F. Linder, and C. Steichele

With 76 Figures and 81 Tables

Springer-Verlag
Berlin Heidelberg New York 1980

PD Dr. med. B. Henningsen
Klinikum der Universität Heidelberg,
Chirurgische Klinik, Kirschnerstraße 1,
D-6900 Heidelberg 1

Prof. Dr. med. Drs. h.c. F. Linder
Klinikum der Universität Heidelberg,
Chirurgische Klinik, Kirschnerstraße 1,
D-6900 Heidelberg 1

Dr. med. C. Steichele
ICI-Pharma, Clinical Research, Postfach 103109,
D-6900 Heidelberg 1

Sponsored by the Swiss League against Cancer

ISBN-13: 978-3-642-81408-2 e-ISBN-13: 978-3-642-81406-8
DOI: 10.1007/978-3-642-81406-8

Library of Congress Cataloging in Publication Data. Main entry under title: Endocrine treatment of breast cancer. (Recent results in cancer research; 71) Proceedings of a symposium held in Heidelberg in fall 1978. Bibliography: p. Includes index. 1. Breast-Cancer-Chemotherapy-Congresses. 2. Hormone therapy-Congresses. 3. Estrogen-Physiological effect-Congresses. 4. Hormone antagonists-Congresses. I. Henningsen, Bodo, 1940– II. Linder, Fritz, 1912– III. Steichele, C., 1929– IV. Schweizerische Nationalliga für Krebsbekämpfung und Krebsforschung. [DNLM: 1. Estrogen antagonists-Therapeutic use-Congresses. 2. Breast neoplasms-Drug therapy-Congresses. W1 RE106P v. 71/WP870 E56 1978] RC261.R35 no. 71 [RC280.B8] 616.9'94'008s [616.9'94'49] 79–23333.

Softcover reprint of the hardcover 1st edition 1980

2125/3140–543210

Preface

Progress in basic research has made it necessary to redetermine the possibility of classic endocrine therapy for the treatment of patients with breast cancer.

Exemplary, close cooperation between biochemistry and animal and clinical research led to a truly interdisciplinary and international exchange of ideas and experience at a symposium held in autumn 1978 in Heidelberg. We owe our thanks to ICI-Pharma for the kind support of this symposium.

The participation of Charles Huggins in the meeting as honorary chairman signified to all participants the meaning of this joint endeavour. It was the same Charles Huggins who through experimental work laid the foundation stone for endocrine therapy of prostate and breast cancer, and who applied his findings clinically.

Thousands of patients owe to him relief from their suffering. He contributed greatly to the attempt to find and stabilize the endocrine therapy for breast cancer, for which we thank him sincerely. We hope that the following contributions will similarly serve the well-being of our patients.

December 1979 F. Linder

Foreword

The principal thrust of the studies presented in this volume is that certain synthetic compounds designated antiestrogens have practical value in the clinical treatment of many women with advanced mammary cancer. Under stated conditions, the administration of antiestrogens induces a remission of the malignant disease. The antiestrogens are nontoxic. They are effective in causing regression, of cancer of the breast in some cases. The antiestrogens themselves are estrogenic, but with endocrine properties quite from those of estradiol and other powerful estrogens.

Hormone-responsive cancer cells can be destroyed by hormone deprivation or by hormone surplus – too little or too much, the methods are poles apart (Huggins, 1979). For an example, extinction of hormone-responsive mammary cancer is brought about both by ovariectomy and – dramatically – by administration of estrogens. Heddow et al. (1944) found that large doses of powerful estrogens can have an ameliorative action in human mammary cancer. A paradox seemed to be involved since, in some circumstances, estrogens were apparently activating agents for cancer of the breast. In one room the surgeons were removing sources of estrogenic hormones while nearby the physicians were prescribing estrogens for mammary cancer. The vexatious paradox was solved by experimental studies (Huggins, 1979). The growth-promoting activity of the most potent estrogens (estrone; estradiol; diethylstilbestrol) on the uterus of the rat can be blocked to an appreciable extent by certain antagonists. The inhibition of estrogen-induced uterine growth by the antagonistic substances is impressive and very useful in clinical medicine, but the suppression of estrogenic action is never complete.

The estrogen inhibitors are of two sorts: (a) certain naturally occurring estrogens including estriol and closely related hormonal congeners; hormones in this class are impeded estrogens (Huggins and Jensen, 1955); (b) synthetic compounds whose structure is reminiscent of chlorotrianisene (Tace), a powerful estrogen; compounds in this class are designated antiestrogens. Both sorts of inhibitors have considerable effectiveness in causing regression of certain mammary cancers, of man and animals, under stated conditions.

1) *Impeded Estrogens.* Possible competitive interaction, in vivo at the cellular level, of the three major naturally occurring estrogens was first investigated by Hisaw, Velardo and Goolsby (1953). The estrogens, estradiol-17, estrone, and estriol were tested in every combination for effects each might have on the others vis-à-vis steroid-induced growth of the uterus in the ovariectomized rat; the estrogens were injected simultaneously but at separate sites. The uterine growth induced by minimal effective doses of estradiol or estrone was reduced approximately 50% when estriol was injected simultaneously (Huggins and Jensen, 1955). When estradiol and estrone were administered at the same time there was neither reduction or summation of their growth-promoting effects on the uterus. Despite antiestrogenic activity, the impeded estrogens in large doses are themselves estrogens.

2) *Antiestrogens.* Compounds in this class are chemical analogs of tris(p-methoxyphenyl)chloroethylene. The antiestrogens are usually known by trivial names, they comprise tamoxifen, chloramiphene, nafoxidine, and similar compounds. Holtkamp et al. (1960) administered the antiestrogen chloramiphene to young rats by daily subcutaneous injections. The compound interrupted the estrus cycles and produced metestrus. In animals injected with chloramiphene the weight of the uterus was around 60% of uninjected controls. When mated with normal male rats the females did not become pregnant. All of the antiestrogens are antifertility agents.

In large doses tamoxifen and related compounds are estrogenic; in small quantities they are antiestrogens as well. In this respect the antiestrogens are similar to estriol in their physiologic effect.

References

1. Haddow, A., Watkinson, J. M., Paterson, E., Koller, P. C.: Influence of synthetic oestrogens upon advanced malignant disease. Brit. Med. J. *2,* 393–398 (1944)
2. Hisaw, F. L., Velardo, J. T., Goolsby, C. M.: Competitive interaction of estrogens on uterine growth in rats. Fed. Proc. *12,* 68 (1953)
3. Holtkamp, D. E., Greslin, J. G., Root, C. A., Lerner, L. J.: Gonadotrophin inhibiting and anti-fecundity effects of chloramiphene. Proc. Soc. Exptl. Biol. Med. *105,* 197–201 (1960)
4. Huggins, C. B.: Experimental leukemia and mammary cancer: induction, prevention and cure. Chicago, London: The University of Chicago Press (1979)
5. Huggins, C., Jensen, E. V.: The depression of estrone-induced uterine growth by phenolic estrogens with exygenated functions at positions 6 or 16: The impeded estrogens. J. Exptl. Med. *102,* 335–346 (1955)

Charles B. Huggins[1]

1 Charles Brenton Huggins has been a member of the faculty of the University of Chicago since 1927. From 1951 to 1969 he was director of the Ben May Laboratory for Cancer Research and he has been the William B. Ogden Distinguished Service Professor since 1962. In 1966 he won the Nobel Prize in medicine and physiology for his work on carcinoma of the prostate.

Contents

List of Contributors

P. Alberto
Clinique Médicale Universitaire, Genève (Switzerland)

J. C. Allegra
National Cancer Institute, Bethesda, MD (USA)

L. Barrelet
Centre Hospitalier Universitaire Vandois, Lausanne (Switzerland)

G. Bastert
Klinikum der Johann Wolfgang Goethe-Universität, Frankfurt am Main (Federal Republic of Germany)

R. Becher
Universitätsklinikum der Gesamthochschule Essen, Essen (Federal Republic of Germany)

K. W. Brunner
Inselspital, Universität Bern, Bern (Switzerland)

F. Cavalli
Ospedale San Giovanni, Bellinzona (Switzerland)

J. Dæhnfeldt
The Fibiger Laboratory, Copenhagen (Denmark)

C. J. Dix
The University of Leeds, Leeds (Great Britain)

J. R. Durant
The University of Alabama, Comprehensive Cancer Center, Birmingham, AL (USA)

B. Fisher
The University of Pittsburgh, School of Medicine, Pittsburgh, PA (USA)

H. H. Fiebig
Klinikum der Albert-Ludwigs-Universität, Freiburg (Federal Republic of Germany)

N. Firusian
Universitätsklinikum der Gesamthochschule Essen, Essen (Federal Republic of Germany)

H. P. Fortmeyer
Klinikum der Johann Wolfgang Goethe-Universität, Frankfurt am Main (Federal Republic of Germany)

W. Geiger
Universitäts-Frauenklinik, Köln (Federal Republic of Germany)

B. Henningsen
Klinikum der Universität Heidelberg, Heidelberg (Federal Republic of Germany)

K. B. Horwitz
The University of Texas, Health Science Center, San Antonio, TX (USA)

R. Jakesz
1. Chirurgische Universitätsklinik, Wien (Austria)

E. V. Jensen
The University of Chicago, Ben May Laboratory for Cancer Research, Chicago, IL (USA)

W. Jonat
Kliniken der Freien Hansestadt Bremen, Bremen (Federal Republic of Germany)

C. Jordan
The University of Leeds, Leeds (Great Britain)

P. W. Jungblut
Max-Planck-Institut für Zellbiologie, Wilhelmshaven (Federal Republic of Germany)

W. F. Jungi
Kantonsspital, St. Gallen (Switzerland)

K. Klinga
Klinikum der Universität Heidelberg, Heidelberg (Federal Republic of Germany)

R. Kolb
1. Chirurgische Universitätsklinik, Wien (Austria)

H.-J. Künzig
Universitäts-Frauenklinik, Köln (Federal Republic of Germany)

D. Kummer
Eberhard Karls-Universität, Tübingen (Federal Republic of Germany)

M. E. Lippman
National Cancer Institute, Bethesda, MD (USA)

J. Løber
Finsen Institute, Copenhagen (Denmark)

H. Maass
Kliniken der Freien Hansestadt Bremen, Bremen (Federal Republic of Germany)

G. Martz
Universitätsspital, Zürich (Switzerland)

W. L. McGuire
The University of Texas, Health Science Center, San Antonio, TX (USA)

J. W. Meakin
The Princess Margaret Hospital and the University of Toronto, Toronto (Canada)

R.-T. Michel
Klinikum der Johann Wolfgang Goethe-Universität, Frankfurt am Main (Federal Republic of Germany)

H. T. Mouridsen
Finsen Institute, Copenhagen (Denmark)

K. E. Naylor
The University of Leeds, Leeds (Great Britain)

J. P. Obrecht
Kantonsspital, Basel (Switzerland)

S. Öhl
Universitätsklinikum der Gesamthochschule Essen, Essen (Federal Republic of Germany)

T. Palshof
The Fibiger Laboratory, Copenhagen (Denmark)

W. Piotrowski
Neurochirurgische Klinik, Mannheim (Federal Republic of Germany)

G. Prestwich
The University of Leeds, Leeds (Great Britain)

H. Reiner
1. Chirurgische Universitätsklinik, Wien (Austria)

G. A. F. Ritchie
Imperial Chemical Industries Ltd., Macclesfield, Cheshire (Great Britain)

C. Rose
The Fibiger Laboratory, Copenhagen (Denmark)

B. Runnebaum
Klinikum der Universität Heidelberg, Heidelberg (Federal Republic of Germany)

W. Schein
Vincent-T.-Lombardi Cancer Research Center, Georgetown University, Washington, D. C. (USA)

D. Schmähl
Deutsches Krebsforschungszentrum, Heidelberg (Federal Republic of Germany)

H. Schmidt-Matthiesen
Klinikum der Johann Wolfgang Goethe-Universität, Frankfurt am Main (Federal Republic of Germany)

P. Schmidt-Rhode
Universitäts-Frauenklinik, Köln (Federal Republic of Germany)

K. D. Schulz
Universitäts-Frauenklinik, Köln (Federal Republic of Germany)

J. Stjernswärd
(Ludwig Breast Cancer Study Group) Inselspital, University of Bern, Bern (Switzerland)

B. A. Stoll
St. Thomas' Hospital, London (Great Britain)

J. S. Strobl
National Cancer Institute, Bethesda, MD (USA)

S. Thorpe
The Fibiger Laboratory, Copenhagen (Denmark)

R. K. Wagner
Max-Planck-Institut für Zellbiologie, Wilhelmshaven (Federal Republic of Germany)

P. Weymar
Universitäts-Frauenklinik, Köln (Federal Republic of Germany)

J. E. Wittliff
University of Louisville, School of Medicine and The Cancer Center, Louisville, KY (USA)

Acknowledgement

The editors wish to thank Mrs. Ingrid Beyrow for her invaluable help in preparing this volume.

Introduction

B. Henningsen

Klinikum der Universität Heidelberg, Chirurgische Klinik, Kirschnerstraße 1,
D-6900 Heidelberg 1 (FRG)

At various conferences held during the last few years, breast cancer has been an important subject of discussion. Therapeutic guidelines for primary and secondary treatment have been published by associations of surgeons and gynaecologists, and the need for cooperation has already found its expression in an interdisciplinary approach.

In view of the enormous flood of published treatment results and treatment modalities it seemed appropriate to select one sub-section, i.e., endocrine therapy, and to consider it in more detail. Before the current place of endocrine therapy in the treatment of breast cancer could be determined it was necessary to assess the value of newly developed biochemical assay methods and treatment modalities.

More and more attention has been given to the remarkable advances achieved with chemotherapy in the treatment of advanced breast cancer. While in the past it was generally applied only as "ultima ratio", chemotherapy has now become one of the most interesting therapies, especially since the introduction of combination chemotherapy by Cooper and the subsequent development of various modifications. Indeed, a remarkable step forward was achieved, in that remission rates could be raised from about 20% to 60% or even 80%.

The worldwide discussion on adjuvant chemotherapy added to the diversion of general attention from other treatment modalities.

The traditional methods of ablative and additive endocrine therapy of breast cancer seemed to be declining in importance. Compared with the high remission rates following chemotherapy, a remission rate of 30% achievable with unselected endocrine therapy was considered by many workers to be too low.

Consequently many efforts were made to develop practicable methods of selective endocrine therapy with accordingly higher remission rates. Morphological criteria were of no further help. Neither did the determination of the nuclear sex produce the desired result. Although the "discriminant function" developed by Bulbrook may give some indication as to the hormonal dependence of tumours, this approach was not successful because it involves a very demanding procedure.

The decisive step was taken by Jensen and his group, who succeeded in demonstrating that the determination of hormone receptors in tumour tissues produced results of clinical relevance. In the meantime, various methodological approaches for oestrogen, gestagen, and androgen assays have been developed, which allow differentiation between receptor-rich and receptor-poor tumours. While in receptor-poor tumours practically no response to hormonal manipulation can be observed, objective remission from endocrine treatment can be obtained in about 60% of the cases with receptor-rich tumours. The clinical application of this experience is beginning to gain ground. However, there are still organisational problems, which will have to be overcome.

This new understanding of the mode of action of oestrogens at the cellular level stimulated the search for substances that would be able to block the receptor functions und thus the hormonal activity.

Among the agents discovered, which were classified as anti-oestrogens, special attention is given to tamoxifen, a triphenylethylene derivative, which has now been tested worldwide in more than 1000 documented patients.

Thus two positive innovations in the field of endocrine therapy of breast cancer have to be discussed:

First, the possibilities of a more selective approach by means of hormone receptor assay in tumour tissue, and second, the new modality of treatment available thanks to the development of receptor-blocking substances with anti-oestrogenic activity.

Consequently a book on new approaches to endocrine therapy of breast cancer should give answers to the following four important questions:

1) Are hormonal receptor assays as important as reported?
2) Has the place of endocrine therapy relative to that of chemotherapy changed as a result of the developments mentioned?
3) Does the development of anti-oestrogens demand a re-evaluation of the other ablative or additive endocrine therapies?
4) Is it now necessary to resume the apparently closed discussion on adjuvant endocrine therapy and to consider it under new aspects?

To answer these questions it was necessary to convene leading international research groups and to learn their experience. In this connection it was also of considerable importance to have interdisciplinary discussions in order to avoid one-sided assessment.

On behalf of the Editors I would like to express here our sincere thanks to all contributing authors for their cooperation.

Special thanks, however, go to all those who so generously made it possible to hold and present the discussions required.

I. Improved Biochemical Characterization of Breast Cancer

1. Improved Biochemical Characterization of Breast Cancer as a Guide to Hormonal Treatment

R. K. Wagner and P. W. Jungblut

Max-Planck-Institut für Zellbiologie, Postfach 1009, D-2940 Wilhelmshaven (FRG)

From a theoretical point of view one would expect all oestrogen receptor-positive (ER+) mammary carcinomas to respond to endocrine therapy. However, it is well known that this is not the case, since only 55%–60% of these tumours respond to endocrine measures while 40%–45% do not (JENSEN et al., 1972; ENGELSMAN et al., 1973; MCGUIRE, 1975). The latter tumours are therefore called nonresponding ER+ breast cancers. This group of breast cancers is currently a challenging problem. The question therefore arises as to whether the presence or absence of oestrogen receptor (ER) alone is an adequate parameter for the determination of the hormone dependency of breast cancers or whether it must be supported by further criteria.

Since several physiological phenomena can exert a marked influence on cytoplasmic receptor levels, we believe that the ER alone is not the ideal marker for hormone sensitivity. These phenomena summarised in Table 1, Point 1, "endogenous hormone levels", need little comment. It is certain that cytoplasmic receptor concentrations are inversely related to steroid hormone levels in the plasma to which the tissue is exposed (WAGNER, 1977). We have observed fluctuations in the ER content that are not dependent on the ovaries (point 2) in several mammalian target tissues (HUGHES et al., 1976). An apparent circadian rhythm (point 2a) influences the uterine ER concentrations of ovariectomised rats, and a seasonal variation (point 2b) has been found in uteri of immature calves and ovariectomised pigs and in breast cancer biopsies from postmenopausal women. Finally, a steroid hormone-independent fluctuation of cytoplasmic ER (point 3) has been observed in the uteri of ovariectomised/hypophysectomised rats. Figure 1 shows two examples of the seasonal variation. In experiments where we measured the uterine ER in ovariectomised pigs every month during 1975 (Fig. 1a), the receptor concentration was significantly lower in August, September, and

Table 1. Physiological influences on cytoplasmic receptor concentrations

1. Endogenous hormone levels
2. Ovarian-independent variations:
   a. Circadian
   b. Seasonal
3. Steroid hormone-independent fluctuations

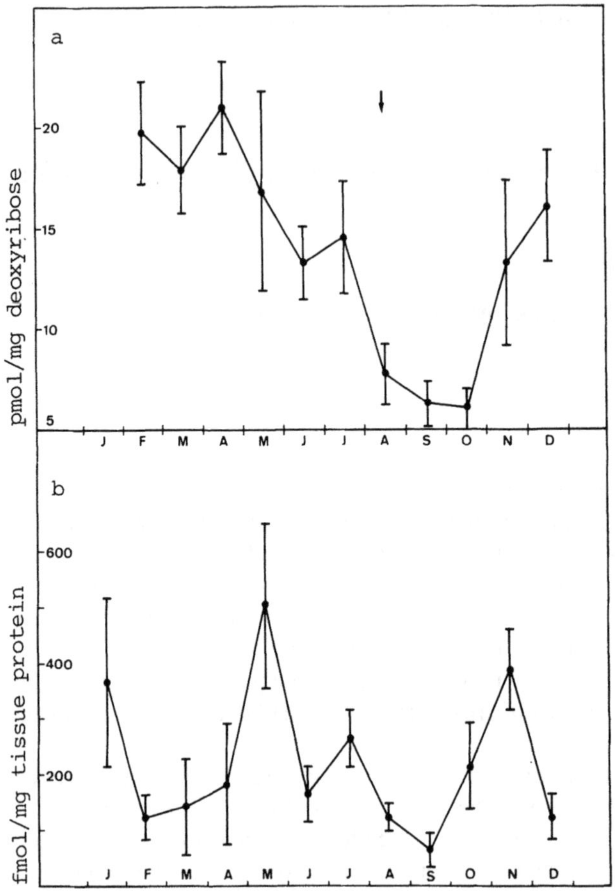

Fig. 1a, b. Seasonal variation in E2R content of uteri of ovariectomised pigs (**a**) and primary mammary tumours of postmenopausal women (**b**)

October than in the other months. A similar phenomenon was observed in uteri of immature calves.

Figure 1b shows the results of 84 receptor analyses in primary breast cancers containing measurable receptor concentrations. This graph shows two maxima, in May and November, i.e., 6 months apart, and two minima, February through April and August through October, which are also 6 months apart. This would suggest that the ER concentration in breast cancer of postmenopausal women varies with a 6-month periodicity. This variation is significant according to the Kruskel-Wallis H-test.

Figure 2 compares our data with those obtained by F. A. G. Teulings in Rotterdam (1976, personal communication) and by A. J. M. Koenders and Th. J. Benraao in Nijmegen (1977, personal communication), who recently analysed their data on postmenopausal cancers. They obtained almost identical patterns. It is especially interesting that the receptor low in August, September, and October coincides in three different species: namely calf, pig, and human.

It would be interesting to know what mechanism induces these fluctuations of the receptor levels in target tissues. There are indications that it might be attributable to the release of adrenal steroids, which are peripherally aromatised. It is well known that the adrenal does not secrete at a constant rate and that there are circadian as well as seasonal fluctuations in steroid secre-

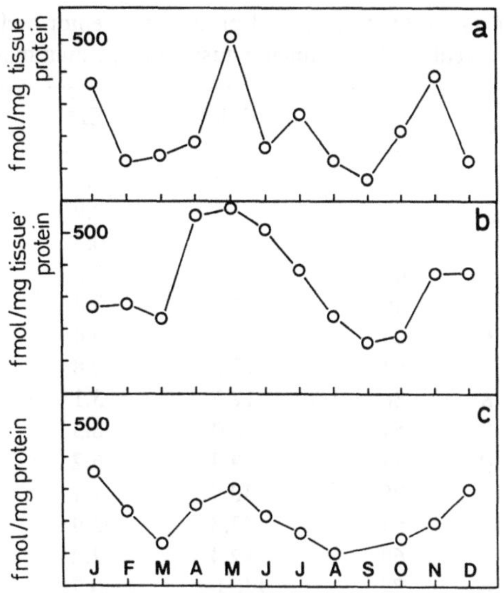

Fig. 2a–c. Seasonal fluctuation in cytosol oestradiol receptor in postmenopausal breast cancer biopsies, as recorded in 84 patients in the Wilhelmshaven study conducted in 1970–1976 (**a**), 80 patients in the Rotterdam study conducted in 1973–1976 (**b**), and 110 patients in the Nijmegen study conducted in 1975–1977 (**c**)

Table 2. Oestrogen- and progesteron receptor and nuclear oestradiol content of premenopausal human mammary cancer in comparison to premenopausal uteri

	Age	Day of cycle	E2R[a]	E2[a]	PR[a]
Mammary carcinomas					
1	35	12	0.0	0.0	0.0
2	41	–	1.6	0.0	0.0
3	37	8	0.3	1.4	0.0
4	40	–	4.4	0.7	0.0
5	46	–	2.6	22.3	5.5
6	41	5	8.4	3.2	8.8
7	45	4	11.5	0.8	51.3
Normal uteri					
1	32	12	6.7	15.3	35.7
2	40	14	13.6	4.7	11.5
3	44	18	7.7	3.6	13.9
4	36	22	10.3	1.4	24.9
5	37	23	4.1	1.1	7.4

[a] Femtomoles per microgram of deoxyribose.

tion (CURTIS, 1974). But it cannot be excluded that the receptor concentrations of target tissues might be modulated by "intrinsic" rhythmic variations.

Considering that cytoplasmic receptor levels are influenced by endogenous hormones as well as by rhythmic fluctuations of unknown origin, it is clear that "normal baseline" levels of receptors in target tissues do not exist. This fact considerably reduces the value placed on the

Table 3. Oestrogen- and progestin receptor and nuclear oestradiol content in 14 postmenopausal human mammary cancers

	Age	E2R[a]	E2[a]	PR[a]
1	72	25.8	0.0	0.0
2	80	7.3	0.9	0.0
3	56	7.4	0.7	0.0
4	69	3.2	2.2	0.0
5	56	3.9	0.8	0.0
6	64	5.4	0.4	5.6
7	54	17.2	0.8	5.6
8	86	12.7	3.1	3.3
9	54	6.0	8.3	43.4
10	74	29.3	6.2	13.3
11	78	30.9	1.1	11.1
12	54 ♂	32.3	2.9	46.5
13	69	12.4	2.2	3.2
14	78	140.0	0.7	8.9
15	64	0.0	1.4	6.8

[a] Femtomoles per microgram of deoxyribose.

quantitative ER assay as a sole indicator of hormone sensitivity. This assay must therefore be complemented by further criteria.

Since in hormone-dependent breast cancers endogenous oestradiol is transported to the nucleus, where it is accumulated and retained, additional determination of the nuclear oestradiol content is the test most likely to lead to a considerable improvement in the prognostic value of the receptor assay.

In addition, the cytoplasmic progestin receptor level should be measured, since its synthesis in hormone-responsive cancer appears to depend on ER action (Horwitz and McGuire, 1975).

In a preliminary study we have measured these three parameters simultaneously in some normal human uteri and in a series of primary breast cancers.

Table 2 shows a comparison between premenopausal mammary carcinomas and normal premenopausal uteri: as expected, all uteri contained relatively high amounts of ER, oestradiol in the nuclear fraction, and progestin receptor.

However, the mammary carcinomas show quite diverse patterns: case 1 contains neither receptors nor nuclear oestradiol, thus indicating a failure in steroid binding.

Case 2 contains ER, but no oestradiol is accumulated in the nuclear fraction. The transport of the hormone to the nucleus is obviously impeded.

The next two cases contain ER and oestradiol in the nuclear fraction, but these tumours are apparently released from oestrogen control, since although oestradiol is accumulated in the nucleus, progestin receptor is not present.

The next three cancers show a pattern similar to that observed in the normal uterus.

A similar pattern was found in 14 primary mammary cancers of postmenopausal women (Table 3). Case 1 contains high amounts of ER only. The next four cases also contain considerable amounts of oestradiol in the nuclear fraction but progestin receptor is absent. All other cases show the normal pattern seen in the uterus.

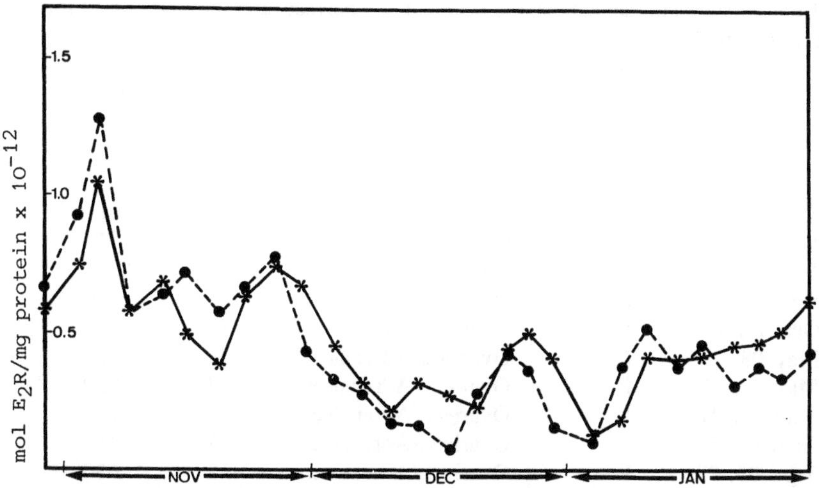

Fig. 3. Oestradiol receptor levels in uteri from rats subjected to ovariectomy alone (*——*) and rats subjected to ovariectomy and hypophysectomy (●——●)

Case 15 is remarkable in that we could not detect any ER, although oestradiol is accumulated in the nuclear fraction. Since we have a second cancer with a similar pattern, it is possible that this situation characterises the few cases in which a response to hormone ablative therapy was observed although ER was not measured. This could be explained either by experimental error or by the presence of undetectable amounts of oestradiol receptor, and underlines the importance of having more than one parameter for assessing hormone sensitivity.

The results presented in Tables 2 and 3 suggest that the presence of ER in breast cancer specimens alone is not a reliable indicator of the determination of hormone sensitivity. In some of these tumours the hormone is not transported to the nucleus, while in other cases, where nuclear oestradiol accumulation still occurs, the oestradiol-induced enhancement of transcription and translation is impaired. These tumours belong properly in the group of the so-called nonresponding ER+ carcinomas.

Thus, we are hopeful that the assessment of these three parameters will improve the prognostic value of the biochemical characterization of breast cancer.

A striking fact noted in the data just presented is that most of the postmenopausal cancers contained surprisingly high nuclear oestradiol concentrations (see Table 3). The question of the source of this oestradiol therefore arises.

Since oestrogen production in the ovaries declines rapidly after the menopause this oestradiol must be of adrenal origin, either due to direct synthesis or due to precursors that undergo peripheral aromatisation. This, of course, has striking consequences for the therapeutic measures to be taken in the case of carcinomas that are potentially hormone-responsive. A complete withdrawal of endogenous hormones by ablative surgery or by a chemical blockade of the adrenal cortex seems to be essential for successful treatment of these oestrogen-stimulated tumours (JUNGBLUT et al., 1977).

However, our latest results make it seem doubtful that even complete hormone withdrawal is fully effective (JUNGBLUT et al., 1976).

It now seems possible that receptor proteins can function without the steroid hormone. Figure 3 shows an example of a steroid hormone-independent fluctuation of ER in uteri of

Table 4. Receptor and oestradiol content[a] in purified uterus nuclei of ovariectomised or ovariectomised/adrenalectomised pigs

Date	Number of animals	Ablative treatment	Days post op.	Binding sites per nucleus	Molecules oestradiol per nucleus
Sept. 13, 76	1	Ovariectomy	47	2,690	1,480
Dec. 20, 76	3	Ovariectomy	56	3,010	1,270
Jan. 26, 77	3	Ovariectomy	63	2,910	1,210
Sept. 12, 77	1	Ovariectomy	47	2,170	210
Oct. 17, 77	1	Ovariectomy	53	2,230	600
May 03, 77	1	Ovariect./Adrenalect.[b]	33	2,480	480[b]
May 03, 77	1	Ovariect./Adrenalect.	33	2,230	0
May 03, 77	1	Ovariect./Adrenalect.	33	1,230	0
Sept. 05, 77	1	Ovariect./Adrenalect.	12	1,180	0
Sept. 05, 77	1	Ovariect./Adrenalect.	12	1,030	0
Sept. 05, 77	1	Ovariect./Adrenalect.	10	1,430	0
Sept. 05, 77	1	Ovariect./Adrenalect.	10	1,180	0

[a] Detection limit for binding sites and oestradiol, 60/nucleus; interassay variation, 6%.
[b] Hypertrophied remnants of adrenal cortex found.

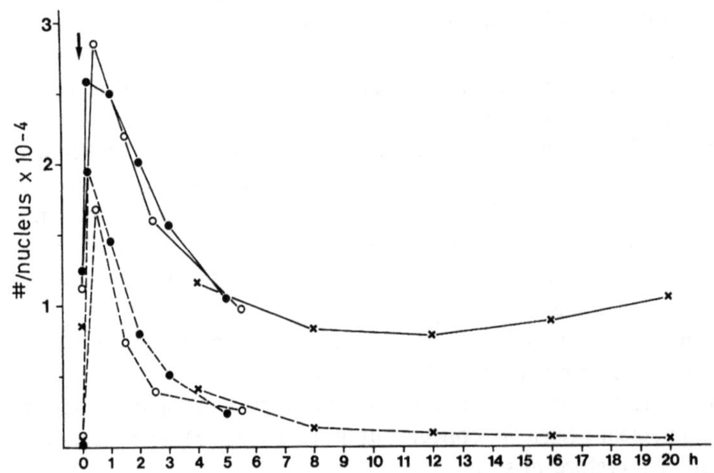

Fig. 4. Receptor and hormone content of pig uterus nuclei after intrauterine oestradiol pulse. ○——○, binding sites on 14 Nov. 1977; ●——●, binding sites on 13 Feb. 1978; ×——×, binding sites on 6 Mar. 1978; ○---○, molecules E2 on 14 Nov. 1977; ●---●, molecules E2 on 13 Feb. 1978; ×---×, molecules E2 on 6 Mar. 1978

ovariectomised/hypophysectomised rats. In these animals steroid hormones are virtually absent, but ER is still synthesised and shows an irregular fluctuation with a periodicity of 6–9 days. This receptor turnover in animals totally deprived of steroid hormones indicates that a receptor protein can regulate at least the transcription of its own messenger in the absence of steroid hormone.

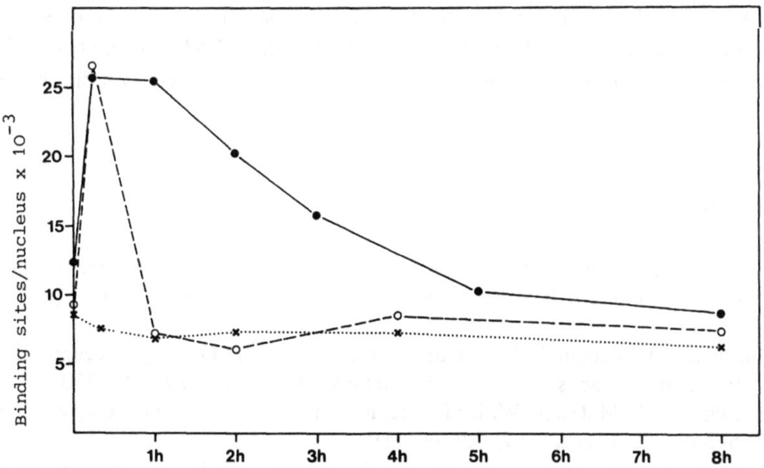

Fig. 5. Nuclear ER pattern after pulses of oestradiol (●——●), oestrone (○– – –○), or TAM (x - - - - - - x) in the pig-uterus system. Dosage was 20 ml 1 × 10^{-6} *M* IU in each case

Another experimental fact that supports this concept is shown in Table 4: in five experiments with purified uterine nuclei from ovariectomised pigs we determined both the total nuclear receptor content and the amount of oestradiol accumulated in the nuclei. On average there was three times more oestradiol receptor than oestradiol in the nuclei. In pigs that had also been adrenalectomised we found considerable amounts of nuclear receptor in six cases, but oestradiol was not detectable. Since oestradiol can be extracted quantitatively while extraction of nuclear receptor cannot be performed without losses, there are only two possible explanations for this phenomenon: the first one is that oestradiol and receptor leave the nucleus – after entering it together – at different rates, and the second is that the receptor enters the nucleus alone. The first seems highly improbable, since even 33 days after adrenalectomy the nuclear receptor is still present (Table 4). From our recent kinetic studies we know that receptor and oestradiol leave the nucleus at a similar rate, as shown in Fig. 4. In these experiments ovariectomised pigs received an intrauterine oestradiol injection. The animals were killed at different times after the oestrogen pulse, and the uteri were excised and used for a preparation of highly purified nuclei. Oestradiol and oestradiol receptor were determined in each batch of nuclei. Besides the parallel increase and decrease in the earlier stages (0–8 h), this experiment also showed that in the later stages (8–20 h) the nuclear receptor level increased again while the nuclear oestradiol content was still declining. Thus this experiment shows that the receptor can enter the nucleus without the assistance of the hormone. The presence of nuclear receptor in uteri of totally hormone-deprived pigs is also explained by this mechanism.

In addition, this steroid-free receptor is able to induce oestrogen-specific synthetic events, since progesterone receptor was detected in the uteri of all ovariectomised/adrenalectomised pigs.

From all these data it can be concluded that complete hormone withdrawal alone is not a totally effective treatment for hormone-responsive cancers, but must be supplemented by an antihormonal treatment that incapacitates the receptor.

The question therefore arises, as to whether tamoxifen (TAM) is such an ideal antihormone. Recently we have tested TAM in our pig-uterus system and found, as shown in Fig. 5, that

TAM (if applied at the same concentration as oestradiol or oestrone) is not able to transfer receptor from the cytoplasm to the nucleus. Since TAM competes with oestradiol at the receptor-binding site its biological effect might be explained by a blockade of the nuclear ER transfer.

References

Curtis, G. C.: Long-term changes in corticosteroid excretion. In: Biorhythms and human reproduction. Ferin, M., Halberg, F., Richart, R. M., Vande Wiele, L. (eds.), p. 417. Chichester: Whiley 1974

Engelsman, E., Persijn, J. P., Korsten, C. B., Cleton, F. J.: Oestrogen receptor in human breast cancer tissue and response to endocrine therapy. Br. med. J. *1973 II,* 750

Horwitz, K. B., McGuire, W. L.: Predicting response to endocrine therapy in human breast cancer: a hypothesis. Science *189,* 726 (1975)

Hughes, A., Jacobson, I., Wagner, R. K., Jungblut, P. W.: Ovarian-independent fluctuations of oestradiol receptor levels in mammalian tissues. Mol. Cell. Endocrinol. *5,* 379 (1976)

Jensen, E. V., Block, G. E., Smith, S., Kayser, K., DeSombre, E. R.: Estrogen receptors and hormone dependency. In: Target tissues and neoplasia. Doa, T. L. (ed.), p. 23. Chicago: Univ. Chicago Press 1972

Jungblut, P. W., Gaues, J., Hughes, A., Kallweit, E., Sierralta, W., Szendro, P., Wagner, R. K.: Activation of transcription-regulating proteins by steroids. J. Steroid Biochem. *7,* 1109 (1976)

Jungblut, P. W., Hughes, A., Sierralta, W., Wagner, R. K.: A proposal for assessment of hormone sensitivity and consequent endocrine therapy of breast cancer. Eur. J. Cancer *13,* 1201 (1977)

McGuire, W. L.: Current status of estrogen receptors in human breast cancer. Cancer *36,* 638 (1975)

Wagner, R. K.: Critical evaluation of receptor assays in relation to tumors. In: Research on steroids, Vol. 7, Chapter 17A, p. 205. Transactions of the Seventh Meeting of the International Study Group for Steroid Hormones. Vermeulen, A. et al. (eds.). Amsterdam: Elsevier 1977

2. *Steroid Receptor Determinations in Mammary Carcinoma in Women*

B. Runnebaum and K. Klinga

Klinikum der Universität Heidelberg, Frauenklinik, Voßstraße 9, D-6900 Heidelberg 1 (FRG)

It is now accepted that the determination of specific steroid-binding proteins in mammary carcinoma tissue allows a forecast of the success of endocrine therapy (Jensen et al., 1971; Savlov et al., 1974; Maass et al., 1975). The content of receptor protein varies and depends on the tumour tissue itself, e.g., primary tumour or metastases, on the endocrinological condition of the woman, and finally on the method of determination. It is important for the clinician to know whether the mammary carcinoma has definite steroid-binding proteins, especially oestradiol receptors (ER), or not. The limit of analytical detection is about 3 fmol/mg cytosol protein. We describe carcinomata as ER-positive if more than 5 fmol oestradiol/mg cytosol protein is bound. In the endocrine treatment of mammary carcinoma, it is striking that ER-positive tumours have shown remission in only about 60% of the cases. It seems therefore that the determination of the ER alone is not sufficient as a marker. In the search for other markers it has been shown that the determination of progesterone receptors (PR) in addition to ERs allows a more accurate statement on the hormone dependence of the tumour.

The PR content appears to be under the influence of the oestrogens, and is detectable in about 60% of ER-positive (ER+) cases. The rate of response is higher after endocrine therapy when both ERs and PRs are present (McGuire et al., 1977). There is no confirmed evidence as to the importance of dihydrotestosterone receptors in mammary carcinoma. In this paper, two methods for the determination of the various steroid receptors are discussed. The transporting and storage of the samples are of decisive importance. The tissue should be placed on ice immediately after the operation, and conveyed to the laboratory in a refrigerating vessel. If immediate processing is not possible the tissue is frozen at −25° C. Storage for more than 4 weeks should be avoided. The prepared carcinoma tissue is homogenised while cooling under liquid nitrogen in a microdismembrator and extracted with three to four times the amount of Tris buffer. After centrifugation the cytosol is incubated at saturation concentration with ^{3}H-labelled steroids. Unspecific binding is ascertained by competitive inhibition. The receptor-bound steroids are separated from the free steroids either by agar gel electrophoresis (Wagner, 1972) or by the second method with dextran charcoal suspension, according to the guidelines of the EORTC Breast Cancer Cooperative Group (1973). Electrophoresis permits a good separation of the ER complex from other protein complexes. Each incubation yields 25 gel fractions. With the controls, 50 fractions per receptor assay are obtained. The gel fractions cannot be counted until after about 6 h. The receptor content is evaluated the next day. For the charcoal method 1 ml charcoal suspension is added, shaken for 30 min and then centrifuged for 10 min, the radioactivity of the supernatant is counted, and the receptor content

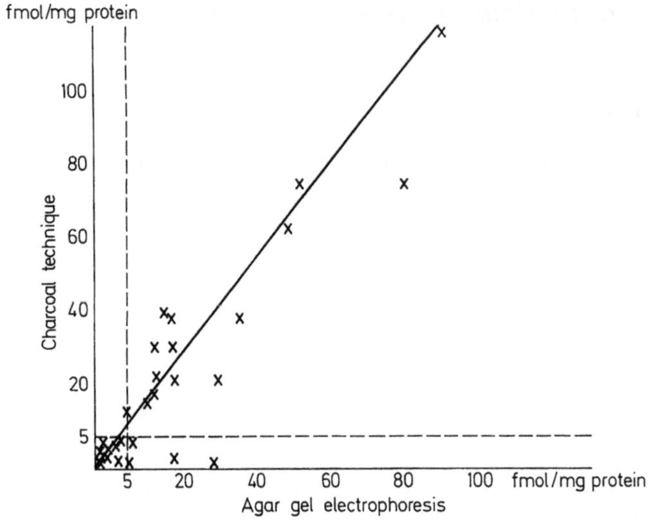

Fig. 1. Comparison of agar gel electrophoresis with the charcoal adsorption method in the determination of oestradiol receptors in 27 cases of mammary carcinoma. $y = 1.095 \times + 0.1042$; $r = 0.9023$; $n = 27$

is evaluated on the same day. In both methods the quantity of steroid bound to the receptors is related to the protein content of the cytosol after deduction of the unspecifically bound fraction. The protein content is determined by the method of LOWRY et al. (1951), and usually lies between 2 and 15 mg protein/ml cytosol. By means of serial dilution, it has been established that electrophoretic receptor determination of solutions with less than 3 mg protein/ml can lead to false-negative results. Because of the relatively high expenditure of work and time and the lower sensitivity with dilute extracts, agar gel electrophoresis is

Table 1. Steroid receptors in mammary carcinoma

Receptor	No. of tumours examined	Positive	Negative
17β-oestradiol	235	148 (63.0%)	87 (37.0%)
Dihydrotestosterone	36	12 (33.3%)	24 (66.7%)
Progesterone	24	12 (50.0%)	12 (50.0%)

Table 2. Dependence of the oestradiol receptor content in mammary carcinoma on the age of the patient

Age	30	31–40	41–50	51–60	61–70	71–80	81
No.	4	24	51	49	67	34	6
Positive (%)	50.0	50.0	51.0	69.4	70.1	79.4	100.0
Negative (%)	50.0	50.0	49.0	30.6	29.9	20.6	0.0

unsuitable as a routine clinical method, and it is inferior to the charcoal method. Figure 1 shows a comparison of the two methods in 27 ER determinations in mammary carcinoma tissue. There is good correlation of the values obtained, with a correlation coefficient of 0.9.

The results of our receptor determinations are presented in Table 1. Of 235 ER determinations, 63% were receptor-positive and 37% receptor-negative. As can be seen from Table 2, the receptor content is age-dependent. In the premenopausal group the receptor-negative proportion of 50% is higher than that in the postmenopausal group, with only 30%. Androgen receptor was determined in 36 tumour extracts. Only 33% of cases were receptor-positive. Because of the low binding of dihydrotestosterone it is often difficult to determine the boundary between positive and negative. No connection could be detected between ER and DHT receptors. The difficulties that arise in the determination of PR through cortisol-binding globulin are well known (Horwitz and McGuire, 1975). Separation of the PR complex from the corresponding CBG complex is impossible with the agar gel method. For this reason we use the synthetic progestin R5020 (Philibert and Raynaud, 1973), which is not bound by CBG. In 24 cases, half the tumours were PR-positive when determined electrophoretically. The data collected so far with the charcoal adsorption method show that the PR-positive fraction is lower.

Our investigations have shown that the charcoal adsorption method is a rapid and sufficiently accurate procedure for the routine determination of ERs and PRs in mammary carcinoma. For the assessment of hormone dependence of mammary carcinoma simultaneous determination of ERs and PRs is appropriate.

References

EORTC Breast Cancer Cooperative Group: Standards for the assessment of estrogen receptors in human breast cancer. Eur. J. Cancer *9,* 379 (1973)

Horwitz, K. B., McGuire, W. L.: Specific progesterone receptors in human breast cancer. Steroids *25,* 497–505 (1975)

Jensen, E. V., Block, G. E., Smith, S., Kyser, K., DeSombre, E. R.: Estrogen receptors and breast cancer response to adrenalectomy. Nat. Cancer Inst. Monogr. *34,* 55–79 (1971)

Lowry, O. H., Rosebrough, N. J., Farr, A. L., Randall, R. J.: Protein measurement with the Folin phenol reagent. J. Biol. Chem. *193,* 265 (1951)

Maass, H., Engel, B., Trams, G., Nowakowski, H., Stolzenbach, G.: Steroid hormone receptors in human breast cancer and the clinical significance. J. Steroid Biochem. *6,* 743–749 (1975)

McGuire, W. L., Horwitz, K. B., Pearson, O. H., Segaloff, A.: Current status of estrogen and progesterone receptors in breast cancer. Cancer *39,* 2934–2947 (1977)

Philibert, D., Raynaud, J. P.: Progesterone binding in the immature mouse and rat uterus. Steroids *22,* 89–98 (1973)

Savlov, E. D., Wittliff, J. L., Hilf, R., Hall, T. C.: Correlations between certain biochemical properties of breast cancer and response to therapy. Cancer *33,* 303–309 (1974)

Wagner, R. K.: Characterization and assay of steroid hormone receptors and steroid-binding serum proteins by agar gel electrophoresis at low temperature. Hoppe-Seylers Z. Physiol. Chem. *353,* 1235–1245 (1972)

3. *Steroid Receptor Determination by Means of Agar Gel Electrophoresis*

D. Kummer

Chirurgische Universitätsklinik, Calwer Straße 7, D-7400 Tübingen (FRG)

Since 1974 hormone receptor analysis has been carried out according to the method of WAGNER (1972) and WAGNER and JUNGBLUT (1976) on 171 human mammary carcinomata at the University Hospital of Tübingen, Department of Surgery. In most cases only the levels of oestradiol receptors (ER) were measured; in the last 34 patients, however, cellular binding proteins for progestin and testosterone have also been determined (PHILIBERT and RAYNAUD, 1973).

The method of measurement with agar gel electrophoresis initially presented difficulties, until the apparatus had been modified by the provision of a cold plate, making it possible to keep the gel plate temperature lower than 5° C during the run. Immediately after completion of the operation the tissue was homogenised in an ice-bath. The 200 000 G supernatant was incubated for 2 h in an ice bath at a concentration of labelled steroids of 2×10^{-8} M.

The nonspecific steroid binding was measured on an extract that had been heated for 1 h at 45° C. The specific receptor protein–steroid complex migrated to the anode in the cooled electrophoresis apparatus. For further details of the method see WAGNER and JUNGBLUT (1972).

In addition to carcinomata, benign mammary tumours were also analysed. Out of 11 fibroadenomas, eight (= 73%) had oestradiol receptor concentrations of 15–90 fmol/mg protein. According to the histological findings, the three adenomas without receptors were re-

Table 1. Hormone receptor analyses of mammary tumours during 1974–1978 at the University Hospital of Tübingen, Department of Surgery

Histological findings	ER detectable	ER not detectable
Fibrocystic mastopathy (*n* = 14)	100%	0%
Fibroadenomas (*n* = 11)	73% (100%)	27% (0%)
Mammary carcinomata:		
Primary tumours (*n* = 171)	48%	52%
Of these		
Adenocarcinomata (*n* = 12)	100%	0%

gressively transformed. All 14 tissue samples of fibrocystic mastopathy investigated showed oestradiol receptor concentrations of 10–30 fmol (Table 1).

In seven cases of 171 with mammary carcinomata lymph node tissue with metastatic involvement was also investigated, in addition to the primary tumour. Hormone receptor analysis always yielded identical values. If the primary carcinoma contained oestradiol receptors these were also detectable in the lymph node metastases, and vice versa.

A dependency on the grade of histological differentiation of the carcinoma could be demonstrated insofar as all 12 adenocarcinomas among the 171 malignant tumours showed an oestradiol receptor concentration of up to 240 fmol/mg protein. In total, 48% of the investigated carcinomata were oestradiol-positive, and 52% oestradiol-negative. This relationship shifted slightly as a function of age; thus in 42 patients under 50 years only 36% of the carcinomas had oestradiol receptors, whilst in 38 patients over 70 years 47% were oestradiol-positive.

So far, 34 mammary carcinomas have been analysed in which receptors for oestradiol, progestin, and testosterone were determined. The results were as follows:

In the oestradiol-positive carcinomata of this group, 39% were progestin-positive; progesterone receptors (PgR) were never found in oestradiol-negative tumours. Testosterone-binding protein was demonstrable in 52% of the oestradiol-positive carcinomata. Two of the 34 mammary tumours (= 6%) had only testosterone receptors.

The therapeutic implications of these hormone-receptor analyses at the above mentioned clinic are based on the clinical experience of McGuire (1975), McGuire et al. (1977), and Maass et al. (1975).

Depending on the menopausal status of the patient, an ablative or additive hormonal therapy is carried out in women with metastatic carcinomata in whom hormone receptors have been demonstrated in the primary tumour or metastases. Otherwise, in the absence of receptors, polychemotherapy is used for the treatment of metastases.

Since a period of only 4 years has been surveyed, we can as yet make no statement on the clinico-therapeutic correlation. However, we beleave that sufficient clinical experience has been gained at other medical centres to justify our decision to base hormonal therapy of metastatic carcinomata on the results of receptor analysis.

References

Maass, H., Engel, B., Nowakowski, H., Stolzenbach, G., Trams, G.: Steroid hormone receptors in human breast cancer and clinical correlations. Arch. Geschwulstforsch. *45,* 423–429 (1975)

McGuire, W. L.: Current status of estrogen receptors in human breast cancer. Cancer *36,* 638–644 (1975)

McGuire, W. L., Horwitz, K. B., Pearson, O. H., Segaloff, A.: Current status of estrogen and progesterone receptors in breast cancer. Cancer *39,* 2934–2947 (1977)

Philibert, D., Raynaud, J. P.: Progesterone binding in the immature mouse and rat uterus. Steroids *22,* 89–98 (1973)

Wagner, R. K.: Characterization and assay of steroid hormone receptors and steroid-binding serum proteins by agar gel electrophoresis at low temperature. Hoppe-Seylers Z. Physiol. Chem. *353,* 1235–1245 (1972)

Wagner, R. K., Jungblut, P. W.: Oestradiol- and dihydrotestosterone receptors in normal and neoplastic human mammary tissue. Acta Endocrinol. (Kbh.) *82,* 105–120 (1976)

4. *Estrogen Receptor Determination Predicts Response to Tamoxifen Therapy*

J. C. Allegra and M. E. Lippman

Medicine Branch, National Cancer Institute, National Institutes of Health, Building 10, Room 6B02, Bethesda, MD 20014 (USA)

Introduction

Tamoxifen (TAM, ICI 46,474) is a nonsteroidal antiestrogen of the triphenylethylene family. The clinical use of TAM was first reported in 1971 (COLE et al., 1971), and early clinical trials suggested that TAM was useful in the treatment of metastatic breast cancer (COLE et al., 1971; WARD, 1973; COLE et al., 1972). These studies yielded response rates ranging between 15% and 60% with minimal toxicity.

Estrogen receptors (ER) are found in approximately 50% of breast tumor specimens obtained from metastases (MCGUIRE et al., 1975). The presence of significant ER concentrations in a tumor specimen is associated with a response rate of about 60% to endocrine therapy, while its absence greatly decreases the likelihood of response to endocrine therapy (MCGUIRE et al., 1977).

The present study provides a preliminary analysis of response rate to TAM therapy as a function of ER status.

Materials and Methods

Receptor Assays

Biopsies of metastatic or inoperable localized breast cancer were trimmed of excess fat and nontumorous tissue and divided, one portion being submitted for confirming pathology in all cases. Samples for ER assay were kept on ice and then frozen in liquid nitrogen within 20 min. ER assays were performed as previously described (LIPPMAN and HUFF, 1976). When the sample was adequate, Scatchard analyses were performed to quantify the number of binding sites; otherwise assays were performed in duplicate at one or two concentrations of estradiol chosen to exceed several times the expected equilibrium dissociation constant. Data were analyzed by computer-assisted methods (AITKEN and LIPPMAN, 1977). A positive ER assay was recorded when 10 fmol ^{3}H-estradiol or more bound to each 1 mg cytoplasmic protein. No adjustment of this value for menopausal status was used.

Patients

Twenty-six patients with metastatic or surgically unresectable primary breast cancer had ER assays performed on a specimen obtained immediately before the institution of TAM therapy.

TAM was administered orally twice a day at various dosages ranging from 2 mg/m^2 to 100 mg/m^2. In all cases, response was assessed according to standardized response criteria (BREAST CANCER TASK FORCE TREATMENT COMMITTEE, 1977). In brief, complete response required the disappearance of all measurable disease, including healing of all bone lesions and a return of the patient to a premorbid performance status. Partial response required a shrinkage of at least 50% of all measurable disease. Though a given lesion might not regress to this extent, regression averaged over all lesions had to be equal to or greater than 50%. No new lesions could appear and no growth could be observed in a preexistent lesion. For purposes of this study, no patient was classified as having achieved a partial response unless improvement was maintained for 2 months or more. Only patients with complete or partial responses are termed objective responders. Any patient not achieving this degree of improvement was termed a nonresponder.

Statistical Analyses

Comparisons of proportions were performed by the contingency χ^2-test with continuity correction. Comparison of continuous or ordered polychotomous distributions was performed by the Wilcoxon rank sum test adjusted for ties (LEHMANN, 1975). This test requires no distributional assumptions of the data, as would a *t*-test. All significance levels correspond to two-sided statistical tests.

Results

Twenty-six patients were evaluable in this study. For a patient to be evaluable, a biopsy and an adequate ER assay performed immediately prior to therapy with TAM were required. Some characteristics of these patients are shown in Table 1. The ER-positive (ER+) and -negative

Table 1. Characteristics of the patients treated with TAM as a function of estrogen receptor status

	ER+	ER−
Number of patients	19	7
Mean ER value		
(fmols/mg cytoplasmic protein)	98	0.9
Median age	53	51
Menopausal status		
Premenopausal	1	4
Postmenopausal	18	3
Karnofsky performance status (mean ± SEM)	88 ± 6	90 ± 5
Disease-free interval (median, months)	16	18
Number of sites involved		
1	3 (16%)	1 (14%)
2	10 (53%)	2 (29%)
≥ 3	6 (32%)	4 (57%)
Prior therapy		
Endocrine	7 (37%)	1 (14%)
Chemotherapy	10 (53%)	6 (86%)

(ER–) groups are essentially identical with respect to age, Karnofsky performance index, disease-free interval, and number of sites involved with metastatic tumor. Ninety percent of the patients in the ER+ group had received prior systemic therapy, and all of the patients in the ER– group had been previously treated. Eighteen of 19 patients in the ER+ group were postmenopausal, as against four of seven in the ER– group. The mean ER value, expressed as femtomoles per milligram of cytoplasmic protein, is 98 for the ER+ patients and 0.9 for the ER– group.

Sites of involvement by metastatic breast cancer for ER+ and ER– patients were similar. In the ER+ group, six of the nineteen patients had visceral dominant disease, as against four of the seven ER– patients. This difference is not statistically significant.

Overall, 11 of 19 (58%) patients whose tumors were ER+ responded to TAM therapy, as against none of the seven patients in the ER– group ($p < 0.05$). In the ER+ group four of six patients with visceral dominant disease responded, compared with seven of thirteen patients with soft tissue and bone dominant disease. Thus patients with visceral metastases whose tumors were ER+ had a similar response rate to antiestrogen therapy to that seen in patients with nonvisceral metastases.

Discussion

The response rate to endocrine therapy in patients with metastatic breast cancer is approximately 30%. In 1971, ER was found in human breast cancer tissues and it was suggested that ER status might be useful in predicting tumor regression after endocrine manipulation (JENSEN et al., 1971). Over the past 7 years there has been a proliferation of reports correlating response to endocrine treatment with ER status. In 1974 these were summarized at an international workshop (MCGUIRE et al., 1975). These collected data show that patients whose tumors possess ER have a response rate of 50%–60%, while tumors that lack ER have a response rate of less than 10%. There have been only a few studies attempting to correlate ER status with response to antiestrogen therapy, however. Recently, data were reported correlating ER status and response to TAM therapy (MORGAN et al., 1976; KIANG and KENNEDY, 1977; O'CONNOR et al., 1978). KIANG and KENNEDY reported on 59 postmenopausal patients with metastatic breast cancer. Overall, the response rate to TAM was 32%, but this increased to 60% in patients whose tumors were ER+. No patient whose tumor was ER– responded. Our data are in agreement with those reported by these authors. Of our patients whose tumors were ER+, 58% responded, while we obtained a 0% response rate in ER– tumors.

Our data also show that response rates are high in ER+ tumors regardless of site of involvement with metastatic disease. Indeed, visceral metastases respond as well as skin or bone dominant disease. This differs from the traditional viewpoint, which is that visceral involvement is refractory to endocrine therapy. It appears that ER status has an overwhelming influence on response rate and that the relative insensitivity of visceral metastasis to endocrine therapy probably reflects the distribution of ER+ and ER– tumors at these sites.

References

Aitken, S., Lippman, M. E.: A simple computer program for quantification and Scatchard analysis of steroid receptor proteins. J. Steroid Biochem. *8*, 77–94 (1977)

Breast Cancer Task Force Treatment Committee, National Cancer Institute: Breast cancer: Suggested protocol guidelines for combination chemotherapy trials and for combined modality trials. U.S. Department of Health, Education and Welfare Publication No. (NIH) 77-1192 (1977)

Cole, M. P., Jones, C. T. A., Todd, I. D. H.: A new anti-oestrogenic agent in late breast cancer. An early clinical appraisal of ICI 46,474. Br. J. Cancer *25,* 270–275 (1971)

Cole, M. P., Jones, C. T. A., Todd, I. D. H.: The treatment of advanced carcinoma of the breast with the anti-oestrogenic agent tamoxifen (ICI 46,474) – a series of 96 patients. Adv. Antimicrob. Antineoplas. Chemother. *2,* 529–531 (1972)

Jensen, E. V., Block, G. E., Smith, S., Kyser, K., De Sombre, E. R.: Estrogen receptors and breast cancer response to adrenalectomy. Natl. Cancer Inst. Monogr. *34,* 55 (1971)

Kiang, D. T., Kennedy, B. J.: Tamoxifen (antiestrogen) therapy in advanced breast cancer. Ann. Intern. Med. *87,* 687–690 (1977)

Lehmann, E. H.: Non-parametrics: Statistical methods based on ranks. p. 208. San Francisco: Holden-Day Inc. 1975

Lippman, M. E., Huff, K. K.: A demonstration of androgen and estrogen receptors in human breast cancer using a new protamine sulfate assay. Cancer *38,* 868–874 (1976)

McGuire, W. L., Carbone, P. P., Sears, M. E., Escher, G. C.: Estrogen receptors in human breast cancer: An overview. In: Estrogen receptors in human breast cancer. McGuire, W. L., Carbone, P. P., Volmer, E. P. (eds.), pp. 1–7. New York: Raven Press 1975

McGuire, W. L., Horwitz, K. B., Pearson, O. H., Segaloff, A.: Current status of estrogen and progesterone receptors in breast cancer. Cancer *39,* 2934–2947 (1977)

Morgan, L. R., Schein, P. S., Woolley, P. V., Hoth, D., Macdonald, J., Lippman, M., Posey, L. E., Beazley, R. W.: Therapeutic use of tamoxifen in advanced breast cancer: correlation with biochemical parameters. Cancer Treat. Rep. *60,* 1437–1443 (1976)

O'Connor, T., Rosenbaum, C., Cardellicchio, D., Cohen, J. L., Stolbach, L.: Estrogen receptor (ER) predicts tamoxifen (Tam) response in advanced breast cancer (Br). Proc. Ann. Meet. Am. Soc. Clin. Oncol. *19,* 374 (1978)

Ward, H. W. C.: Anti-oestrogen therapy for breast cancer: a trial of tamoxifen at two dose levels. Br. Med. J. *1973 I,* 13–14

5. *Estrogen Receptor Status and the Disease-Free Interval in Breast Cancer*

J. C. Allegra and M. E. Lippman

Medicine Branch, National Cancer Institute, National Institutes of Health, Building 10, Room 6B02, Bethesda, MD 20014 (USA)

Introduction

Most patients with breast cancer initially present with locally resectable disease. Unfortunately, at least half these patients will eventually die of disseminated disease, proving that clinical resectability and cure are far from synonymous terms. Obviously many patients have clinically occult or microscopic metastases at the time of initial surgical intervention. Aside from suggesting the eventual clinical outcome there has been little need for accurate prediction of which patients would eventually have recurrences. With the recent exciting development of effective adjuvant regimens the need for careful and precise patient selection for systemic therapy has become mandatory. While several factors, such as tumor size, tumor location, histologic grade, local lymphatic invasion, and patient weight are of some value, axillary lymph node status has provided the best estimate of tumor recurrence rate, ranging to over 90% if four or more axillary lymph nodes are involved by tumor. Unfortunately, this is an insufficiently accurate guide to which patients have recurrences. Up to one-third of axillary lymph node-negative patients will eventually die of disseminated disease, while only one-half of patients with one node involved with the tumor will succumb to their disease.
Several lines of evidence have suggested that estrogen receptor (ER) determinations may be a substantial aid in clinical assessment of the likelihood of eventual disease recurrence. ER-negative (ER–) tumors have been shown to have high thymidine labeling indices and therefore more rapid proliferative rates than ER-positive (ER+) tumors (Meyer et al., 1977). It has been reported that patients with ER– tumors have a shorter survival than patients with ER+ tumors (Walt et al., 1976). Recently, Knight et al. (1977, 1978) have shown that patients with ER+ tumors have a longer disease-free interval and also a longer survival than patients with ER– tumors. This report analyzes the association between ER status and the disease-free interval, as measured from the time of mastectomy until first recurrence.

Patients and Methods

Receptor Assays

Biopsies of primary tumors at the time of mastectomy and of metastatic lesions were trimmed of excess fat and nontumorous tissue and divided, with a portion submitted for confirming pathology in all cases. Samples for ER assay were kept on ice and then frozen in liquid nitrogen within 20 min. Steroid hormone receptor assays were performed as previously described (LIPPMAN and HUFF, 1976). When the samples were adequate, Scatchard analyses were performed to quantify the number of binding sites; otherwise assays were performed in duplicate at one or two concentrations of 17β-estradiol chosen to exceed the expected equilibrium dissociation constant by several times. Data were analyzed by computer-assisted methods (AITKEN and LIPPMAN, 1977). An ER assay was taken to be positive if 10 fmol ^{3}H-estradiol binding per mg cytoplasmic protein was found.

Patients

From July, 1974 until September, 1977, mastectomy was performed in 182 women for resectable breast cancer; 110 women had biopsies of metastatic lesions. All patients were from Georgetown University, Howard University, George Washington University, and the National Cancer Institute. Clinical information was obtained from the patient records. Recurrence of disease was documented by liver, bone, and brain scans, chest X-ray, and bone survey. Biopsies were usually performed if metastatic lesions were easily accessible. ER status did not influence the frequency or extent of follow-up examinations. Of the patients, 83% were followed for at least 1 year; 70% for at least 18 months; 42% for at least 2 years; 22% for at least 30 months, and 9% for at least 3 years. The median follow-up was 23 months.

Statistical Analysis

Comparisons of proportions were performed by the contingency χ^2-test with continuity correction. Comparisons of continuous or ordered polychotomous distributions were performed by the Wilcoxon rank-sum test adjusted for ties (LEHMANN, 1975). This latter test requires no distributional assumptions of the data, as would a t-test. All significance levels are of the two-sided type.

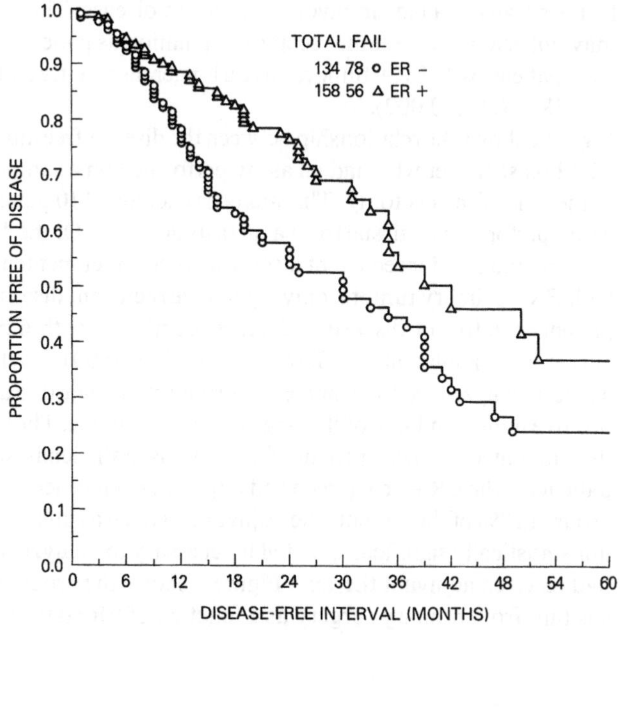

Fig. 1. The relationship between the disease-free interval and ER status in patients with breast cancer. O——O, ER–; Δ——Δ, ER+

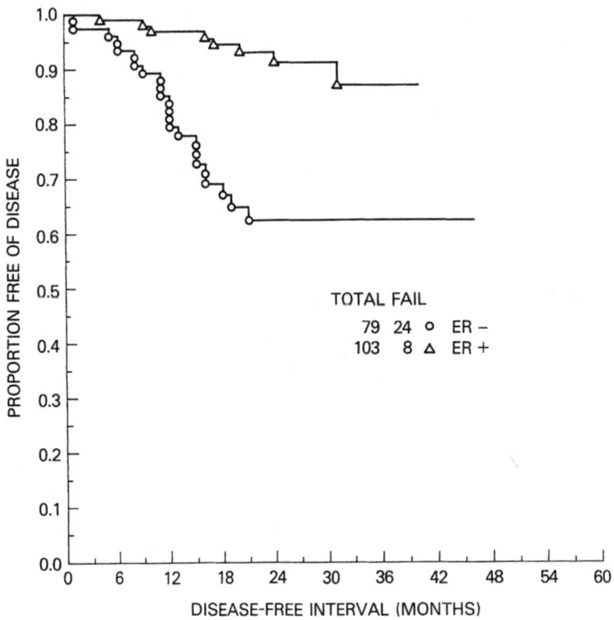

Fig. 2. The relationship between the disease-free interval and ER status in patients with breast cancer. This figure includes only patients who had an assay performed on their primary tumor at the time of mastectomy and excludes patients who had an assay performed on tissues from a metastatic lesion. O——O, ER−; Δ——Δ, ER+

Results

Figure 1 illustrates the relationship between disease-free interval and ER status in 292 patients with breast cancer. In this overall analysis, we included patients who had an assay performed on their primary tumor at the time of mastectomy and also patients who had an assay performed on metastatic lesions. The inclusion of patients with an assay performed on a metastasis leads to a bias in favor of recurrent disease. That is, patients who have not recurred may not belong to the same receptor population as patients who have recurred. Even with this bias, patients with ER+ tumors have a longer disease-free interval than patients whose tumors are ER− ($P < 0.002$).

Figure 2 shows the relationship between the disease-free interval and ER status in 182 patients with breast cancer who had an assay performed on a sample taken from their primary tumor at the time of mastectomy. This analysis excludes 110 patients included in Fig. 1 who had an assay performed on tissue from a metastatic lesion. Of the 182 patients, 79 had ER− primary tumors, and thus far recurrent disease has been documented in 24 patients. Of the 103 patients with ER+ primary tumors, only eight have recurrent disease. Ninety-one percent of the ER+ patients are free of disease at 2 years, compared with 62% of the ER− patients. The two curves are significantly different at the $P < 0.001$ level.

Table 1 analyzes the ER+ and ER− groups with regard to age, menopausal status, number of positive nodes, and size of the largest primary nodule. The two groups are similar and none of the differences in these prognostic factors is statistically significant. Twenty-five percent of patients in the ER+ group received adjuvant chemotherapy, compared with 32% in the ER− group. In 8% of the patients the adjuvant status was unknown. Although these differences are not statistically significant, we felt it necessary to analyze our data excluding all patients who had received adjuvant therapy. Figure 3 shows the proportion of patients free of disease versus time from primary surgery as a function of ER status for the 108 patients who did not re-

Table 1. Comparison of the ER+ and ER− groups with regard to factors that may affect the disease-free interval

	ER+ (%)	ER− (%)
Age	(N = 103)	(N = 79)
< 30	1	7
30–39	12	13
40–49	13	26
50–59	36	35
60–69	24	10
≥ 70	15	8
Menopausal status		
Premenopausal	21	46
Postmenopausal	79	54
Size of the largest primary nodule		
< 2 cm	47	52
> 2 cm	53	48
Number of positive axillary nodes		
0	61	41
1–3	15	31
≥ 4	24	28

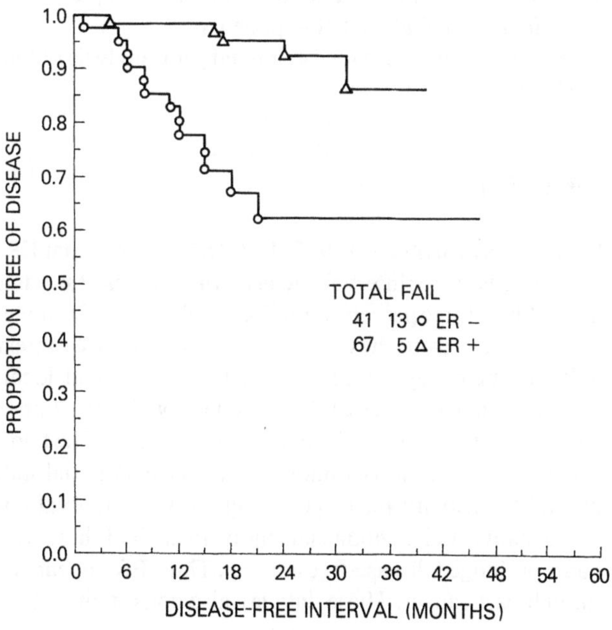

Fig. 3. The relationship between the disease-free interval and ER status in patients with breast cancer. This figure includes only patients who had an assay performed on their primary tumor at the time of mastectomy and who did not receive adjuvant chemotherapy. O——O, ER−; Δ——Δ, ER+

Table 2. The relationship between ER status and disease-free interval as a function of nodal status, tumor size and menopausal status

	Rate of recurrence	
	ER+	ER−
Axillary nodal status		
0	5/52	8/30 ($P < 0.02$)
1–3	0/13	6/23 ($P = 0.08$)
4	2/20	7/21 ($P = 0.05$)
Tumor size		
< 2 cm	4/36	7/30 ($P < 0.04$)
> 2 cm	1/40	10/28 ($P < 0.001$)
Menopausal status		
Premenopausal	1/20	14/32 ($P < 0.01$)
Postmenopausal	4/76	7/37 ($P < 0.01$)

ceive adjuvant chemotherapy. Of these patients, 41 were in the ER− group and 13 have recurrent disease, compared with 5 of 67 patients in the ER+ group with recurrent disease ($P < 0.001$). This analysis shows that the ER status influences the disease-free interval in patients who are not receiving adjuvant chemotherapy.

Table 2 shows the effect of ER status on disease-free interval as a function of other prognostic factors that could affect the disease-free interval. Axillary nodal status, tumor size, and menopausal status are examined. In all categories, ER+ patients have a significantly lower recurrence rate than patients whose tumors are ER−. Thus, it appears unlikely that differences in known prognostic variables can explain the improved disease-free interval in ER+ patients compared with that in ER− patients.

At present our data are too preliminary for analysis of the effect of ER status on patient survival.

Discussion

Recently, Knight et al. (1977, 1978) have shown that ER positivity is associated with a prolonged disease-free interval and also with increased survival. These authors examined 145 patients. Sixty-three percent were ER+ and 37% had primary tumors that were ER−. Not only did the ER+ group have a prolonged disease-free interval, but also this association was independent of age, nodal status, tumor size and location, and postoperative therapy.

Our data agree with these results. Patients with ER+ tumors have a prolonged disease-free interval compared with patients with ER− tumors. The two groups were similar with respect to age, menopausal status, tumor size, and axillary nodal status. In addition, the relationship between ER positivity and prolonged disease-free interval was present irrespective of tumor size, nodal status, and menopausal status. In each of these categories, patients with ER+ tumors had a prolonged disease-free interval. Thus, ER appears to be an independent prognostic factor in breast cancer. These data are also consistent with reported data showing that ER− tu-

mors have high thymidine labeling indices and rapid proliferative rates. Both of these factors could lead to the shorter disease-free interval characteristic of ER− tumors.
Finally, these data have certain implications for the treatment of breast cancer. If ER status is indeed associated with a prolonged disease-free interval, then it seems logical to stratify future adjuvant therapy trials according to receptor status, as is now done for other prognostic factors such as tumor size and axillary nodal status. Second, caution would be required in comparing disease-free interval in patients receiving adjuvant chemotherapy with disease-free interval in an historical control group, unless ER status is known for both groups. Third, these studies clearly encourage the extension of adjuvant therapy trials to axillary lymph node-negative ER− patients, because of their high rate of recurrence. Finally, the low rate of recurrence in ER+ patients, together with the very high incidence of ER positivity in postmenopausal patients, may contribute to the failure of adjuvant regimens to show any significant advantage in older women, given the relatively short periods of follow-up thus far analyzed.

References

Aitken, S., Lippman, M. E.: A simple computer program for quantification and Scatchard analysis of steroid receptor proteins. J. Steroid Biochem. *8,* 77–94 (1977)

Knight, W. A., Livingston, R. B., Gregory, E. J., McGuire, W. L.: Estrogen receptor as an independent prognostic factor for early recurrence in breast cancer. Cancer Res. *37,* 4669–4671 (1977)

Knight, W. A., Livingston, R. B., Gregory, E. J., Walder, A. I., McGuire, W. L.: Absent estrogen receptor and decreased survival in human breast cancer. Proc. Ann. Meet. Am. Soc. Clin. Oncol. (Abstract) #C-342 (1978)

Lehman, E. H.: Non parametrics: Statistical methods based on ranks. p. 208. San Francisco: Holden-Day 1975

Lippman, M. E., Huff, K. K.: A demonstration of androgen and estrogen receptors in human breast cancer using a new protamine sulfate assay. Cancer *38,* 868–874 (1976)

Meyer, J. S., Rao, B. R., Stevens, S. C., White, W. L.: Low incidence of estrogen receptor in breast carcinomas with rapid rates of cellular replication. Cancer *40,* 2290–2298 (1977)

Walt, A. J., Singhakaowinta, A., Brooks, S. C., Cortez, A.: The surgical implications of estrophile protein estimations in carcinoma of the breast. Surgery *80,* 506–512 (1976)

6. *Clinical Predictive Criteria for Response to Endocrine Treatment and the Receptor Status*

H. Maass and W. Jonat

Kliniken der Freien Hansestadt Bremen, Zentralkrankenhaus St. Jürgen-Straße, Frauenklinik, Abteilung II, St. Jürgen-Straße, D-2800 Bremen 1 (FRG)

Oestrogen receptors have a well-established value in prediction of the response to endocrine treatment in advanced breast cancer. Recent data have given evidence that the receptor status could also be of value for predicting the chemotherapeutic effect. This was first pointed out by LIPPMAN et al. (1978). A similar trend had been observed in the prospective trial being conducted by KING (1978) and our own data also give the same impression (JONAT and MAASS, 1978) (Table 1).

Table 1. ER status versus remission rate after cytotoxic agents

Receptor assay	JONAT	LIPPMAN	KING
ER+	6/14[b] (43)[a]	3/25 (12)	11/19 (58)
ER–	20/28 (71)	34/45 (76)	8/12 (67)

[a] Numbers in parentheses are response rates (percentage).
[b] Number of patients with remission/total number of patients.

Table 2. Clinical course of oestrogen receptor-positive versus ER-negative patients under endocrine treatment

	No.	Objective remission	No change Partial remission R. of another lesion	Previous remission	No effect
ER+	53	34 = 64%	5	7	7 = 13%
ER–	52	3	4	2	43 = 83%

Table 3. ER-receptor status in metastases of human breast carcinoma. (KORSTEN et al., 1974; LEUNG et al., 1974)

Site of biopsy	ER+	ER–
Soft tissue	42%	58%
Viscera	61%	39%
Bone	55%	45%
Liver	87%	13%

Table 4. Influence of interval between menopause and beginning of hormone therapy. (Modified from HEUSON, 1974)

	A.M.A.[a]	C.B.C.G.[b]	STOLL[c]
Interval (years)	Remission (%)	Remission (%)	Remission (%)
0–4	12	7	7
5–9	38	29	23
>9	37	20	26

[a] A.M.A., Council on Drugs (1960).
[b] C.B.C.G., COOPERATIVE BREAST CANCER GROUP (1964).
[c] STOLL (1973).

Contradictory findings were reported by FRENNING's group to the American Society of Clinical Oncology in April, 1978, however. Therefore, we need further information on this very important point, especially insofar as it concerns the selection of patients for adjuvant trials.

On the other hand, the fact that about 40% of receptor-positive patients with metastatic breast cancer have no objective response to endocrine treatment is one of the main problems, although the remission rates in this group selected for receptor status are absolutely comparable to those after chemotherapy. If we include patients with partial remission (less than 50% of bulk) and no change in their disease there have been over 75% clinically favourable responses in our material (Table 2).

Nevertheless, this correlation is not yet satisfactory. We know that quantification of oestrogen-receptor content and determination of other receptors can lead to better results, these parameters are needed, probably together with certain morphological examinations, for better characterisation of the tumour.

There have been clinical experiences with prognostic factors that have not been in full agreement with the receptor status. The prognostic criterion of the length of the disease-free interval seems to be in line with the receptor findings. JENSEN (1978) and KNIGHT et al. (1977) observed a shorter disease-free interval in patients with no or a very low oestrogen-receptor content in their tumours. In our material we did not find a significant difference, but nevertheless there probably is a link.

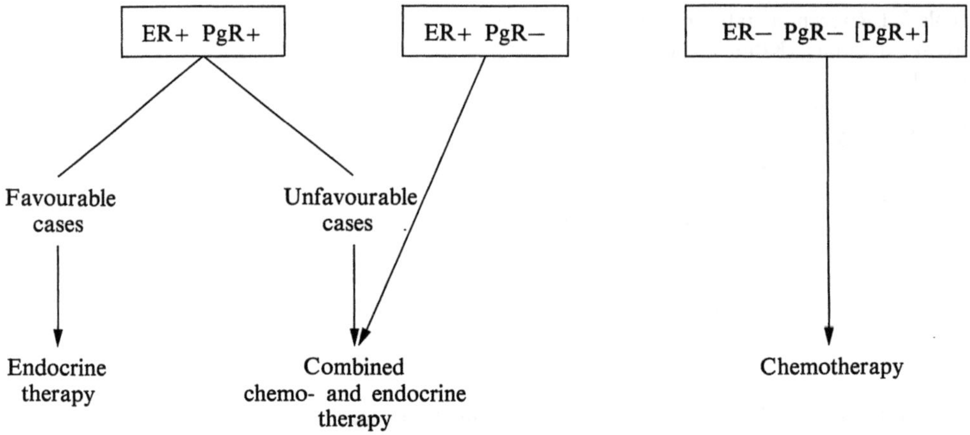

Fig. 1. Treatment of advanced breast cancer. ER, oestrogen receptor; PgR, progesterone receptor

The other important clinical parameter for response to endocrine manipulations is the site of metastases. We all know that patients with visceral metastases, especially of liver and brain, are poor responders to any kind of endocrine therapy. This is obviously not reflected in the receptor status. Table 3 shows the data of LEUNG et al. (1974) and KORSTEN et al. (1974), who published a reasonable number of receptor determinations from liver metastases. The rate of "positives", especially among liver lesions, is disproportionately high. This is in contrast to our clinical experience and knowledge.

The third clinical parameter is the duration of menopause. Patients in the first 5 years after menopause are very poor responders to ablative and additive endocrine treatments. This well-known fact is demonstrated in Table 4. The reason for it is unknown. We do not know whether there are any data available on the endocrine milieu of these patients, for example expressed as a discriminant function.

The oestrogen receptor data give no explanation for this phenomenon. Figure 1 does not differentiate the ER-positive cases according to the menopausal status of patients with primary breast cancer. The women who are in the early years of menopause show quantitative ER contents comparable to those of elderly patients. It cannot be excluded that patients who develop metastases during this phase of their lives may have a higher proportion of receptor-negative metastatic lesions, but it seems unlikely.

In conclusion, there are patients who are not suitable for endocrine treatment only, regardless of their positive receptor status. In consequence they are candidates for a combined hormonal and cytotoxic therapy. If we exclude these ER-positive patients with unfavourable prognosis from our trials we should achieve better correlations in the remaining subjects.

References

Cooperative Breast Cancer Group: Progress report: Results of studies of the Cooperative Breast Cancer Group 1961–1963. Cancer Chemother. Rep. *41,* 1 (1964)

Council on Drugs: Androgens and estrogens in the treatment of disseminated mammary carcinoma. Retrospective study of nine hundred forty-four patients. Report to the Council. JAMA *172,* 1271 (1960)

Jensen, E.: Presented at the First Innsbruck Winter Conference on Biochemistry in Clinical Medicine, Jan. 1978. Innsbruck, Austria (to be published)

Jonat, W., Maass, H.: Some comments on the necessity of receptor determination in human breast cancer. Cancer Res. *38,* 4305–4306 (1978)

King, R.: Presented at the First Innsbruck Winter Conference on Biochemistry in Clinical Medicine. Jan. 1978 Innsbruck, Austria (to be published)

Knight, III, W. A., Livingston, R. B., Gregory, E. J., McGuire, W. L.: Estrogen receptor as an independent prognostic factor for early recurrence in breast cancer. Cancer Res. *37,* 4669–4671 (1977)

Korsten, G. B., Engelsman, E., Persijn, J. P.: Clinical value of estrogen receptors in advanced breast cancer. In: Estrogen receptors in human breast cancer. McGuire, W. L., Carbone, P. P., Vollmer, E. P. (eds.), pp. 93–105. New York: Raven Press 1974

Leung, S. B., Moseley, H. S., Davenport, C. E., Krippaehne, W. W., Fletcher, W. S.: Estrogen receptor in prediction of clinical responses to endocrine ablation. In: Estrogen receptors in human breast cancer. McGuire, W. L., Carbone, P. P., Vollmer, E. P. (eds.), pp. 107–129. New York: Raven Press 1974

Lippman, M. E., Allegra, J. C., Thompson, E. B., Simon, R., Barlock, A., Green, R. N. L., Huff, K. K., Do, H. M. T., Aitken, S. C., Warren, R.: The relation between estrogen receptors and response rate to cytotoxic chemotherapy in metastatic breast cancer. N. Engl. J. Med. *298,* 1223–1228 (1978)

Stoll, B. A.: Hypothesis: breast cancer regression under oestrogen therapy. Br. Med. J. *1973 III,* 446

II. Antiestrogens in Experimental Breast Cancer

7. *Anti-Oestrogen Action in Experimental Breast Cancer*

V. C. Jordan, K. E. Naylor, C. J. Dix, and G. Prestwich

Department of Pharmacology, Medical and Dental Building, University of Leeds, Leeds LS2 9JT (U.K.)

The pharmacological response to a drug is dependent upon efficient absorption after administration, followed by distribution to the site of action. The duration of the pharmacological effect is directly related to the biological half-life of the parent drug and its active metabolites. At the molecular level, the tissue response is the result of an interaction of the drug and its metabolites with a biochemical target or receptor.

In laboratory animals tamoxifen (1-p-β-dimethylaminoethoxyphenyl-trans-1,2-diphenylbut-1-ene) is metabolically hydroxylated to mono- and dihydroxytamoxifen (Fromson et al., 1973), and it has been shown that these metabolites are pharmacologically active in the rat (Jordan et al., 1977a). Structural derivatives of tamoxifen that cannot undergo metabolic para-hydroxylation are only weakly anti-oestrogenic in the rat (Clark and Jordan, unpublished observation), so that the ability to be hydroxylated seems to be an advantage for tamoxifen's activity in vivo.

Since the properties of tamoxifen in laboratory animals may be the net result of a complex interaction of the parent drug and its metabolites with either oestrogen target tissues or hormone-dependent cancers, we describe the pharmacology of tamoxifen and its metabolite monohydroxytamoxifen (Fig. 1) in the present review.

Uterine Effects of Tamoxifen and Monohydroxytamoxifen

Classic tests (e.g., vaginal cornification and uterine wet weight) for assay of oestrogenic and anti-oestrogenic activity have shown tamoxifen to be an anti-oestrogen with a partial oestrogen-agonist activity in immature (Harper and Walpole, 1967; Jordan, 1976a) and ovariectomised rats (Jordan and Koerner, 1976). Monohydroxytamoxifen has similar

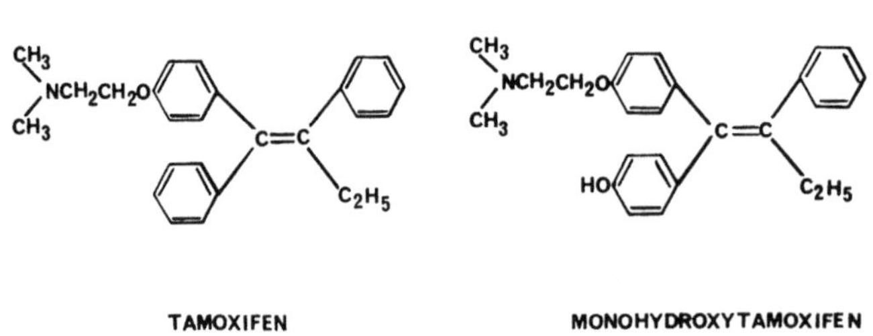

Fig. 1. Structure of tamoxifen and its metabolite monohydroxytamoxifen

Fig. 2. Effect of administration (sc in 0.1 ml arachis oil) of 0.08 μg oestradiol alone (○) or oestradiol and various doses of the anti-oestrogens monohydroxytamoxifen (●) or tamoxifen (■) to immature rats for 3 days on uterine wet weight. Animals were killed on day 4. Results are means ± SEM (*bars*), with ten rats in each treatment group. (Data from JORDAN, V. C. et al., 1978b)

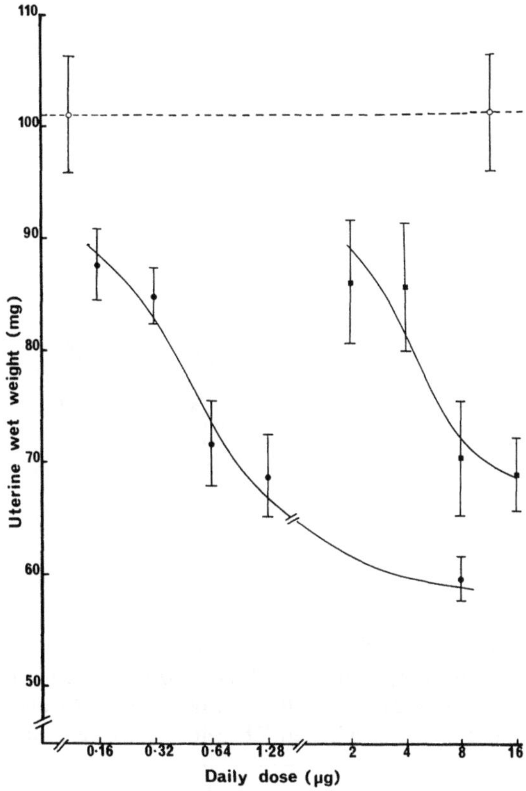

pharmacological properties but it is more potent than tamoxifen. (JORDAN et al., 1977a). This is illustrated in Fig. 2. To facilitate some understanding of the reasons for the application of anti-oestrogens in the treatment of hormone-dependent cancer it is perhaps pertinent to review the various cellular and subcellular effects of oestrogens and compare these effects with those observed with tamoxifen and monohydroxytamoxifen.

Since the pioneering work of JENSEN and JACOBSEN (1962) on the binding of ^{3}H-17β-oestradiol in immature rat oestrogen target tissues (uterus and vagina), intense interest has focussed upon the initiation and control of oestrogen-dependent events. Oestradiol is believed to stimulate uterine growth by selectively binding to oestrogen-receptor (ER) proteins located in the cell cytoplasm, which are then translocated in association with the steroid to the nucleus where RNA and DNA synthesis is initiated (JENSEN and DESOMBRE, 1973).

Tamoxifen and monohydroxytamoxifen inhibit the binding of ^{3}H-oestradiol in vitro to the 8S cytoplasmic ER protein derived from human (HUNTER and JORDAN, 1975; JORDAN and KOERNER, 1975a; JORDAN et al., 1977a) and animal (JORDAN and KOERNER, 1975b; POWELL-JONES et al., 1975; JORDAN and DOWSE, 1976) oestrogen target tissues. The antagonism of oestrogen binding has been shown to be competitive (SKIDMORE et al., 1972). Recently, studies with ^{3}H-tamoxifen have demonstrated direct binding to the rat uterine 8S ER (JORDAN and PRESTWICH, 1977a; CAPONY and ROCHEFORT, 1978).

The administration of tamoxifen or monohydroxytamoxifen depletes the cytoplasmic ER pool in a dose-dependent manner (JORDAN et al., 1978b) by translocating the resulting complexes to the nucleus (JORDAN et al., 1977b; KOSEKI et al., 1977a).

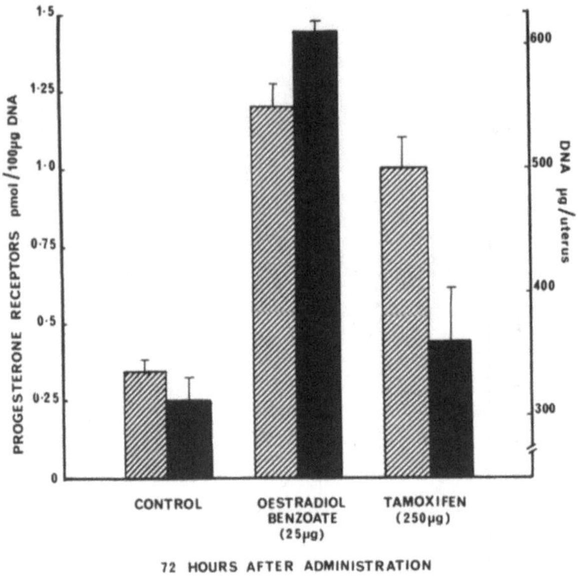

Fig. 3. The effect of sc injection of oestradiol benzoate (25 μg in 0.5 ml 0.9% saline) and tamoxifen (250 μg in 0.5 ml 0.9% saline) on immature rat uterine progesterone receptor content (pmol/100 μg DNA: ▨) and uterine DNA (μg/uterus: ■) content. Progesterone receptors were determined with ^{3}H-R5020 according to the method described by VU HAI and MILGROM (1978), and DNA was determined by the method of BURTON (1956) with calf uterine DNA standards 72 h after administration. Results represent mean ± SEM of groups of four determinations. (Data from JORDAN, V. C. et al. in press)

Table 1. The effect of sc administration of oestradiol benzoate (25 μg in 0.1 ml arachis oil) or monohydroxytamoxifen (25 μg in 0.1 ml arachis oil) to immature female rats on endometrial thickness and mitosis. Uteri were obtained 24, 48, and 72 h after administration. Colchicine (100 μg in saline) was administered 7 h before sacrifice to facilitate mitotic counts

Treatment (hours after administration)	Endometrial thickness[a] (μm ± SEM) (n = 20)	Mean % of endometrial mitoses (± SEM) n = 50
Control	14.4 ± 0.4	0
Oestradiol benzoate		
24 h	25.3 ± 0.7	0.18 ± 0.18
48 h	42.9 ± 1.4	22.9 ± 0.93
72 h	25.6 ± 0.66	9.22 ± 0.88
Monohydroxytamoxifen		
24 h	27.1 ± 0.95	0
48 h	44.3 ± 1.13	0.07 ± 0.07
72 h	55.7 ± 1.06	0.47 ± 0.19

[a] All treatments significantly ($P < 0.001$ by Student's *t*-test) increased endometrial thickness over that in controls.

Tamoxifen produces a partial rise in uterine wet weight but only slightly increases the uterine DNA content in ovariectomised (JORDAN, 1976a) or immature (JORDAN et al., 1977b) rats. The inability to stimulate a rise in uterine DNA content is unaffected if the administered dose of tamoxifen is increased. Injection of 25μg (CLARK et al., 1978) or 250 μg tamoxifen (Fig. 3) does not increase the uterine DNA content. In contrast, oestradiol or oestradiol benzoate does increase rat uterine DNA content. These observations have been confirmed histologically (JORDAN et al., 1980). Oestradiol benzoate produces an increase in endometrial cell division, resulting in hyperplasia, whereas tamoxifen increases endometrial cell size with virtually no cell division. The principle is illustrated in Table 1, where the effects of oestradiol benzoate and monohydroxytamoxifen on endometrial cell thickness and mitosis are compared.

Although uterine cell division is inhibited by anti-oestrogens, protein synthesis seems to be initiated in the hypertrophied cells. Tamoxifen (JORDAN and PRESTWICH, 1977b; KOSEKI et al., 1977b; Fig. 3) and monohydroxytamoxifen (JORDAN and PRESTWICH, 1978; DIX and JORDAN, 1978) produce rises in the concentration of rat uterine progesterone receptors. Therefore the anti-oestrogen—ER complex has produced a separation of the biological functions of uterine protein synthesis and DNA synthesis.

The anti-oestrogen-stimulated rises in uterine progesterone receptors may have important implications for the future clinical management of endometrial carcinoma and the resulting metastases. Tamoxifen inhibits the binding of ^{3}H-oestradiol to ERs derived from human uterine adenocarcinomata (JORDAN and KOERNER, 1975a), which suggests that anti-oestrogens might be expected to inhibit oestrogen-stimulated growth. If tamoxifen could also sensitise the carcinomata to the pharmacological effects of progestin therapy then a careful clinical study of all the practical therapeutic regimens should be undertaken. It is interesting to note that a combination of nonsteroidal anti-oestrogens and progestins has a synergistic effect on the growth inhibition of rat uterine adenocarcinoma cells in tissue culture (SEKIYA and TAKAMIZAWA, 1976).

Effect of Tamoxifen and Monohydroxytamoxifen on Dimethylbenzanthracene (DMBA)-Induced Mammary Carcinomata

Mammary carcinomata induced by a single oral administration of DMBA to 50-day-old Sprague Dawley rats were first described by HUGGINS et al. (1961). Tumours appear 60—200 days after carcinogen administration. The initiation of tumour induction requires a stable hormone environment, since ovariectomy (DAO, 1962) and a variety of antihormone (HEUSON et al., 1971) and pharmacological therapies (KLEDZIK et al., 1974) will inhibit or retard the appearance of tumours. The majority of established DMBA-induced tumours regress following ovariectomy or hypophysectomy (STERENTAL et al., 1963), and the tumours in ovariectomised rats regrow in response to oestradiol or prolactin administration (PEARSON et al., 1972). The model is complicated by the fact that oestradiol can stimulate prolactin release (CHEN and MEITES, 1970), and the precise mechanism of hormonal control of the tumours has remained obscure. The possibility that both prolactin and oestradiol are necessary for tumour homeostasis has been suggested (SINHA et al., 1973; LEUNG and SASAKI, 1975), and this thesis can be defended at the subcellular level since both ERs (KING et al., 1965; MOBBS, 1966) and prolactin (TURKINGTON, 1974; KELLY et al., 1974) receptors have been shown to be present in the tumours.

Tamoxifen is effective in preventing the initiation (JORDAN, 1974; 1976b) and inhibiting the growth of hormone-dependent DMBA-induced rat mammary carcinomata (NICHOLSON and GOLDER, 1975; JORDAN and DOWSE, 1976; JORDAN and JASPAN, 1976a; JORDAN and KOERNER, 1976). The effectiveness of daily administration of tamoxifen on the growth of mammary tumours on a single rat is illustrated in Fig. 4. Each tumour responds individually, about 10%—15% of a tumour population being completely unresponsive. The antitumour activity appears to be reversible; once the anti-oestrogenic effects disappear after a short course of therapy, i.e., when the compound is cleared from the body, some of the tumours continue to

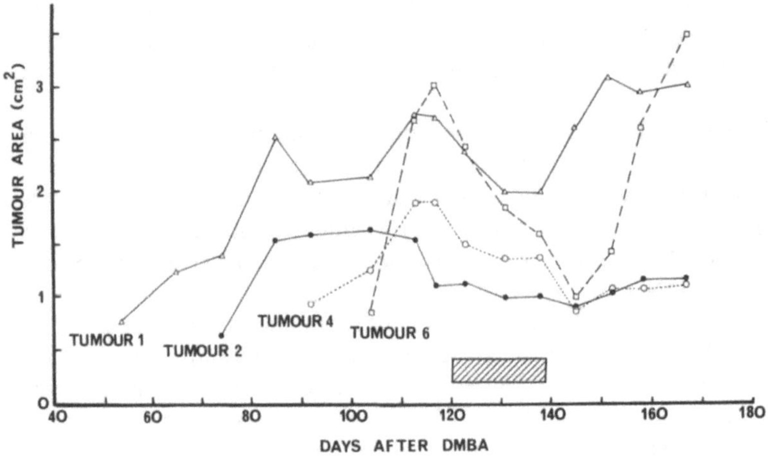

Fig. 4. Effect of daily sc administrations of tamoxifen (50 μg in 0.1 ml arachil oil) on the growth of DMBA-induced mammary carcinomata in a single female rat. Tumours were measured weekly with calipers in two dimensions; length (l) and width (w). Tumour area was calculated according to the formula $\pi \times \frac{1}{2} \times w/2$. Oestrous cycles stopped during tamoxifen therapy (▨) and resumed 1 week after the cessation of treatment. (Data from JORDAN, V. C., 1976a)

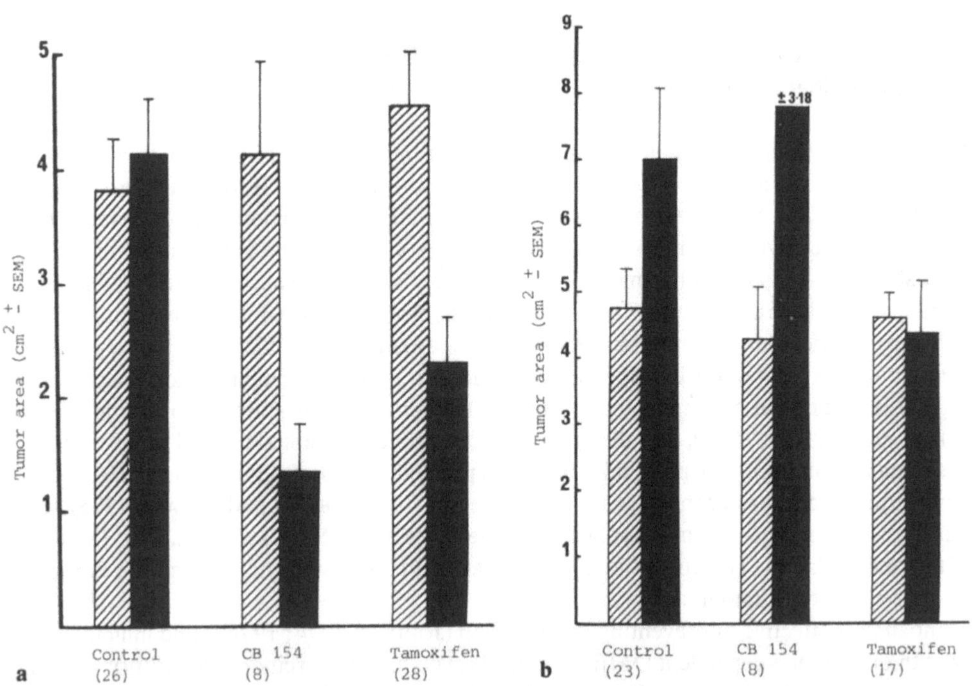

Fig. 5a, b. Effect of CB154 (bromocryptine) or tamoxifen on the growth of DMBA-induced tumours < 200 days after DMBA (**a**) or > 200 days after DMBA (**b**). Compounds (CB154 1.5 mg; tamoxifen 50 μg) were administered daily and the mean tumour areas compared before (▨) and after 3 weeks of therapy (■). The number of tumours followed is shown in parentheses. Comparisons by means of Student's *t*-test before and after therapy (**a**): CB154 and tamoxifen $P < 0.01$. All other values $P > 0.05$

grow. Tumour 6, for example, regressed rapidly during tamoxifen therapy but started to regrow when therapy was stopped. In a continuation of the experiment not shown in the figure, this tumour regressed upon ovariectomy but regrew during the daily administration of oestradiol.

The age of the tumour after DMBA seems to have important implications for the successful outcome of antihormone therapy. Young tumours, used for experiments no later than 200 days after DMBA, usually regress in response to 3 weeks of therapy with either tamoxifen or an inhibitor of prolactin release such as CB154 (Fig. 5a). In contrast, older tumours (more than 200 days after DMBA) appear to be refractory to the effects of antihormone therapy (Fig. 5b).

Possible Modes of Action of Tamoxifen

Tamoxifen could potentially have an effect at one or all of three major sites, thereby modifying the hormonal environment in which the tumour is growing:
1) Chemical oophorectomy by inhibition of the synthesis of ovarian steroids,
2) Inhibition of oestrogen-stimulated prolactin release from the pituitary,
3) Blockade of ERs in the mammary tumour so that direct oestrogenic effects are inhibited (whilst the direct effects of prolactin may be modified).
Each of these mechanisms will be considered in turn.

1) Chemical Oophorectomy

Tamoxifen has been found to reduce the circulating levels of oestradiol in the rat (WATSON et al., 1975) by inhibiting the synthesis of oestradiol in the ovary (WATSON and ALAM, 1976; WATSON and HOWSON, 1977). Reductions in the peripheral levels of circulating oestradiol during tamoxifen therapy have been reported in animals with DMBA-induced tumours (JORDAN and KOERNER, 1976). Clearly a reduction in the levels of oestradiol would reduce the direct effects of oestradiol on the tumour and may also modify oestrogen-stimulated release of prolactin from the pituitary.

2) Inhibition of Oestrogen-Stimulated Prolactin Release

Nonsteroidal antioestrogens partially inhibit oestrogen-stimulated rises in plasma prolactin (HEUSON et al., 1971, JORDAN et al., 1975) but whereas tamoxifen will produce a dose-related decrease in the rise in oestradiol-stimulated uterine wet weight in ovariectomised rats, this trend is not paralleled by the circulating levels of prolactin (Table 2). Tamoxifen will only produce about a 50% reduction in the circulating prolactin levels and is unable to reduce plasma levels to those observed in ovariectomised rats.

Results in intact animals have been confusing. Tamoxifen inhibits (or delays) the pro-oestrous surge of prolactin (JORDAN et al., 1975), but studies in rats with DMBA-induced tumours have failed to show a uniform decrease in circulating prolactin levels (NICHOLSON and GOLDER, 1975; JORDAN and KOERNER, 1976). It is interesting to note that in one study (JORDAN and KOERNER, 1976) a group of rats whose tumours continued to grow during tamoxifen treatment had a high circulating level of prolactin. This finding is consistent with the report that perphenazine, a stimulator of prolactin secretion, can reverse tumour regression by tamoxifen (MANNI et al., 1977). An interesting parallel can perhaps be drawn with the effects of pharmacological doses of oestrogen on the growth of DMBA-induced tumours. Oestradiol

Table 2. Mean (± SEM) uterine wet weights and plasma prolactin levels of ovariectomised rats treated for 8 days with sc injections of oestradiol alone or in combination with increasing doses of tamoxifen (8 rats per group) (Data from JORDAN, V. C. and KOERNER, S., 1976)

Tamoxifen μg/day	Oestradiol μg/day	Uterine wet weight (mg)	Plasma prolactin level (ng/ml)
–	–	152 ± 7^{c}	22.8 ± 5.7^{c}
–	5	515 ± 19	304.4 ± 48.4
12.5	5	443 ± 19^{b}	240.8 ± 27.3
50.0	5	378 ± 27^{c}	179.4 ± 16.8^{a}
200.0	5	290 ± 11^{c}	183.1 ± 4.7^{a}
800.0	5	252 ± 13^{c}	172.9 ± 27.9^{a}

[a–c] Levels of significance compared with oestradiol-treated rats, by Student's *t*-test: [a] $P < 0.05$; [b] $P < 0.02$; [c] $P < 0.001$; other values $P > 0.05$.

benzoate alone or in combination with ergocornine, an inhibitor of prolactin release, provokes tumour regression (QUADRI et al., 1974) and reduces prolactin binding in tumour tissue (KLEDZIK et al., 1976). The inhibitory effects of oestrogen can be reversed by the simultaneous administration of prolactin (MEITES et al., 1971). This suggests that high doses of oestrogen may interfere directly with the stimulating action of prolactin on mammary tumour tissue, despite the ability of oestrogen to stimulate prolactin release. Tamoxifen may therefore have an action at the hypothalamo–pituitary axis, modifying the secretion of prolactin, or at the level of the tumour cell, modifying the effects of prolactin.

3) Inhibition of Oestrogen Binding

Tamoxifen inhibits the binding of ^{3}H-oestradiol in DMBA-induced tumour tissue determined either in vivo (JORDAN, 1976b; JORDAN and DOWSE, 1976) or in vitro (NICHOLSON and GOLDER, 1975; JORDAN and JASPAN, 1976a). Figure 6 illustrates the effect of 3 weeks of tamoxifen administration on the binding of ^{3}H-oestradiol in vivo. The levels of radioactivity in uterus and vagina were significantly reduced in tamoxifen-treated animals and the levels of radioactivity in DMBA-induced tumours were reduced to those found in nontarget tissue (heart). At the subcellular level, the binding of ^{3}H-oestradiol to the 8S ER protein derived from DMBA-induced tumours is inhibited by tamoxifen (POWELL-JONES et al., 1975; JORDAN and DOWSE, 1976). Oestradiol and tamoxifen translocate ERs from the cytoplasm to the nucleus, but unlike oestradiol tamoxifen cannot sustain rises in RNA polymerase activity in the tumours (NICHOLSON et al., 1977).

JENSEN et al. (1971) have suggested that the presence of the ER in human breast cancer may indicate the dependence of the tumour on oestrogen. Since DMBA-induced tumours exhibit a spectrum of oestrogen binding activities (MOBBS, 1966), we applied JENSEN's concept to experimental rat mammary cancer in an attempt to rationalise the heterogeneous responses to tamoxifen. Rats with established DMBA-induced tumours (approximately 2 cm^2 in cross-sectional area) were biopsied and the ER concentrations were determined (JORDAN and JASPAN, 1976a). Three types of tumour response occurred to three weeks of tamoxifen (50 μg/day) therapy (Fig. 7). At low levels of oestrogen binding (< 12 fmol/mg cytosol protein) the tumours either remained static or continued to grow during therapy. As the ER

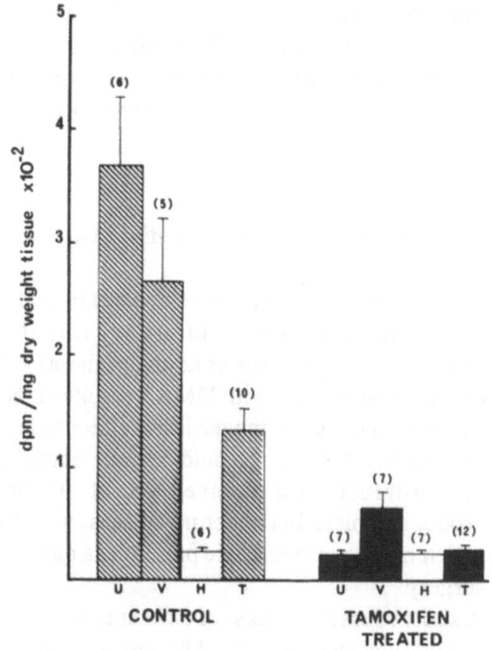

Fig. 6. Binding of 6,7 ^{3}H-oestradiol (30 μCi) in vivo in rat uterus (U), vagina (V), and heart (H), and in DMBA-induced tumour (T) samples. Animals were treated with either arachis oil (control) or tamoxifen (200 μg daily) for 3 weeks to produce a significant reduction in tumour area ($P < 0.05$). Animals were killed 4 h after ^{3}H-oestradiol administration and tissues were dried, weighed, and burnt in a Packard Tricarb tissue oxidizer to determine the levels of radioactivity. The numbers of samples are shown in parentheses. Comparisons by Student's t-test between treated and control groups gave the following results: U, $P < 0.001$; V, $P < 0.01$; T, $P < 0.001$; H, $P > 0.05$. (Data from JORDAN, V. C. and DOWSE, L. J., 1976)

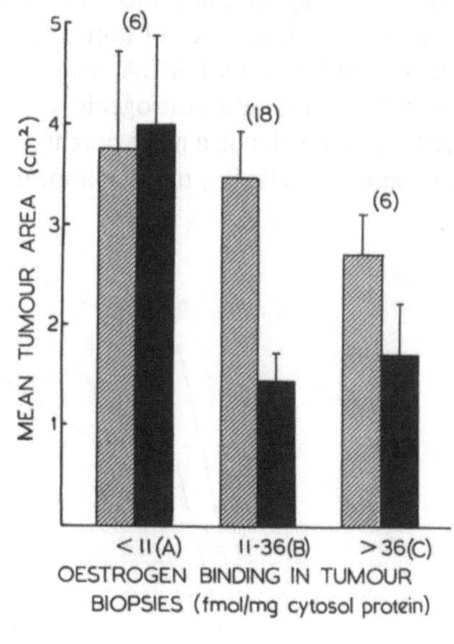

Fig. 7. The types of DMBA-induced tumour response to 3 weeks of tamoxifen therapy (50 μg/day), based on the ER concentration in biopsy samples taken prior to therapy. Details of the ER assay with a sensitive Sephadex LH20 column method for separation of bound and free ^{3}H-oestradiol are in JORDAN and JASPAN (1976a). Tumours were measured before (▨) and after (■) therapy. The numbers of tumours are shown in parentheses. Comparisons of before and after therapy by Student's t-test: group B $P < 0.001$; other groups $P > 0.05$. (Data from JORDAN, V. C. and JASPAN, T., 1976b)

concentration in the biopsy samples increased (12–36 fmol/mg cytosol protein) there was a greater probability of increasing tumour regression. At high concentrations of ERs (> 36 fmol/mg cytosol protein) the mean tumour response was < 50% regression and not complete tumour regression, which might be expected if all the tumour cells were oestrogen-dependent. In these tumours it is possible that the dose of tamoxifen was inadequate to provoke regression or, alternatively, that the tumours contained a low concentration of cells with abnormally high levels of ERs. It is also possible that an inadequate inhibition of prolactin release might aid tumour survival.

In conclusion, it appears that tumours containing low ER levels do not respond to tamoxifen therapy, whilst tumours with more ERs are highly likely to respond to tamoxifen therapy.

Anti-Oestrogens as a Potential Adjuvant Therapy

Although the simultaneous administration of tamoxifen and DMBA reduces the numbers of rat mammary tumours (JORDAN, 1974; JORDAN, 1976b), the model is unsatisfactory for the study of anti-oestrogens as adjuvant therapy. It is possible that simultaneous administration of the anti-oestrogen with DMBA results in the alteration of the receptive nature of the breast tissue so that the carcinogen is less effective in producing a cellular insult. We have formed the opinion that the model would be more acceptable if animals were used 30 days after DMBA administration. It is assumed that at this time the carcinogen will have been effective in producing microfoci of deranged cells, which would be analogous to the clinical situation in which micrometastases are present in a patient after the primary tumour has been removed at surgery.

A short course (4 weeks) of different doses of tamoxifen produced a dose-related decrease in tumour incidence (Fig. 8). Although tumour production was initially decreased by increasing doses of tamoxifen, it is important to note that the majority of animals developed tumours eventually. Their appearance was thus delayed rather than inhibited.

A comparison of equal doses of tamoxifen and monohydroxytamoxifen, administered between 30 and 60 days after DMBA, demonstrated that the pharmacological properties of antitumour activity and anti-oestrogenic activity were not paralleled in this assay. Although monohydroxytamoxifen is a more potent anti-oestrogen than tamoxifen, it was less effective than tamoxifen in delaying tumour appearance (Fig. 9). Since it was possible that mono-

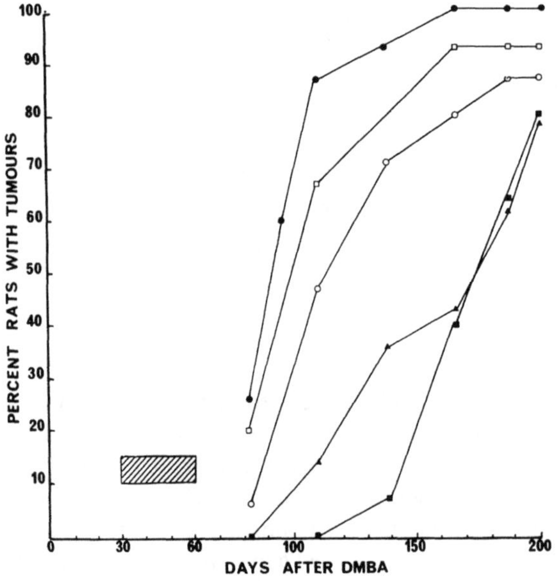

Fig. 8. The effect of sc administration of different daily doses of tamoxifen (0.2, 3, 50, or 800 μg/day in 0.1 ml arachis oil 5 days per week) between 30 and 60 days (▨) after DMBA on the percentage of rats (15 per group) developing tumours by 200 days after DMBA. Controls received arachis oil alone. All tumours were identified histologically as adenocarcinomata. ●——●, controls; □——□, rats treated with 0.2 μg tamoxifen/day; ○——○, 3 μg/day; ▲——▲, 50 μg/day; ■——■, 800 μg/day

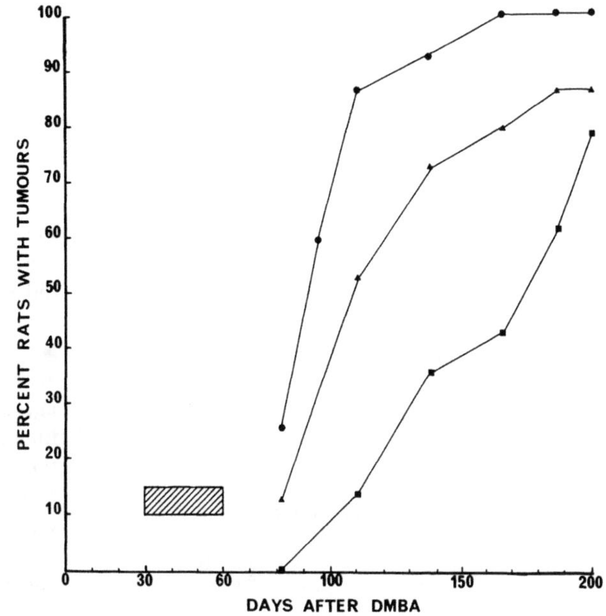

Fig. 9. The effect of daily SC administration (5 days per week) of either monohydroxytamoxifen (▲——▲; 50 μg) in 0.1 ml arachis oil or tamoxifen (■——■, 50 μg in 0,1 ml arachis oil) between 30 and 60 days (▨) after DMBA on the percentage of rats (15 per group) developing tumours by 200 days after DMBA. Controls (●——●) received arachis oil alone. All tumours were identified histologically as adenocarcinomata

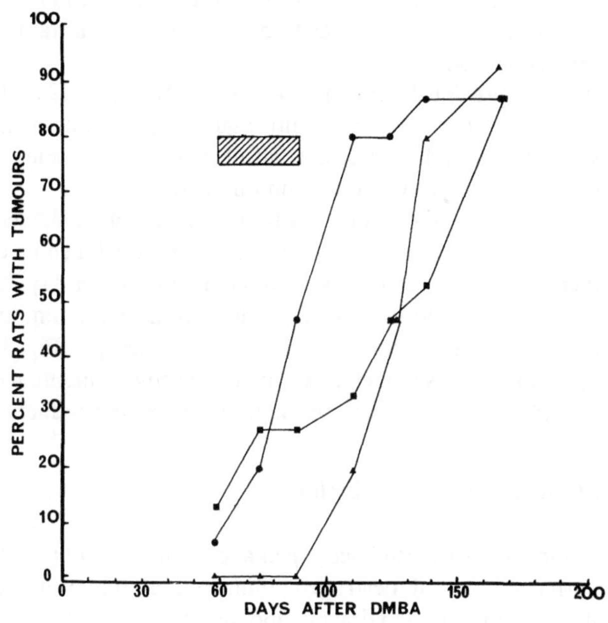

Fig. 10. The effect of daily SC administration (5 days per week) of either monohydroxytamoxifen (▲——▲; 50 μg in 0.1 ml arachis oil) or tamoxifen (■——■; 50 μg in 0.1 ml arachis oil) between 60 and 90 days after DMBA (▨) on the percentage of rats (15 per group) developing tumours. Controls (●——●) received arachis oil alone. All tumours were identified histologically as adenocarcinomata

hydroxytamoxifen had no antitumour activity and that anti-oestrogenic activity was unimportant in this model, we decided to treat animals with the same drug regimens, but this time between 60 and 90 days after DMBA, i.e., when the first palpable tumours were appearing. If monohydroxytamoxifen was an active antitumour agent then tumours in the treated group would not appear as early as controls. With this experimental design monohydroxytamoxifen effectively delayed tumour production, whilst tamoxifen appeared to be less active (Fig. 10).

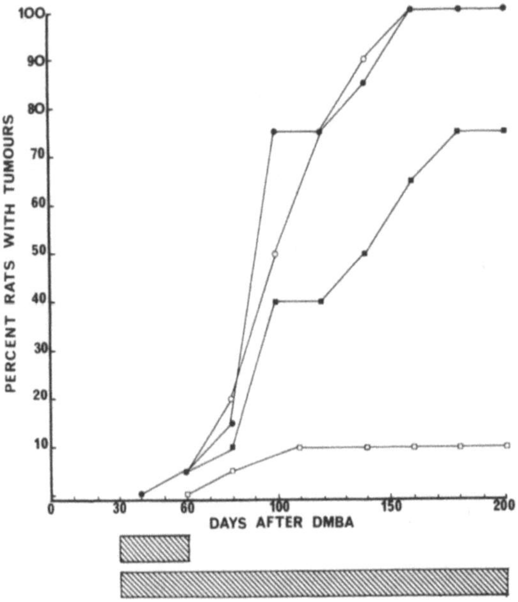

Fig. 11. The effect of daily sc administration (5 days per week) of tamoxifen (50 μg in 0.1 ml arachis oil) for a short period (30–60 days after DMBA ■——■) or continuously (30–200 days after DMBA □——□) on the percentage of rats (20 per group) developing tumours. The experiments were undertaken at different times and the related controls (○——○ and ●——●) received arachis oil alone. All tumours were identified histologically as adenocarcinomata. ▧ treatment periods

After treatment ceased, tumours appeared rapidly in animals previously treated with monohydroxytamoxifen, whereas tumour appearance in tamoxifen-treated animals was perhaps slightly slower.

We have previously shown (Jordan and Naylor, 1978) that the uterine effects produced by monohydroxytamoxifen are not maintained as long as the effects produced by tamoxifen, suggesting that the biological half-life (as well as potency) of a particular anti-oestrogen is an important property for antitumour activity.

Finally, since a short course of tamoxifen therapy only delayed the appearance of tumours in the adjuvant therapy model, we then compared a short course of therapy with continuous therapy. Groups of rats were treated either from day 30 to day 60 after DMBA or from day 30 to day 200 after DMBA. The appearance of tumours was almost completely inhibited in animals during continuous tamoxifen therapy (Fig. 11). In conclusion, it is clearly an advantage in this model for adjuvant therapy to maintain blood levels of tamoxifen for a prolonged period to effectively suppress tumour production.

Summary and Conclusions

Tamoxifen is a partial oestrogen agonist in the rat and inhibits oestrogen-stimulated vaginal cornification and oestrogen-stimulated uterine wet weight increases. Monohydroxytamoxifen, the reported first metabolite of tamoxifen, is a more potent anti-oestrogen. At the cellular level, oestradiol increases endometrial mitosis, whereas both tamoxifen and monohydroxytamoxifen cause endometrial cells to hypertrophy without undergoing division. Although anti-oestrogens inhibit cell division, the uterus is metabolically active, since the concentration of progesterone receptors is increased. This potential sensitisation of uterine cells to the pharmacological effects of progestins may have important implications for the future application of combinations of anti-oestrogens and progestins in the treatment of endometrial carcinoma and the resultant metastases.

Tamoxifen inhibits the initiation and growth of DMBA-induced rat mammary carcinomata. Young tumours appear to be more sensitive to the effects of antihormone therapies and older tumours are refractory to treatment. The growth of DMBA-induced tumours is dependent upon the effects of oestrogens and prolactin. Anti-oestrogens may modify the hormonal environment of the tumour by reducing ovarian oestrogen synthesis, by inhibiting oestrogen-stimulated pituitary prolactin release, or by inhibiting oestrogen binding in tumour tissue. Tumours with a low ER concentration do not respond to tamoxifen therapy.

Although anti-oestrogens are effective in controlling the growth of the majority of established tumours, it is difficult to achieve complete tumour remission. This situation is not unlike the clinical experience with anti-oestrogen therapy in advanced breast cancer. Clearly it would be an advantage to treat animals with a small tumour load to achieve a cure. We have described a model for adjuvant therapy in which tamoxifen administration on days 30–60 after DMBA produced an early dose-related inhibition of tumour incidence. Tumour production was only delayed, however, rather than inhibited. Monohydroxytamoxifen was less active than tamoxifen in this model, and it is concluded that high-potency anti-oestrogens with long biological half-lives have an advantage as antitumour agents. Continued administration of tamoxifen on days 30–200 after DMBA almost completely inhibited the appearance of tumours. The data suggest that short courses of antihormone therapy as adjuvant therapy may ultimately be ineffective in controlling hormone-dependent metastases and prolonged treatment cycles may have to be considered.

Acknowledgements

Studies undertaken at the Worcester Foundation for Experimental Biology, Shrewsbury, Massachusetts, U.S.A., were supported by AID contract CSD 2837; by contract N01-CB-43967 from the Division of Cancer Biology and Diagnosis, National Cancer Institute, DHEW and by ICI United States Inc. Studies at the University of Leeds, England, were supported by grants from the Yorkshire Cancer Research Campaign and ICI Ltd. (Pharmaceuticals Division).

References

Burton, K.: A study of the conditions and mechanism of the diphenylamine reaction for the colorimetric estimation of deoxyribonucleic acid. Biochem. J. *62,* 315–323 (1956)

Capony, F., Rochefort, H.: High-affinity binding of the antiestrogen [^{3}H] tamoxifen to the 8S oestradiol receptor. Mol. Cell. Endocrinol. *11,* 181–198 (1978)

Chen, C. L., Meites, J.: Effect of estrogen and progesterone on serum and pituitary prolactin levels in ovariectomized rats. Endocrinology *86,* 503–505 (1970)

Clark, E. R., Dix, C. J., Jordan, V. C., Prestwich, G., Sexton, S.: A comparison at the cellular and subcellular levels, of the effects of tamoxifen and oestradiol benzoate on the immature rat uterus. Br. J. Pharmacol. *62,* 442P-443P (1978)

Dao, T. L.: The role of ovarian hormones in initiating the induction of mammary cancer in rats by polynuclear hydrocarbons. Cancer Res. *22,* 973–981 (1962)

Dix, C. J., Jordan, V. C.: Contrasting subcellular responses to monohydroxytamoxifen and oestradiol benzoate in the immature rat uterus. Br. J. Pharmacol. *64,* 375P–376P (1978)

Fromson, J. M., Pearson, S., Bramah, S.: The metabolism of tamoxifen (ICI 46,474). 1. In laboratory animals. Xenobiotica *3,* 693–710 (1973)

Harper, M. J. K., Walpole, A. L.: A new derivative of triphenylethylene: effect on implantation and mode of action in rats. J. Reprod. Fertil. *13,* 101–119 (1967)

Heuson, J. C., Waelbroeck, C., Legros, N., Gallez, G., Robyn, C., L'Harmite, N.: Inhibition of DMBA-induced mammary carcinogenesis in the rat by 2Br-α-ergocryptine (CB 154), an inhibitor of prolactin secretion, and by nafoxidine (U-11, 100A), an estrogen antagonist. Gynecol. Invest. *2,* 130–137 (1971)

Huggins, C., Grand, L. C., Brillantes, F. P.: Mammary cancer induced by a single feeding of polynuclear hydrocarbons and its suppression. Nature *189,* 204–207 (1961)

Hunter, R. E., Jordan, V. C.: Detection of the 8S oestrogen binding component in human uterine endometrium during the menstrual cycle. J. Endocrinol. *65,* 457–458 (1975)

Jensen, E. V., DeSombre, E. R.: Estrogen-receptor interactions. Science *182,* 126–134 (1973)

Jensen, E. V., Jacobson, H. I.: Basic guides to the mechanism of estrogen action. Recent Prog. Horm. Res. *18,* 318–414 (1962)

Jensen, E. V., Block, G. E., Smith, S., Kyser, K., DeSombre, E. R.: Estrogen receptors and breast cancer response to adrenalectomy. Natl. Cancer Inst. Monogr. *34,* 55–70 (1971)

Jordan, V. C.: Antitumor activity of the antiestrogen ICI 46,474 (tamoxifen) in the dimethylbenzanthracene (DMBA)-induced rat mammary carcinoma model. J. Steroid Biochem. *5,* 354 (1974)

Jordan, V. C.: Antiestrogenic and antitumor properties of tamoxifen in laboratory animals. Cancer Treat. Rep. *60,* 1409–1419 (1976a)

Jordan, V. C.: Effect of tamoxifen (ICI 46,474) on initiation and growth of DMBA-induced rat mammary carcinomata. Eur. J. Cancer *12,* 419–424 (1976b)

Jordan, V. C., Dowse, L. J.: Tamoxifen as an anti-tumour agent: effect on oestrogen binding. J. Endocrinol. *68,* 297–303 (1976)

Jordan, V. C., Jaspan, T.: Tamoxifen as an antitumour agent: oestrogen binding as a predictive test for tumour response. J. Endocrinol. *68,* 453–460 (1976a)

Jordan, V. C., Jaspan, T.: Oestrogen binding as a predictive test for DMBA-induced tumour response to tamoxifen therapy. In: Chemotherapy. Vol. 7. Hellman, K., Connors, T. A. (eds.), p. 89. New York: Plenum Press 1976b

Jordan, V. C., Koerner, S.: Tamoxifen (ICI 46,474) and the human carcinoma 8S oestrogen receptor. Eur. J. Cancer *11,* 205–206 (1975a)

Jordan, V. C., Koerner, S.: Inhibition of oestradiol binding to mouse uterine and vaginal oestrogen receptors by triphenylethylenes. J. Endocrinol. *64,* 193–194 (1975b)

Jordan, V. C., Koerner, S.: Tamoxifen as an antitumor agent: role of oestradiol-17β and prolactin. J. Endocrinol. *68,* 305–311 (1976)

Jordan, V. C., Naylor, K. E.: The antitumour activity of tamoxifen and monohydroxytamoxifen: a comparative study in the rat. Br. J. Pharmacol. *64,* 376P-377P (1978)

Jordan, V. C., Prestwich, G.: Binding of [^{3}H] tamoxifen in rat uterine cytosols: a comparison of swinging bucket and vertical tube rotor sucrose density gradient analysis. Mol. Cell. Endocrinol. *8,* 179–188 (1977a)

Jordan, V. C., Prestwich, G.: An investigation by sucrose density gradient analysis of the interaction of ligands with steroid hormone receptors. In: Multiple molecular forms of steroid hormone receptors. Agarwal, M. K. (ed.), p. 245. Amsterdam: Elsevier, North-Holland 1977b

Jordan, V. C., Prestwich, G.: Effect of non-steroidal antioestrogens on the concentration of rat uterine progesterone receptors. J. Endocrinol. *76,* 363–364 (1978)

Jordan, V. C., Koerner, S., Robison, C.: Inhibition of oestrogen stimulated prolactin release by antioestrogens. J. Endocrinol. *65,* 151–152 (1975)

Jordan, V. C., Collins, M. M., Rowsby, L., Prestwich, G.: A monohydroxylated metabolite of tamoxifen with potent antioestrogenic activity. J. Endocrinol. *75,* 305–316 (1977a)

Jordan, V. C., Dix, C. J., Rowsby, L., Prestwich, G.: Studies on the mechanism of action of the nonsteroidal antioestrogen tamoxifen (ICI 46,474) in the rat. Mol. Cell. Endocrinol. *7,* 177–192 (1977b)

Jordan, V. C., Dix, C. J., Naylor, K. E., Prestwich, G., Rowsby, L.: Non-steroidal antiestrogens: their biological effects and potential mechanisms of action. J. Toxicol. Environ. Health *4*, 363–390 (1978a)

Jordan, V. C., Rowsby, L., Dix, C. J., Prestwich, G.: Dose related effects of non-steroidal antioestrogens and oestrogens on the measurement of cytoplasmic oestrogen receptors in the rat and mouse uterus. J. Endocrinol. *78*, 71–81 (1978b)

Jordan, V. C., Prestwich, G., Dix, C. J., Clark, E. R.: Binding of anti-oestrogens to the oestrogen receptor: the first step in anti-oestrogen action. In: Pharmacological modulation of steroid action. Mainwaring, W. I. P., Genazzini, E., Di Carlo, F. (eds.). New York: Raven Press (in press)

Kelly, P. A., Bradley, C., Shiu, R. P. C., Meites, J., Friesen, H. G.: Prolactin binding to rat mammary tumor tissue. Proc. Soc. Exp. Biol. Med. *146*, 816–819 (1974)

King, R. J. B., Cowan, D. M., Inman, D. R.: The uptake of [6, 7^3H] oestradiol by dimethylbenzanthracene-induced rat mammary tumours. J. Endocrinol. *32*, 83–90 (1965)

Kledzik, G. S., Bradley, C. J., Meites, J.: Reduction of carcinogen-induced mammary cancer incidence in rats by early treatment with hormones or drugs. Cancer Res. *34*, 2953–2956 (1974)

Kledzik, G. S., Bradley, C. J., Marshal, G. A., Campbell, G. A., Meites, J.: Effects of high doses of estrogen on prolactin binding activity and growth of carcinogen-induced mammary cancers in rats. Cancer Res. *36*, 3265–3268 (1976)

Koseki, Y., Zava, D. T., Chamness, G. C., McGuire, W. L.: Estrogen receptor translocation and replenishment by the antiestrogen tamoxifen. Endocrinology *101*, 1104–1110 (1977a)

Koseki, Y., Zava, D. T., Chamness, G. C., McGuire, W. L.: Progesterone interaction with oestrogen and antioestrogen in the rat uterus – receptor effects. Steroids *30*, 169–178 (1977b)

Leung, B. S., Sasaki, G. H.: On the mechanism of prolactin and estrogen actions in 7,12 dimethylbenz(a)anthracene-induced mammary carcinoma in the rat II. In vivo tumor responses and estrogen receptor. Endocrinology *97*, 564–572 (1975)

Manni, A., Trujillo, J. E., Pearson, O. H.: Predominant role of prolactin in stimulating the growth of 7,12 dimethylbenz(a)-anthracene-induced rat mammary tumor. Cancer Res. *37*, 1216–1219 (1977)

Meites, J., Cassell, E., Clark, J.: Estrogen inhibition of mammary tumour growth in rats; counteraction by prolactin. Proc. Soc. Exp. Biol. Med. *137*, 1225–1227 (1971)

Mobbs, B. G.: The uptake of tritiated oestradiol by dimethylbenzanthracene-induced mammary tumours of the rat. J. Endocrinol. *36*, 409–444 (1966)

Nicholson, R. I., Golder, M. P.: Effect of synthetic antiestrogens on the growth and biochemistry of rat mammary tumours. Eur. J. Cancer *11*, 571–579 (1975)

Nicholson, R. I., Davis, P., Griffiths, K.: Early increases in ribonucleic acid polymerase activities of dimethylbenzanthracene-induced mammary tumour nuclei in response to oestradiol-17β and tamoxifen. J. Endocr. *73*, 135–142 (1977)

Pearson, O. H., Molina, A., Butler, T. P., Llerena, L., Nasr, H.: Estrogens and prolactin in mammary cancer. In: Estrogen target tissues and neoplasia. Dao, T. L. (ed.), p. 287. Chicago, London: Univ. Chicago Press 1972

Powell-Jones, W., Jenner, D. A., Blamey, R. W., Davis, P., Griffiths, K.: Influence of antioestrogens on the specific binding in vitro of [^{3}H]oestradiol by cytosols of rat mammary tumours and human breast carcinomata. Biochem. J. *150*, 71–75 (1975)

Quadri, S. K., Kledzik, G. S., Meites, J.: Enhanced regression of DMBA-induced mammary cancer in rats by combination of ergocornine with ovariectomy or high doses of estrogen. Cancer Res. *34*, 499–501 (1974)

Sekiya, S., Takamizawa, H.: The combined effect of non-steroidal anti-oestrogens and sex steroids on the growth of rat uterine adenocarcinoma cells in tissue culture. Br. J. Obstet. Gynaecol. *83*, 183–186 (1976)

Sinha, D., Cooper, D., Dao, T. L.: The nature of estrogen and prolactin effect on mammary tumorigenesis. Cancer Res. *33*, 411–414 (1973)

Skidmore, J. R., Walpole, A. L., Woodburn, J.: Effect of some triphenylethylenes on oestradiol binding in vitro to macromolecules from uterus and anterior pituitary. J. Endocrinol. *52,* 289–298 (1972)

Sterental, A., Dominguez, J. N., Weissman, C., Pearson, O. H.: Pituitary role in the estrogen dependency of experimental mammary cancer. Cancer Res. *23,* 481–484 (1963)

Turkington, R. W.: Prolactin receptors in mammary carcinoma cells. Cancer Res. *34,* 758–763 (1974)

Vu Hai, M. T., Milgrom, E.: Characterization and assay of the progesterone receptor in rat uterine cytosol. J. Endocrinol. *76,* 21–31 (1978)

Watson, J., Alam, M.: Oestrogen synthesis during delayed implantation in the rat. Contraception *13,* 101–107 (1976)

Watson, J., Anderson, F. B., Alam, M., O'Grady, J. E., Heald, P. J.: Plasma hormones and pituitary luteinizing hormone in the rat during the early stages of pregnancy and after post-coital treatment with tamoxifen (ICI 46,474) J. Endocrinol. *65,* 7–17 (1975)

Watson, J., Howson, J. W. H.: Inhibition by tamoxifen of the stimulatory action of FSH on oestradiol-17β synthesis by rat ovaries in vitro. J. Reprod. Fertil. *49,* 375–380 (1977)

8. *Studies on Mechanisms of Estrogen and Antiestrogen Action in Human Breast Cancer*

K. B. Horwitz and W. L. McGuire

The University of Texas, Health Science Center, 7703 Floyd Curl Drive,
San Antonio, TX 78284 (USA)

Introduction

Since the original identification of cytoplasmic estrogen receptors (ER) in human breast cancer (JENSEN et al., 1971), rapid progress has been made towards linking presence of the receptor with endocrine responsiveness of the tumor. It is now known that the likelihood of a successful response to endocrine therapy is increased at least tenfold in patients whose tumors are positive for ER (ER+) (MCGUIRE et al., 1975). However, not all ER-containing tumors respond, and this has led to the concept that ER are necessary but not sufficient markers of hormone dependence. We have demonstrated progesterone receptors (PgR) in human breast tumors (HORWITZ et al., 1975a) and have proposed that this receptor, whose synthesis is known to be controlled by estrogen in the uterus, might serve as a marker of estrogen action in breast cancer (HORWITZ et al., 1975b). Thus, the presence of PgR in a tumor would indicate that the entire sequence involving estrogen binding to cytoplasmic receptor, movement of the receptor complex into the nucleus, and stimulation of a specific end product can be achieved in the tumor cell, and would rule out the existence of a defect beyond the binding step. Though this proposal assumes that PgR are under control of estrogen acting through ER, this priming effect had not been demonstrated in human breast cancer. We have used the MCF-7 human breast cancer cell line to study the response of PgR to estrogens and antiestrogens. The MCF-7 cell line, derived from a patient with metastatic breast cancer (SOULE et al., 1973), is ideally suited to study the mechanism of PgR induction. These cells are in permanent tissue culture, contain ER (BROOKS et al., 1973; HORWITZ et al., 1975a), and are estrogen-responsive (LIPPMAN et al., 1976). Cells grown without estradiol have low PgR levels (HORWITZ et al., 1975a). MCF-7 cells have an unusual ER distribution; unfilled receptor sites can be demonstrated in the cytoplasm (Rc) and are also associated with nuclei (Rn) (ZAVA and MCGUIRE, 1977; ZAVA et al., 1977). This chapter summarizes our recent work in this model system, which shows that PgR are under estrogen control and that PgR synthesis involves the ER. We have also studied the effects of antiestrogens and find that tamoxifen (TAM) is a potent inducer of PgR in these cells. This estrogenic property (LEAVITT et al., 1977) of TAM is masked at very high doses (1 μM), which also inhibit cell growth. Another antiestrogen, nafoxidine (NAF), in contrast, has little if any effect on PgR when tested over a wide dose range. The fact that growth-inhibitory effects of both antiestrogens can be reversed by estradiol (LIPPMAN et al., 1976; ZAVA et al., 1977) suggests that the effects of these compounds are mediated through the ER system.

Furthermore, we describe (HORWITZ and MCGUIRE, 1978a) a complex response system in cells in which ER binding and translocation and turnover of nuclear receptors or their "processing" mediate the induction of PgR by estradiol. Though antiestrogens can bind and translocate Rc and bind Rn, the subsequent nuclear receptor-processing step is partially (TAM) or completely (NAF) impaired (HORWITZ and MCGUIRE, 1978b). This may explain the differential effect of these two antiestrogens on PgR induction.

Estradiol, ER, and PgR Synthesis

Binding, Translocation, and Processing of ER

Estradiol enters the cell and binds to unfilled receptor sites, which are found both in cytosol (Rc) or more or less firmly associated with nuclear components (Rn). The newly formed hormone-receptor complex is rapidly translocated to sites in the nucleus from which it can only be extracted with buffers of high ionic strength (RnE). Bound nuclear receptors then undergo rapid turnover or processing; within 3–5 h, 70% or more of RnE sites are lost from the cells without reappearance of unfilled sites. Much later (a period of several days for PgR induction) we see formation of specific products or effects on growth or DNA synthesis. The data from an experiment in which we follow these movements and changes in ER levels are shown in Fig. 1. The untreated cells (C) have approximately half their unfilled sites associated with the nucleus (Rn) and half in the cytoplasm (Rc). There are no filled nuclear

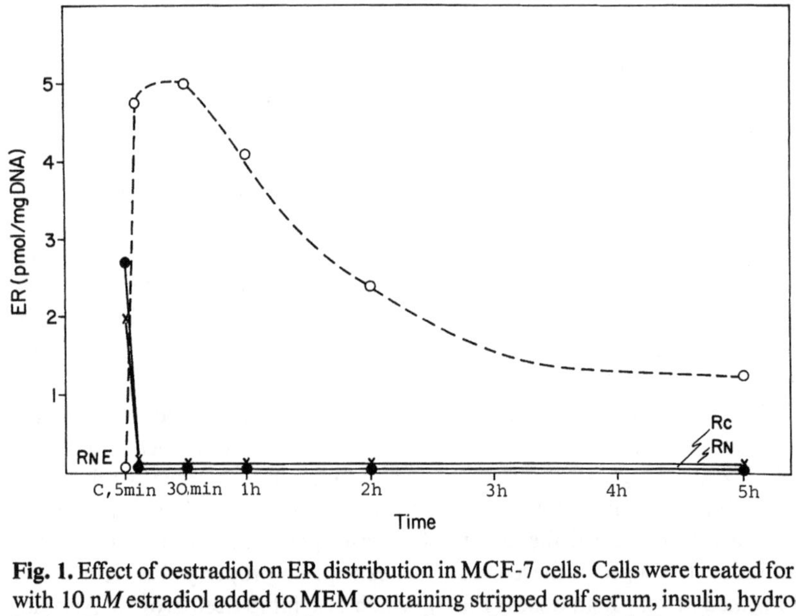

Fig. 1. Effect of oestradiol on ER distribution in MCF-7 cells. Cells were treated for the times indicated with 10 n*M* estradiol added to MEM containing stripped calf serum, insulin, hydrocortisone, and prolactin. Control flasks received the same medium without estradiol. Cytoplasmic and nuclear ER were measured by the single saturating dose protamine assay (ZAVA and MCGUIRE, 1977). Values have been corrected for nonspecific binding. ●, unoccupied cytoplasmic receptors (Rc, 4° C incubation); unoccupied nuclear receptors (Rn, 4° C incubation); ○, occupied nuclear receptors (RnE, 30° C–4° C incubations). (Adapted from HORWITZ, K. B. and MCGUIRE, W. I., 1978c)

sites (RNE). Within 5 min after the addition of 10^{-8} *M* estradiol, Rc and Rn are no longer measurable and all cellular receptors appear in the nucleus bound to estradiol. Starting at about 30 min and continuing for 3–5 h we see a progressive loss of RnE. Processing is essentially complete by 5 h; thereafter RnE levels stabilize at the new steady-state level as long as the cells are kept on oestradiol. If the hormone is removed (Horwitz and McGuire, 1978a) there are several effects: the binding of estradiol as RnE is remarkably prolonged. At least some estrogen (E) always remains bound to nuclear receptors even 8 days after the hormone has been removed. However, in addition, unfilled cytoplasmic and nuclear sites are restored. Restoration of cell ER cannot be explained by loss of E from the nuclear receptor followed by redistribution of the newly emptied sites. Instead, both cytoplasmic receptors (Rc) and nuclear receptors (Rn) are clearly being synthesized de novo, and this synthesis is reflected in the restoration of total cellular ER.

ER Processing and Estradiol Dose

The extent of receptor loss during processing depends on the dose of estradiol, as shown in Fig. 2. The cells grown on estrogen-free medium have approximately equal levels of Rc and Rn. With increasing doses of estradiol there is progressive depletion of these unfilled sites. At 0.1 n*M* only 15% of sites remain unfilled and virtually complete depletion occurs at higher doses. Rc does not remain in the cytoplasm in bound form (RcE, 30° C incubation; not shown) or in cytoplasmic organelles (0.6 *M* KCl extract of high-speed pellet). We conclude that Rc is translocated to the nucleus while Rn sites are filled so that all receptor is in the nucleus in bound form (RnE).

However, the quantity of RnE measured at different doses varies. After a 4-day treatment at the lower doses, though Rc and Rn decrease, there is little accumulation of occupied nuclear receptors (RnE). Instead, levels of total cellular receptors (Rc + Rn + RnE) become progressively lower. At the higher estradiol doses free cytoplasmic and nuclear receptors are entirely depleted but total receptor levels (as RnE) are only 30% of total cell receptors present in controls. There appears to be a limit to amount of receptor loss, however, so that at higher doses RnE accumulation occurs.

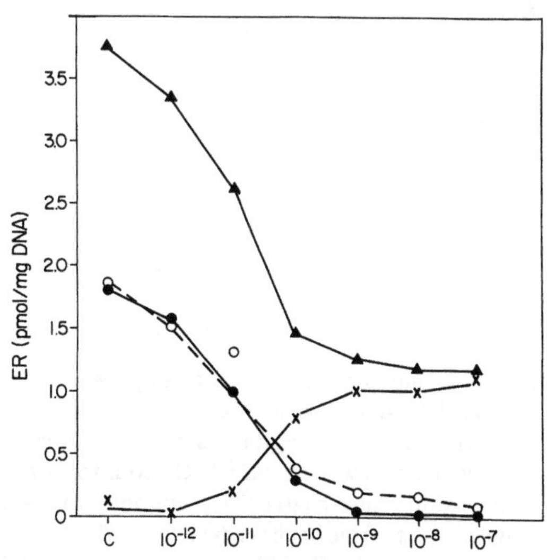

Fig. 2. Effect of estradiol on ER distribution in MCF–7 cells. Cells (four T-75 flasks per treatment group) were treated for 4 days with increasing estradiol concentrations (0.001–100 n*M*) added to MEM containing stripped calf serum, insulin, hydrocortisone, and prolactin. Control flasks received the same medium without estradiol. Cytoplasmic and nuclear ER were measured by the single saturating dose protamine assay. Values have been corrected for nonspecific binding. ●, unoccupied cytoplasmic receptors (Rc, 4° C incubation), ○, unoccupied nuclear receptors (Rn, 4° C incubation); ×, occupied nuclear receptor (RnE, 30° C–4° C incubations); ▲, total cell receptors (Rc + Rn + RnE). (Horwitz, K. B. and McGuire, W. L., 1978a)

ER Processing and PgR Induction

Figure 3 compares the amount of ER that is processed at different estradiol doses with the amount of PgR induced. The extent of free receptor binding and processing parallels PgR induction. Induction is incomplete at low doses if receptor binding and processing is incomplete, reaches a maximum at 0.1 n*M* when RnE processing is maximal, and is not increased further by accumulation of unprocessed RnE. This suggests that processing may be an essential step in the induction of a specific protein by estradiol. These studies with cells of human breast cancer origin show that one response to estradiol treatment is an increase in levels of PgR, as would be predicted from studies of chick oviduct (SHERMAN et al., 1970), rat uterine PgR priming (FABER et al., 1972), and cyclic changes in PgR levels observed in the human endometrium (BAYARD et al., 1975). Our results clearly show that human breast cells that have undergone malignant transformation can continue to synthesize a specific protein under hormone control. Furthermore, these results lend credence to our hypothesis (HORWITZ et al., 1975b) that the presence of PgR in biopsies of human breast tumors indicates that in situ the tumor was exposed to, and was capable of responding to circulating estrogens. Since the tumor, in one instance, has remained hormone-responsive, one might suspect that other estrogen-sensitive effects have also been retained.

We must emphasize, however, that PgR induction is only one product of estrogen action. The data cannot be construed to mean that other estrogen responses will necessarily be present. We find, for instance, that the growth of MCF-7 cells is estrogen-sensitive, but that unlike PgR, the growth is not estrogen-dependent. Thus, effects of estrogens on growth and PgR induction might well be dissociated. We find this to be true in some DMBA-induced tumors as

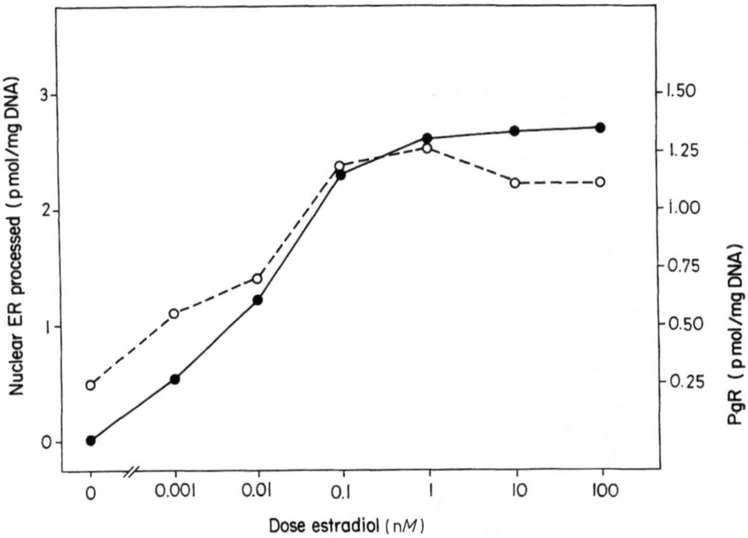

Fig. 3. Comparison of ER processing (●——●) and PgR induction (○----○). Cells were incubated as described in Fig. 2. ER was measured and the amount of ER lost at each dose (control–total) plotted. PgR measured by single saturating dose assay: 200 μl cytosol incubated 4 h at 4° C, in triplicate, with 20 n*M* ^{3}H-R5020 alone or with 100fold excess R5020. After 15 min incubation with dextran-coated charcoal suspension, cytosols were centrifuged, and aliquots of the supernatant counted to determine bound radioactivity. Data shown are corrected for nonspecific binding. (Adapted from HORWITZ, K. B. and MCGUIRE, W. L., 1978a)

well. Occasional tumors grow in castrated rats so that growth can be considered estrogen-autonomous, while tumor PgR levels decline and could therefore be considered estrogen-dependent (HORWITZ and MCGUIRE, 1977). Conversely, we would predict that tumors regressing during high-dose estradiol medication would have elevated PgR levels.

Our studies strongly suggest that estrogen stimulation of PgR involves ER. First, the extent of PgR induction closely parallels both the binding and translocation of Rc and the binding of Rn. Second, PgR induction is correlated with ER processing during estradiol stimulation; when processing ceases PgR levels fall.

The nature of processing is unclear. It may represent loss of the steroid-binding site, or be an active state in which a new equilibrium between receptor degradation and synthesis is achieved (SARFF and GORSKI, 1971; WILLIAMS and GORSKI, 1972), or represent a redistribution of receptor within nuclear binding sites of differing affinities (DEHERTOGH et al., 1973) or specificities (SCHRADER et al., 1972), or sequestration of receptor to sites inaccessible to salt extraction (CLARK and PECK, 1976; RUH and BAUDENDISTEL, 1977). We will return to these questions later. In any event, our data suggest that the processing step is saturable, that peak activation occurs when RnE processing is maximal, and that the RnE accumulated in excess of that processed may be superfluous. That is, a dose of 0.1 n*M* estradiol is equal to 10 n*M* estradiol, despite the fact that for the former some Rc remains, while for the latter some unprocessed RnE remains.

In attempts to extend our understanding of the role of nuclear processing in ER action, we have studied the effects of antiestrogens.

Nafoxidine and Tamoxifen Effects on PgR and ER Processing

ER Compartmentalization and Processing

Tamoxifen (TAM) and nafoxidine (NAF), two nonsteroidal antiestrogens, are potent growth inhibitors of MCF-7 cells when present in high doses (LIPPMAN et al., 1976; HORWITZ et al., 1978; ZAVA et al., 1977). Doses above 50 n*M* are inhibitory for NAF, and doses above 100 n*M* are inhibitory for TAM. These effects are probably mediated through the ER system and are not simply toxic effects of the compounds, since they can be reversed by addition of estradiol at concentrations 100- to 1000fold lower than the antiestrogen.

Estradiol, TAM, and NAF have distinctly different effects on ER in MCF-7 cells. Figure 4 shows the levels of total cytoplasmic and total nuclear receptors in cells during 5 h of hormone or antagonist treatment. Untreated control cells have only unfilled ER. When estradiol (10 n*M*) is added, Rc binds the hormone, and the receptor–hormone complex is rapidly translocated, as shown by the reciprocal increase of receptor in the nucleus (RnE) and decrease in the cytoplasm within 5 min. Rn also binds the hormone rapidly, so that in 5 min all cell receptors are in the nucleus in bound form (RnE); they then fall rapidly to processed levels. In the presence of TAM or NAF, Rc also translocates, and receptor accumulates in the nucleus. This recompartmentalization is slower with antiestrogens than with estradiol. The subsequent processing step is quite different for the antiestrogens. With TAM, processing also results in decreased nuclear receptor levels; however, whereas the decrease represents 30%–50% loss from control levels, it is never as extensive as that seen with estradiol. This processed level is also maintained as long as cells are exposed to TAM. In cells treated with NAF, all cell receptors also accumulate in the nucleus, but no subsequent processing of receptor occurs.

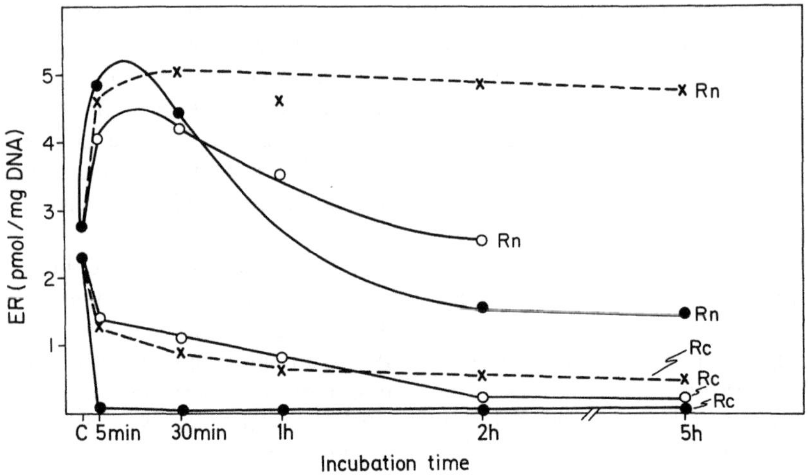

Fig. 4. Kinetics of ER distribution after estradiol or antiestrogen treatment. Cells were treated as in Fig. 1 with estradiol (●, 10 n*M*), TAM (○, 0.1 μ*M*), or NAF (×, 1 μ*M*). ER was measured by protamine sulfate precipitation. (Horwitz, K. B. and McGuire, W. E. 1978b)

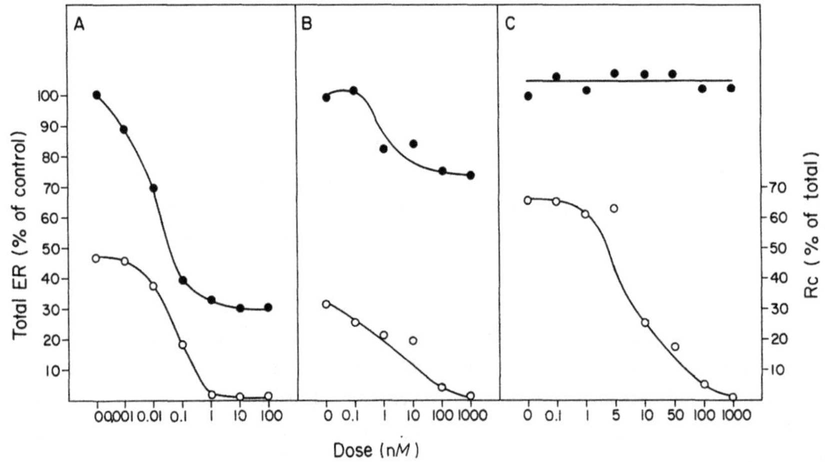

Fig. 5 A–C. Effect of hormone dose on cytoplasmic ER levels (○——○, Rc) and total ER (●——●) in the cell. Cells in T-75 flasks were grown for 4 days with MEM containing 5% stripped calf serum, insulin, hydrocortisone, and prolactin alone, or with varying doses of estradiol (**A**), TAM (**B**), or NAF (**C**). **A** Data from cells in passage #174; **B** from cells in passage #175; **C** from cells in passage #177. In each group the untreated control is shown as ○. Cells from four flasks were pooled and homogenized, and cytoplasmic and nuclear ER were measured by the single saturating dose protamine exchange assay. Total cell ER is the sum of unfilled cytoplasmic (Rc, 4°) and total nuclear sites (filled plus unfilled, 30°). The percentage of the total that represents Rc is also shown. The difference between Rc and total is nuclear receptor. The number of receptors in pmol/mg DNA for control cells are: Rc, 2.0; Rn, 2.1 (**A**); Rc, 1.2; Rn, 2.4 (**B**) and Rc, 3.1; Rn, 1.6 (**C**). (Horwitz, K. B. and McGuire, W. E., 1978b)

Effect of Antiestrogen Dose on ER Processing

As we have shown above, the steady-state level of ER achieved when cells are incubated with estradiol for over 5 h depends on the estradiol dose used.
With increasing doses of TAM, Rc are also progressively depleted. At 100 n*M* more than 95% of Rc are translocated. However, total receptor levels fall to only 70% of control values even at the highest doses (Fig. 5b). No processing at all is seen with NAF, despite complete Rc depletion (Fig. 5c).

Effect of Antiestrogen Dose on PgR Induction

Again, with antiestrogens, as with estradiol, processing parallels PgR induction. Figure 6 shows that TAM is a potent inducer of PgR. While low doses have only minimal effects at intermediate doses, PgR induction equals or exceeds that obtained with estradiol (not shown). When doses are raised further, PgR levels are suppressed even below control levels. This high (1 μ*M*) TAM dose is markedly antiestrogenic: at this dose, but not at lower doses, we see inhibition of cell growth and eventual cell death. NAF (Fig. 7), in contrast to TAM, has little or no

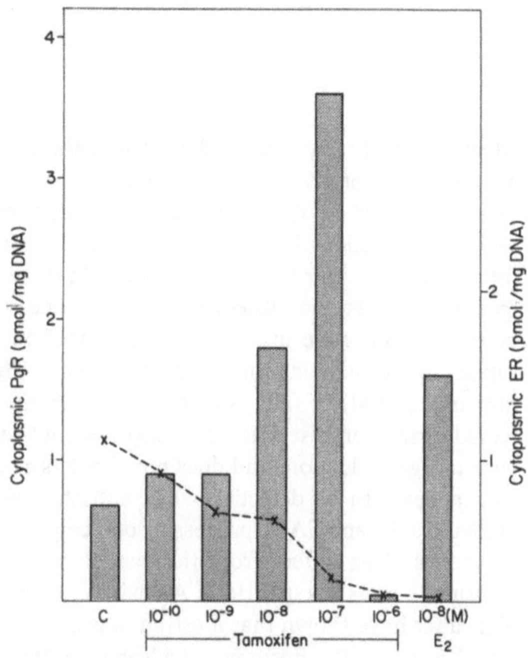

Fig. 6. Cytoplasmic PgR (□) and ER (× --- ×) levels in cells treated with varying doses of TAM (10^{-10}–10^{-6}*M*). Control cells were untreated (none). Cells from four T-75 flasks were pooled and assayed for PgR by the single saturating dose DCC assay: triplicate 100-μl aliquots of cytosols were incubated for 4 h at 4° C with 20 n*M* ^{3}H-R5020 alone or with 100fold excess R5020. After 15 min incubation with a DCC suspension, the charcoal was pelleted and aliquots of the supernatant were counted to determine bound radioactivity. ER was determined by the single saturating dose protamine sulfate assay: 200-μl aliquots of cytosols, in triplicate, were precipitated with 250 μl · 1 mg/ml protamine sulfate. The protamine bound receptor was incubated for 18 h at 4° C with 5n*M* ^{3}H-estradiol with and without 100fold excess DES. Pellets were washed and counted. Data shown are corrected for nonspecific binding. (Horwitz, K. B. et al., 1978)

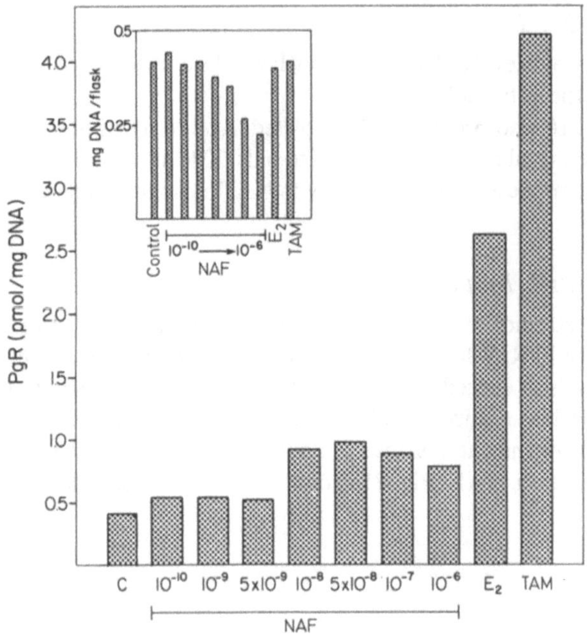

Fig. 7. Effect of varying doses of NAF on growth and PgR in MCF-7 cells. Cells were treated for 5 days with MEM containing 5% stripped calf serum, insulin, hydrocortisone, and prolactin (C) or this medium with the addition of varying doses of NAF (0.1 n*M*–1 μ*M*) with estradiol (E_2, 10 n*M*) or TAM (0.1 μ*M*). Four similarly treated T-75 flasks were pooled, cells were homogenized, and cytosols were assayed for PgR by the single saturating dose DCC assay. Growth was determined by DNA measurement (16) of the 105,000 *g* pellet. (HORWITZ, K. B. et al., 1978)

effect on PgR at any dose studied. The slight increase at high doses may reflect an effect on another receptor (ZAVA, unpublished).

These results show that in breast cancer cells of human origin, the ER system mediates antiestrogen action. Antiestrogens bind and translocate cytoplasmic ER; they also bind the free nuclear receptor present in the cells. In these respects estrogen antagonists resemble estradiol. However, the subsequent nuclear processing reactions of estrogen- and antiestrogen-bound receptors are dissimilar. After estradiol, nuclear hormone-receptor complexes fall rapidly to less than one-third of control values. This pathway of receptor processing is either impaired (TAM) or fails entirely (NAF) for the antiestrogen-receptor complex. Our data would further suggest that processing is an active step in ER function, at least in the special case of PgR induction, and does not simply serve to return receptor to the cytoplasm. This step appears to be defective when antiestrogens bind the receptor.

With estradiol and TAM, processing of receptor occurs despite the continuous presence of the hormones. This differs from the loss of nuclear ER described in the rat uterus (GIANNOPOULOS and GORSKI, 1971; ANDERSON et al., 1975) following a single pulse of estradiol. The latter have shown that if estradiol is administered to the rat so as to maintain elevated blood levels of the hormone, nuclear receptors rise to very high levels. Thus, significant differences are found between the early nuclear reactions of the ER–hormone complex of human tumor cells and those in the rat uterus, the usual model for estrogen action. Other tissue differences in mechanisms of ER action have also been reported (LAZIER and ALFORD, 1977; CIDLOWSKI and MULDOON, 1976), suggesting perhaps that studies of estrogen action in uteri cannot always be extrapolated to other tissues.

Estrogenic and antiestrogenic responses in the rat uterus are characterized as early (< 6 h) or late (24 h) (HARDIN et al., 1976; LAN and KATZENELLENBOGEN, 1976; STORMSHAK et al., 1976), and different control mechanisms may be required for each. Upon initial injection both responses are evoked by antiestrogens (CLARK et al., 1974, KATZENELLENBOGEN and

FERGUSON, 1975, CAPONY and ROCHEFORT, 1975); however, late responses cannot be elicited either by estradiol or by antiestrogens if a primary antiestrogen injection precedes either of these by 24 h (KATZENELLENBOGEN et al., 1977; FERGUSON and KATZENELLENBOGEN, 1977). This has led to models of estrogen action having at least two nuclear binding sites for the ER complex, one of which is accessible to antiestrogen–receptor complexes. These models are further supported by evidence of differential salt extractability of estrogen- and antiestrogen-bound nuclear receptors (CLARK and PECK, 1976; MESTER and BAULIEU, 1975; JULIANO and STANCEL, 1976; RUH and BAUDENDISTEL, 1977) and by their unequal nuclear retention time (CLARK et al., 1973). Our data lend support to the concept of dual nuclear sites of action of estrogen–receptor complexes; they suggest, moreover, that processing of ER occurs at only one ot these. These sites may be temporally as well as structurally distinct, since as we show below, binding to the processing site can be prevented without affecting initial nuclear binding.

Effects of Actinomycin on ER Compartmentalization and Processing

Inhibition of ER Processing

Actinomycin D (AcD) has been a powerful tool in investigations into the biochemistry of nucleic acids and their involvement in replication and transcription (GOLDBERG and FRIEDMAN, 1971). The antibiotic intercalates into double-stranded DNA with its chromophore between successive G-C base pairs; two pentapeptides lie in the minor groove of the double helix (SOBEL and JAIN, 1972). Two binding sites distinguished by different affinities for DNA have been described; both are partially blocked by the presence of chromosomal proteins (KLEIMAN and HUANG, 1971).

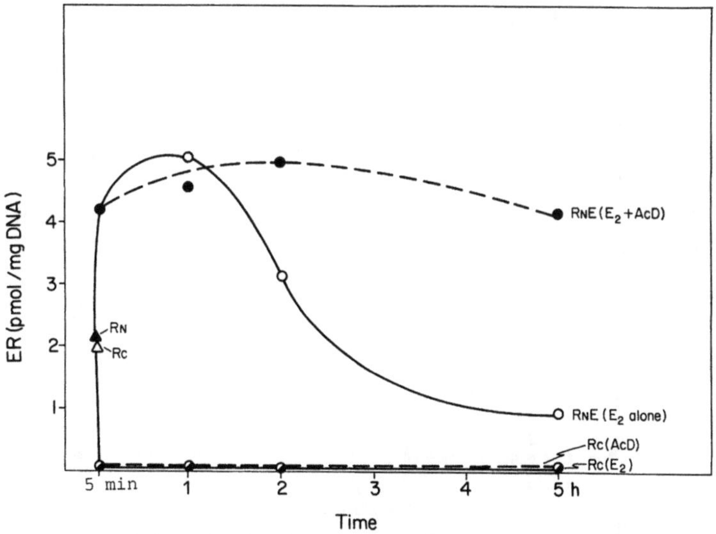

Fig. 8. Effect of continuous actinomycin treatment on processing of MCF-7 ER. Cells were treated at time 0 with 10 n*M* estradiol alone (○, △) or together with 2 μ*M* actinomycin D (●, ▲,). At the indicated times cells were harvested and assayed for ER by protamine sulfate precipitation. Rn, Rc, RnE as described in Fig. 1. (HORWITZ, K. B. and MCGUIRE, W. E., 1978c)

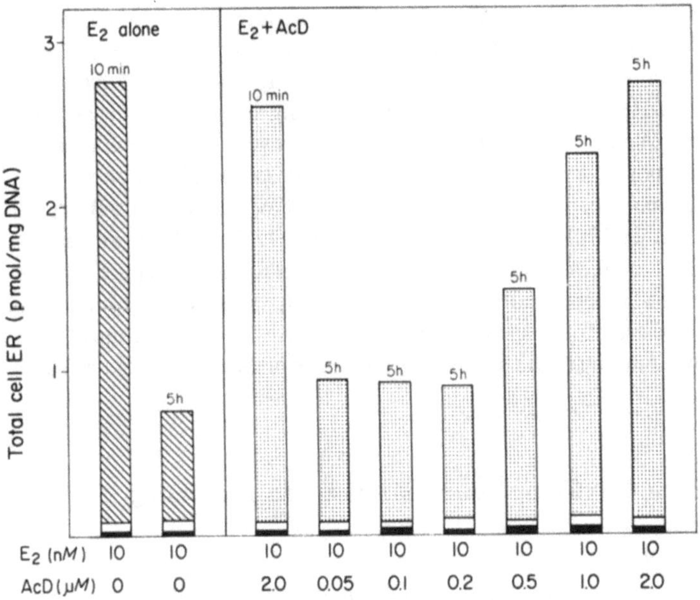

Fig. 9. Effect of AcD dose on extent of nuclear ER processing. Cells were treated for 10 min or 5 h with estradiol (10 n*M*) alone or together with 0.05 n*M* (0.06 μg/ml) to 2 n*M* (2.5 μg/ml) AcD. At the end of incubation cells were harvested, washed, homogenized, and assayed for cytoplasmic and nuclear ER by the single saturating dose protamine method. ■, unoccupied cytoplasmic (4° C); □, unoccupied nuclear receptors (4° C); ▦, ▧, occupied nuclear receptors (30° C—4° C). The bar heights represent total cell receptors (Rc + Rn + RnE), determined in triplicate from four pooled T-75 flasks. (Horwitz, K. B. and McGuire, W. E., 1978c)

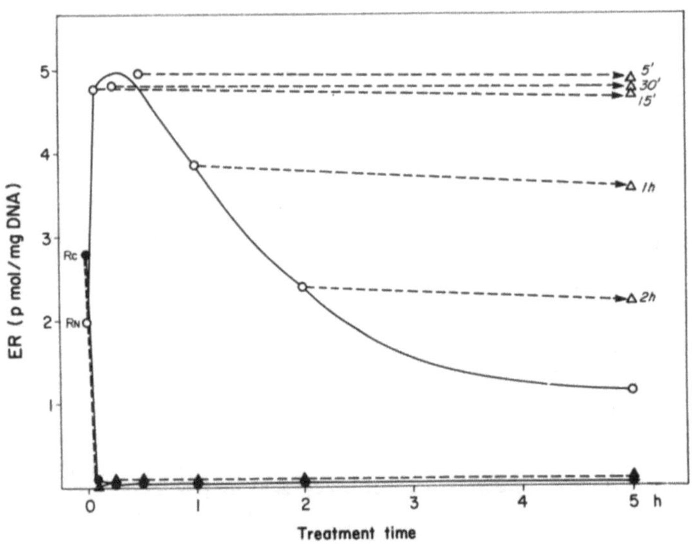

Fig. 10. Effect of delayed AcD treatment on ER levels. MCF-7 cells were treated with 10 n*M* estradiol alone (○, RnE; ○ Rc), or with estradiol followed by AcD given 5 min to 2 h later (△, RnE; △, Rc). Cells were harvested at the end of 5 h of estradiol treatment and assayed for ER as described in Fig. 1. *Dashed lines* represent the changes in ER levels from the time of AcD addition to the end of the experiment. (Horwitz, K. B. and McGuire, W. E. 1978c)

The nature of the inhibitory action of AcD is complex and partially concentration-dependent. Actinomycin D suppresses the synthesis of all cellular RNA fractions by preferentially blocking chain elongation catalyzed by DNA-directed RNA polymerase. However, at low concentrations there is differential inhibition of various RNA classes, ribosomal RNA being the most sensitive (GOLDBERG and FRIEDMAN, 1971). Synthesis of DNA in intact cells or by isolated DNA polymerases is also sensitive to AcD but requires the presence of much higher inhibitor concentrations.

More recently it has been suggested that AcD may inhibit protein synthesis through direct effects on mRNA movement or translation (LEINWALD and RUDDLE, 1977; BASTOS and AVIV, 1977).

Figure 8 shows the effect of the addition of AcD (2 μ*M*) to estradiol-treated cells. In this study cells were treated simultaneously with the hormone and inhibitor, and receptor levels were measured at the indicated times. AcD completely inhibits the normal processing of estrogen-charged nuclear receptor. The result is analogous to the effects of NAF. Interestingly, neither the initial binding of estradiol to unfilled sites nor the translocation of the hormone receptor complex to the nucleus is affected by actinomycin.

These measurements were made with an exchange assay on protamine-precipitated receptor extracted from nuclei with high salt. However, actinomycin does not simply enhance salt extractability of RnE, since a similar loss of ER, and its inhibition by AcD, can be demonstrated when nuclear receptors are labeled directly with ^{3}H-estradiol, thereby obviating the need to extract receptors (not shown) (HORWITZ and MCGUIRE, 1978c).

Dose of AcD and ER Processing

The inhibitory effects of AcD on ER processing are only achieved when it is present in high concentrations (Fig. 9). In this study cells were treated for 10 min or 5 h with estradiol alone or with estradiol plus increasing doses of actinomycin. Ten minutes after estradiol treatment all unfilled sites have disappeared and only estrogen-filled nuclear sites can be measured. This step is not inhibited even by high doses (2.0 μ*M*) of AcD. Five hours later, normal processing has taken place in the absence of the inhibitor or, when it is present, at low doses (0.05–0.2 μ*M*). However, as AcD doses are increased (0.5–2.0 μ*M*) there is progressive inhibition of ER processing.

Actinomycin could be working in at least two ways: its effect could be direct, physically blocking ER access to a specific DNA-binding site, or indirect, by inhibiting RNA and protein synthesis. We have several indirect lines of evidence based on the rate of inhibition and the effects of other inhibitors that suggest that AcD acts directly to block processing.

Rate of AcD Block and Effect of Other Inhibitors

At first, the inhibitory effect of actinomycin is rapid, as shown in Fig. 10. In this study cells were treated with estradiol, while addition of actinomycin was delayed from 5 min to 2 h. The effect of AcD is to fix ER immediately at the levels they had reached before addition of the inhibitor. If estradiol and AcD are added together at the start of treatment (*arrow*), estrogen binding and translocation of Rc and binding to Rn and the initial accumulation of total receptor in the nucleus are not inhibitable. However, all subsequent processing stops. The slight downward slopes of the dotted lines show that the effect on ER processing occurs within 15 min of AcD addition, so that entry of AcD into nuclei must be quite rapid, and an intermediate effect of AcD on protein synthesis is unlikely.

In preliminary experiments we have also tested several other inhibitors of cell function for their effect on ER binding, translocation, and processing during estradiol treatment. At 1 μ*M* all other intercalators and inhibitors tested were ineffective when co-incubated with estradiol; the list includes other inhibitors of transcription (daunomycin, adriamycin, distamycin A, α-amanatin), inhibitors of replication (chloroquine, nalidixic acid, mitomycin C, novobiocin, ethidium bromide), a translation inhibitor (cycloheximide), and inhibitors of other cell processes (colchicine, cytochalasin B). The sole exception was chromomycin A_3. This compound behaves identically with AcD, and like AcD is the only inhibitor that shows specificity for G-C base pairs (GOLDBERG and FRIEDMAN, 1971).

The rate of AcD inhibition and the failure of other intercalators and translation inhibitors to prevent ER processing suggests indirectly that the AcD effect is not due to inhibition of RNA and protein synthesis. However, because of the inhibitors' complex actions the possibility cannot be ruled out that actinomycin is regulating the nuclear exit of receptors by an action distinct from its effect on chromatin, or that it alters the proteins' turnover rate at some extranuclear site. Blocking of transcription is the classic and best-studied effect of this antibiotic, which suggests that inhibition of ER processing may occur because AcD directly blocks ER access to DNA. In that case AcD may distinguish between two RnE-binding sites in nuclei. Newly translocated receptor binds to a site on chromatin or DNA that is insensitive to inhibition. Actinomycin D or chromomycin A_3 stops subsequent processing by preventing RnE insertion at a second base-specific region on DNA. The existence of two receptor-binding sites in nuclei, one for chromatin and another for DNA, has been postulated in the chick oviduct for PgR (SCHRADER et al., 1972). PALMITER et al. (1976), also proposed a two-step nuclear receptor-translocation mechanism involving a rate-limiting movement of steroid receptors from initial nonproductive chromatin-binding sites to productive sites. Alternatively, a model involving only one binding site requires that nuclear ER binds immediately to DNA; AcD may then mechanically prevent ER release from this site. As so little is understood about the mechanism of action of actinomycin, none of these various explanations can be ruled out by our data.

In summary, we have provocative data suggesting that the nuclear estrogen–receptor complex interacts with DNA, that this interaction is required for appropriate receptor turnover or processing, and that processing may be essential for induction of a specific protein by estrogen. If the receptor is improperly inserted into DNA, as for instance when it is bound by NAF, processing fails and the biological effect is blunted.

References

Anderson, J. N., Peck, E. J., Jr., Clark, J. H.: Estrogen induced uterine responses and growth: relationship to receptor estrogen binding by uterine nuclei. Endocrinology *96*, 160–167 (1975)

Bastos, R. N., Aviv, H.: Globin RNA precursor molecules: biosynthesis and processing of erythroid cells. Cell *11*, 641–650 (1977)

Bayard, F., Damilano, S., Robel, P., Baulieu, E. E.: Recepteurs de l'oestradiol et de la progesterone dans l'endometre humain au cours du cycle menstruel. C. R. Acad. Sci. [D] (Paris) *281*, 1341–1344 (1975)

Brooks, S. C., Locke, E. R., Soule, H. D.: Estrogen receptor in a human cell line (MCF-7) from breast carcinoma. J. Biol. Chem. *248*, 6251–6253 (1973)

Capony, F., Rochefort, H.: In vivo effect of antiestrogens on the localization and replenishment of ER. Mol. Cell. Endocrinol. *3*, 233–251 (1975)

Cidlowski, J. A., Muldoon, T. G.: Dissimilar effects of antiestrogens upon estrogen receptors in responsive tissues of male and female rats. Biol. Reprod. *15*, 381–398 (1976)

Clark, J. H., Peck, E. J., Jr.: Nuclear retention of receptor-oestrogen complex and nuclear acceptor sites. Nature *260,* 635–637 (1976)

Clark, J. H., Anderson, J. N., Peck, E. J., Jr.: Estrogen receptor antiestrogen complex: atypical binding by uterine nuclei and effect on uterine growth. Steroids *22,* 707–718 (1973)

Clark, J. H., Peck, E. J., Jr., Anderson, J. N.: Oestrogen receptors and antagonism of steroid hormone action. Nature *251,* 446–448 (1974)

DeHertogh, R., Ekka, E., Vanderheyden, I., Hoet, J. J.: "Unbound" ligand adsorption on dextran-coated charcoal: practical considerations. J. Steroid Biochem. *4,* 313–320 (1973)

Faber, L. E., Sandmann, M. L., Stavely, H. E.: Progesterone binding proteins of the rat and rabbit uterus. J. Biol. Chem. *247,* 5648–5649 (1972)

Ferguson, E. R., Katzenellenbogen, B. S.: A comparative study of antiestrogen action: temporal patterns of antagonism of estrogen stimulated uterine growth and effects on estrogen receptor levels. Endocrinology *100,* 1242–1251 (1977)

Giannopoulos, G., Gorski, J.: Estrogen receptors-quantitative studies on transfer of estradiol from cytoplasmic to nuclear binding sites. J. Biol. Chem. *246,* 2524–2529 (1971)

Goldberg, I. H., Friedman, P. A.: Antibiotics and nucleic acids. Ann. Rev. Biochem. *40,* 775–810 (1971)

Hardin, J. W., Clark, J. H., Glasser, S. R., Peck, E. J., Jr.: RNA polymerase activity and uterine growth: differential stimulation by estradiol, estriol and nafoxidine. Biochemistry *15,* 1370–1374 (1976)

Horwitz, K. B., McGuire, W. L.: Progesterone and progesterone receptors in experimental breast cancer. Cancer Res. *37,* 1733–1738 (1977)

Horwitz, K. B., McGuire, W. L.: Estrogen control of progesterone receptor in human breast cancer: correlation with nuclear processing of estrogen receptor. J. Biol. Chem. *253,* 2223–2228 (1978a)

Horwitz, K. B., McGuire, W. L.: Nuclear mechanisms of estrogen action: effects of estradiol and antiestrogens on estrogen receptors and nuclear receptor processing. J. Biol. Chem. *253,* 8185–8191 (1978)

Horwitz, K. B., McGuire, W. L.: Actinomycin D prevents nuclear processing of estrogen receptor. J. Biol. Chem. *253,* 6319–6322 (1978)

Horwitz, K. B., Costlow, M. E., McGuire, W. L.: MCF-7: A human breast cancer cell line with estrogen, androgen, progesterone and glucocorticoid receptors. Steroids *26,* 785–795 (1975a)

Horwitz, K. B., McGuire, W. L., Pearson, O. H., Segaloff, A.: Predicting response to endocrine therapy in human breast cancer: a hypothesis. Science *189,* 726–727 (1975b)

Horwitz, K. B., Koseki, Y., McGuire, W. L.: Estrogen control of progesterone receptor in human breast cancer: role of estradiol and antiestrogen. Endocrinology *103,* 1742–1751 (1978)

Jensen, E. V., Block, G. E., Smith, S., Kyser, K., DeSombre, E. R.: ER and breast cancer response to adrenalectomy. Natl. Cancer Inst. Monogr. *34,* 55–79 (1971)

Juliano, J. V., Stancel, G. H.: Estrogen receptors in the rat uterus. Retention of hormone-receptor complexes. Biochemistry *15,* 916–920 (1976)

Katzenellenbogen, B. S., Ferguson, E. R.: Estrogen action in the uterus: biological ineffectiveness of nuclear bound estradiol after antiestrogen. Endocrinology *97,* 1–12 (1975)

Katzenellenbogen, B. S., Ferguson, E. R., Lan, N. C.: Fundamental differences in the action of estrogens and antiestrogens on the uterus: comparison between compounds with similar duration of action. Endocrinology *100,* 1252–1259 (1977)

Kleiman, L., Huang, R. C. C.: Binding of actinomycin D to calf thymus chromatin. J. Mol. Biol. *55,* 503–521 (1971)

Lan, N. C., Katzenellenbogen, B. S.: Temporal relationships between hormone receptor binding and biological responses in the uterus: studies with short- and long-acting derivatives of estriol. Endocrinology *98,* 220–227 (1976)

Lazier, C. B., Alford, W. S.: Interaction of the anti-oestrogen nafoxidine hydrochloride with the soluble nuclear oestradiol-binding protein in chick liver. Biochem. J. *164,* 659–667 (1977)

Leavitt, W. W., Chen, T. J., Allen, T. C.: Regulation of progesterone receptor formation by estrogen action. Ann. N.Y. Acad. Sci. *286,* 210–225 (1977)

Leinwald, L., Ruddle, F. H.: Stimulation of in vitro translation of messenger RNA by actinomycin D. Science *197,* 381–383 (1977)

Lippman, M., Bolan, G., Huff, K.: Human breast cancer responsive to androgen in long term tissue culture. Cancer Res. *36,* 4595–4601 (1976)

McGuire, W. L., Carbone, P. P., Sears, M. E., Escher, G. C.: Estrogen receptors: an overview. In: Estrogen receptors in human breast cancer. McGuire, W. L., Carbone, P. P., Vollmer, E. P. (eds.), p. 1. New York: Raven Press 1975

Mester, J., Baulieu, E. E.: Dynamics of oestrogen-receptor distribution between the cytosol and nuclear fraction of immature rat uterus after oestradiol administration. Biochem. J. *146,* 617–623 (1975)

Palmiter, R. D., Moore, P. B., Mulvihill, E. R., Emtage, S.: A significant lag in the induction of ovalbumin messenger RNA by steroid hormones: A receptor translocation hypothesis. Cell *8,* 557–572 (1976)

Ruh, T. S., Baudendistel, L. J.: Different nuclear binding sites for antiestrogen and estrogen receptor complexes. Endocrinology *100,* 420–426 (1977)

Sarff, M., Gorski, J.: Control of estrogen binding protein concentration under basal conditions and after estrogen administration. Biochemistry *10,* 2557–2563 (1971)

Schrader, W. T., Toft, D. O., O'Malley, B. W.: Progesterone binding protein of chick oviduct. VI. Interaction of purified progesterone receptor components with nuclear constituents. J. Biol. Chem. *247,* 2401–2407 (1972)

Sherman, M. R., Corval, P. I., O'Malley, B. W.: Progesterone binding components of chick oviduct. J. Biol. Chem. *245,* 6085–6096 (1970)

Sobel, H. M., Jain, S. C.: Stereochemistry of actinomycin binding to DNA: II. Detailed molecular model of actinomycin-DNA complex and its implications. J. Mol. Biol. *68,* 21–34 (1972)

Sonnenschein, C., Soto, A. M., Cologiore, J., Farookhi, R.: Estrogen target cells. Establishment of a cell line derived from rat pituitary tumor MtT/F_4. Exp. Cell Res. *101,* 15–22 (1976)

Soule, H. D., Vasquez, J., Long, A., Albert, S., Brennan, M. J.: A human cell line from a pleural effusion derived from a breast carcinoma. J. Natl. Cancer Inst. *51,* 1409–1416 (1973)

Stormshak, F., Leake, R., Wertz, N., Gorski, J.: Stimulatory and inhibitory effects of estrogen on uterine DNA synthesis. Endocrinology *99,* 1501–1511 (1976)

Williams, D., Gorski, J.: Kinetic and equilibrium analysis of estradiol in uterus: a model of binding site distribution in uterine cells. Proc. Natl. Acad. Sci. USA *69,* 3464–3468 (1972)

Zava, D. T., McGuire, W. L.: Estrogen receptor. Unoccupied sites in nuclei of a breast tumor cell line. J. Biol. Chem. *252,* 3703–3708 (1977)

Zava, D. T., Chamness, G. C., Horwitz, K. B., McGuire, W. L.: Human breast cancer: Biologically achieve estrogen receptor in the absence of estrogen? Science *197,* 663–664 (1977)

9. Human Breast Cancer in Nude Mice: A Model for Testing Endocrine Treatment[1]

R.-T. Michel, H. Schmidt-Matthiesen, G. Bastert, and H. P. Fortmeyer

Klinikum der Johann Wolfgang Goethe-Universität, Abteilung für Gynäkologie und Onkologie, Theodor-Stern-Kai 7, D-6000 Frankfurt 70 (FRG)

It is clinically well known that addition or deletion of steroids is an effective treatment in about one-third of patients with advanced breast cancer. However, it is difficult to predict the responsiveness of an individual tumour. In vitro assays of oestrogen receptors have proved to yield useful indications of the hormone responsiveness of human breast cancer. Nevertheless, many oestrogen receptor-positive tumours fail to respond to endocrine therapy. Supplementary markers like quantification of oestrogen receptors, differentiation of the 4 S and 8 S receptors, determination of the progesterone receptor, and certain clinical characteristics such as menopausal status, type of metastasis, and disease-free interval are additional aids in the identification of responsive tumours.

When Rygaard and Povlsen (1969) succeeded in transplanting human tumour material to nude mice a new animal model for quasi in vivo testing of human breast cancer became available. With this model we have tested the effect of various endocrine treatments on the tumour growth of serially transplanted human breast cancers and spontaneous mouse breast cancer in nude mice.

Nude mice of a random-bred strain, with a body weight of approximately 25 g and aged 6—7 weeks served as recipients. Tumour slices 0.5 cm in diameter were transplanted under sterile conditions behind the shoulder blade into the area of the mammary gland. Tumours from premenopausal women were transplanted to fertile nude mice, and tumours from postmenopausal women to castrated male or female nude mice. After 3—9 weeks endocrine treatment started. Animals were sacrificed between the 18th and 40th day of treatment. Figure 1 shows a mouse with a human mammary cancer, 7 and 17 weeks after transplantation. Oestrogen receptors, androgen receptors and progesterone receptors were measured by gel electrophoresis according to Wagner (1972). For determination of the progesterone receptor R 5020 was used. Bilateral ovariectomy and adrenalectomy were performed through a double incision. Control animals underwent laparotomy. To investigate the influence on tumour growth oestradiol, testosterone, progesterone and the anti-oestrogen tamoxifen were administered by i.m. injection. Tumours were measured and the product of the two longest perpendicular diameters recorded once a week.

1 The authors wish to thank Professor Jungblut and Dr. Wagner of the Max Planck Institut, Wilhelmshaven, Federal German Republic, for providing the gel electrophoresis equipment and technical assistance.

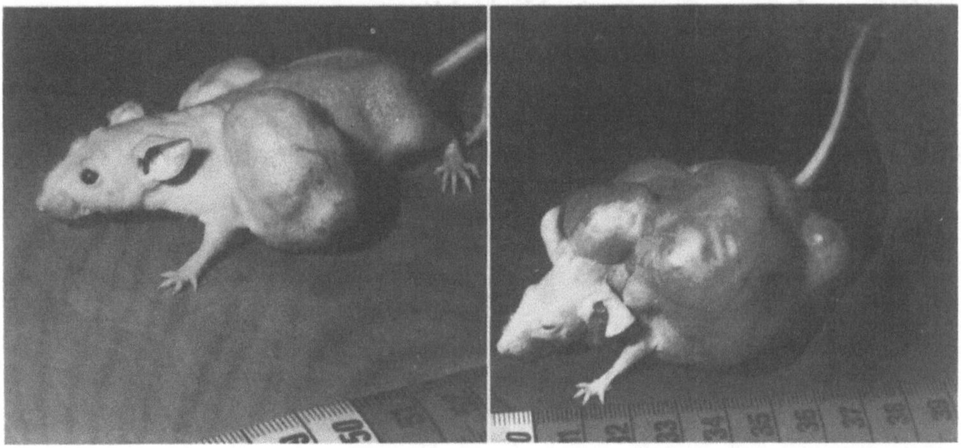

Fig. 1. Nude mouse with human mammary cancer SE 7 weeks (*left*) and 17 weeks (*right*) after heterotransplantation

In the comparison of chromosomal material, histology, and ^{3}H-thymidine labelling index good correlations were demonstrable between the original tumour and its transplants. In studies of endocrine treatment it is of interest whether the original tumour has the same receptor pattern as its transplant.

In Fig. 2 (with diethylstilboestrol [DES] as competitor instead of oestradiol) the oestradiol receptor of an original tumour extract (below) and its transplant (above) is demonstrated by gel electrophoresis.

Table 1 shows several receptor patterns of original tumours and their transplants up to the 13th passage. All tumours have been tested by gel electrophoresis. By quantitation, which we carried out and expressed as fmoles per microgram of DNA, good correlations could be found between the original tumour and its transplants over several passages.

In the next experiment (Fig. 3), the premenopausal tumour SE in the second passage, with a positive oestrogen receptor and a positive testosterone receptor but a negative progesterone receptor, was treated by ovariectomy and testosterone. No difference in tumour growth was demonstrable between the experimental group and the controls.

The same premenopausal tumour SE was also treated with tamoxifen and ovariectomy plus adrenalectomy (Fig. 4). In comparison with the control group a slight decrease of tumour growth can be seen with tamoxifen (this was significant according to the Kruskal-Wallis Test) and a highly significant decrease of tumour growth with ovariectomy plus adrenalectomy. We also checked the effect of ovariectomy plus adrenalectomy plus tamoxifen in a separate study. A slight additional decrease was seen in comparison with the ovariectomy plus adrenalectomy group. But this was not significant. As adrenalectomy is a major operation, the combination of ovariectomy and tamoxifen has been considered an alternative to ovariectomy plus adrenalectomy.

We checked this question with the aid of the same hormone-dependent premenopausal tumour SE.

In this experiment (Fig. 5) ovariectomy plus tamoxifen is not so beneficial as ovariectomy plus adrenalectomy. In the next series we treated the premenopausal hormone-dependent and

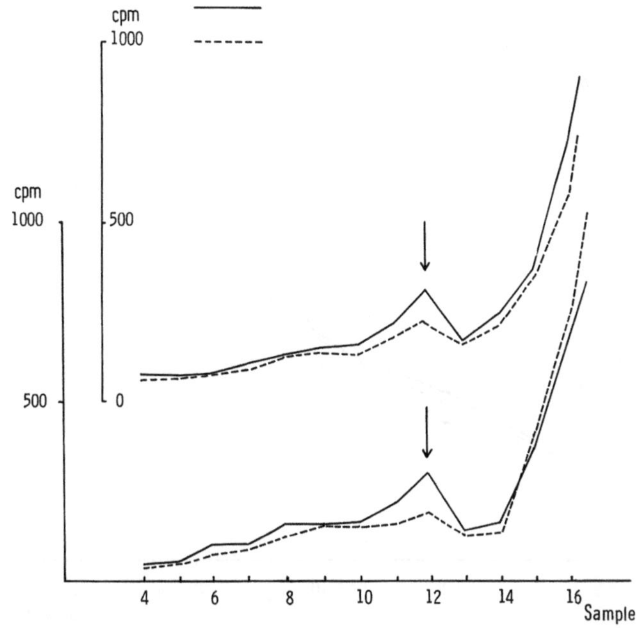

Fig. 2. Agar gel electrophoresis of an original human breast cancer extract (*lower part*) and the same tumour after heterotransplantation (*upper part*). *Dotted line* represents incubation with radioactive oestradiol and excess of cold oestradiol; *continuous line,* incubation with radioactive oestradiol alone. Peaks (*arrows*) indicate oestradiol bound to the cytoplasmic receptor

Table 1. Receptor patterns of original tumors and their transplants in various passages

Patient	Original tumour	1st passage	4th passage	11th passage	13th passage
SE	ER DHTR+ PgR–	ER DHTR+ PgR–	ER DHTR– PgR–	ER DHTR– PgR–	ER DHTR– PgR–
LO	ER DHTR+	ER DHTR+	ER DHTR+		
RO	ER DHTR+	ER DHTR+			
ZA	ER DHTR+	ER DHTR+			
CA	ER DHTR+ PgR+	ER DHTR+ PgR+	ER DHTR+ PgR+		
KA	ER DHTR– PgR–	ER DHTR– PgR–			

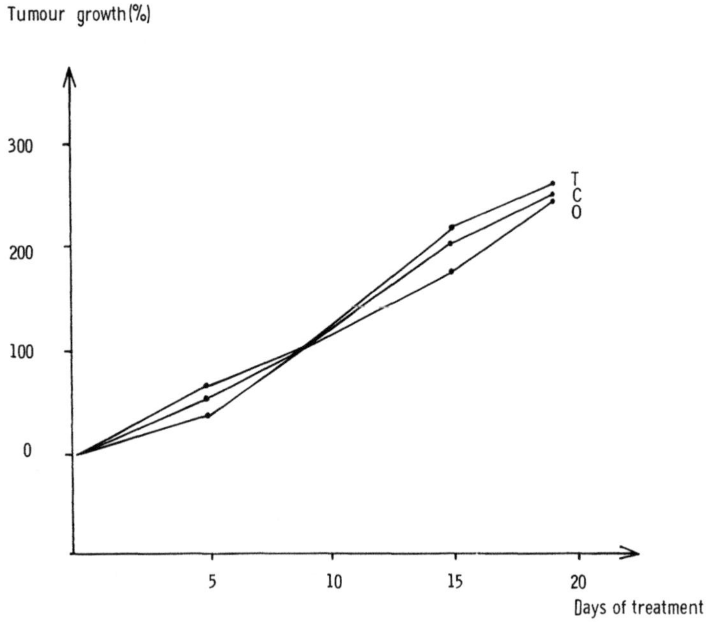

Fig. 3. Premenopausal oestradiol receptor-positive and testosterone receptor-positive human mammary cancer (SE) treated with ovariectomy (O) or testosterone (T). Control results are indicated by C. The experimental group consisted of 44 animals

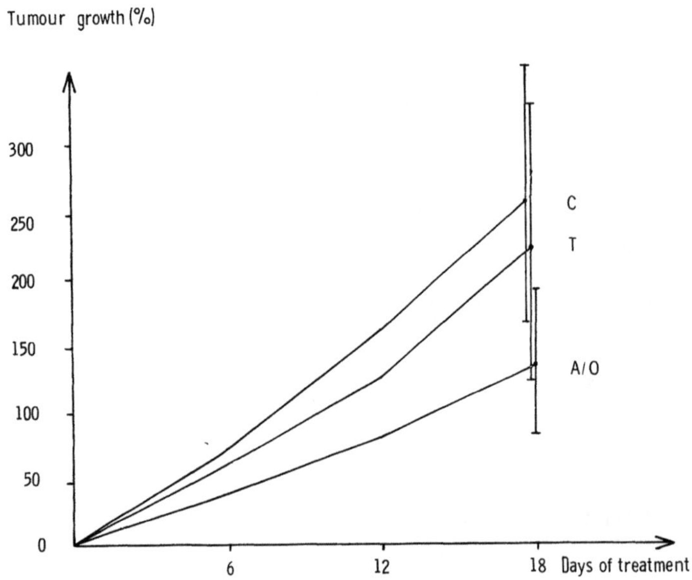

Fig. 4. Premenopausal oestradiol receptor-positive and progesterone receptor-negative human breast cancer (SE) treated with tamoxifen (T: 12 animals) or adrenalectomy plus ovariectomy (A/O: 15 animals). Control results (15 animals) are indicated by C

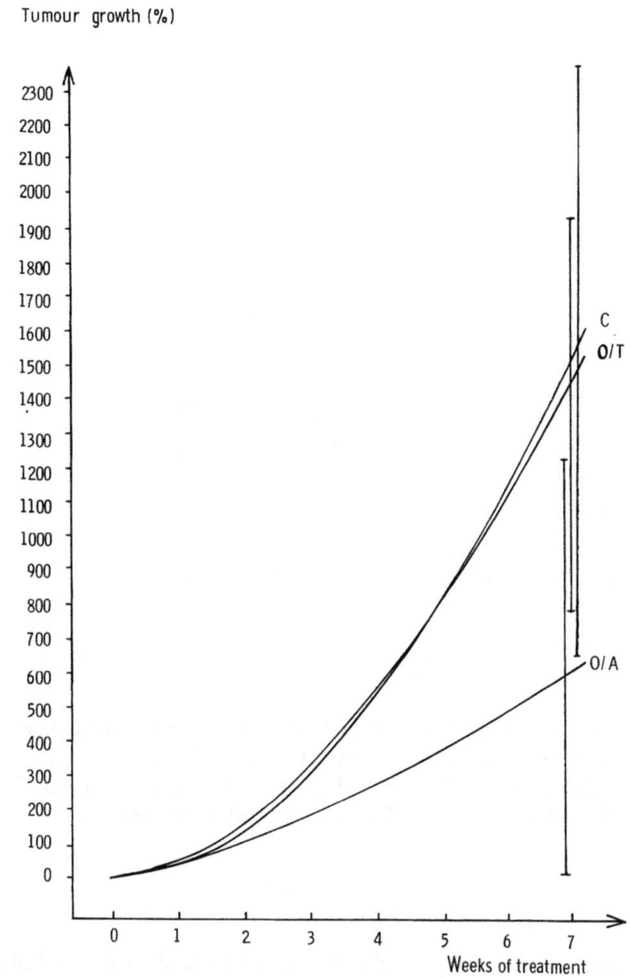

Fig. 5. Premenopausal oestradiol receptor-positive and progesterone receptor-negative human breast cancer (SE) treated with ovariectomy plus tamoxifen (O/T: 19 animals) or ovariectomy plus adrenalectomy (O/A: 16 animals). Control results (23 animals) are indicated by C

cyclophosphamide-sensitive mammary cancer SE with tamoxifen, cyclophosphamide (Endoxan) plus tamoxifen, ovariectomy plus cyclophosphamide plus tamoxifen, and cyclophosphamide alone.

The combined hormonal and cytotoxic treatment was not more effective than cytotoxic treatment alone (Fig. 6). The cytotoxic dose was 20% of the LD_{50} (about 100 mg/kg/week i.p.) in all groups with cyclophosphamide treatment.

In the next experiment (Fig. 7) the postmenopausal human mammary tumour CA, with a positive oestrogen receptor, a negative testosterone receptor, and a positive progesterone receptor, was treated with tamoxifen and oestradiol. Tamoxifen treatment stopped tumour growth, whereas oestradiol treatment resulted in a decrease of tumour size.

The postmenopausal human mammary cancer was also treated with cyclophosphamide, as in the previous experiments, oestradiol plus cyclophosphamide, and tamoxifen plus cyclo-

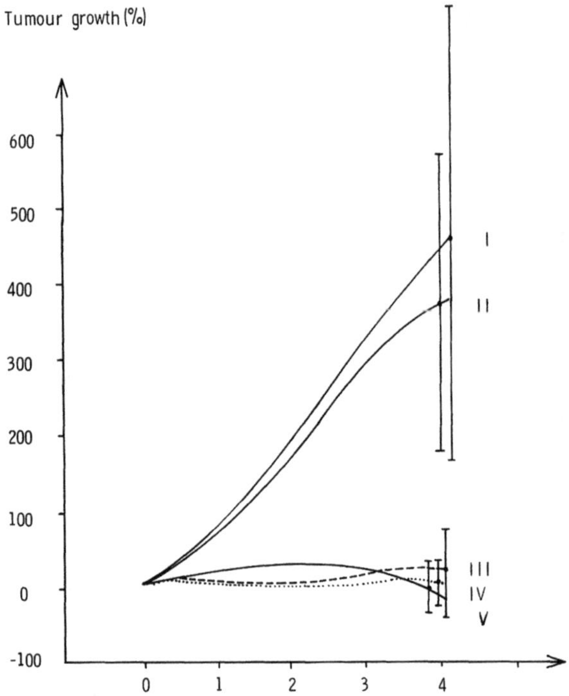

Fig. 6. Combined hormone and cytotoxic treatment of a premenopausal oestradiol receptor-positive, progesterone receptor-negative, and cyclophosphamide (Endoxan)-sensitive human breast cancer (SE). I, controls (18 animals); II, tamoxifen alone (14 animals); III, Endoxan + tamoxifen (20 animals); IV, ovariectomy + Endoxan + tamoxifen (14 animals); V, Endoxan alone (15 animals)

phosphamide (Fig. 8). The tumour has a positive oestradiol and progesterone receptor and is cyclophosphamide-sensitive. As in the premenopausal tumour SE, the combined cytotoxic and hormonal treatment was no more effective than the cytotoxic treatment alone.

In the next series the tumour of a postmenopausal woman with a negative oestradiol receptor and a positive testosterone receptor was treated with testosterone and oestradiol (Fig. 9). No difference in tumour growth was demonstrable in comparison with the controls.

The postmenopausal tumour SI, which was testosterone receptor-positive, oestradiol receptor-negative, and progesterone receptor-negative, was treated with testosterone and oestradiol (Fig. 10). An additional increase in tumour size can be seen with testosterone treatment. We repeated this experiment with about 20 tumours in each group and obtained the same results.

Figure 11 shows the results obtained when a spontaneous breast cancer in a fertile mouse (oestradiol receptor-positive, testosterone receptor-positive, and progesterone receptor-positive) was treated by ovariectomy, tamoxifen, ovariectomy plus adrenalectomy, and ovariectomy plus adrenalectomy plus tamoxifen. Ovariectomy and tamoxifen treatment alone resulted in only a slight decrease of tumour growth, whereas the major ablative procedure, including adrenalectomy and additional treatment with tamoxifen, resulted in a significant decrease of tumour growth.

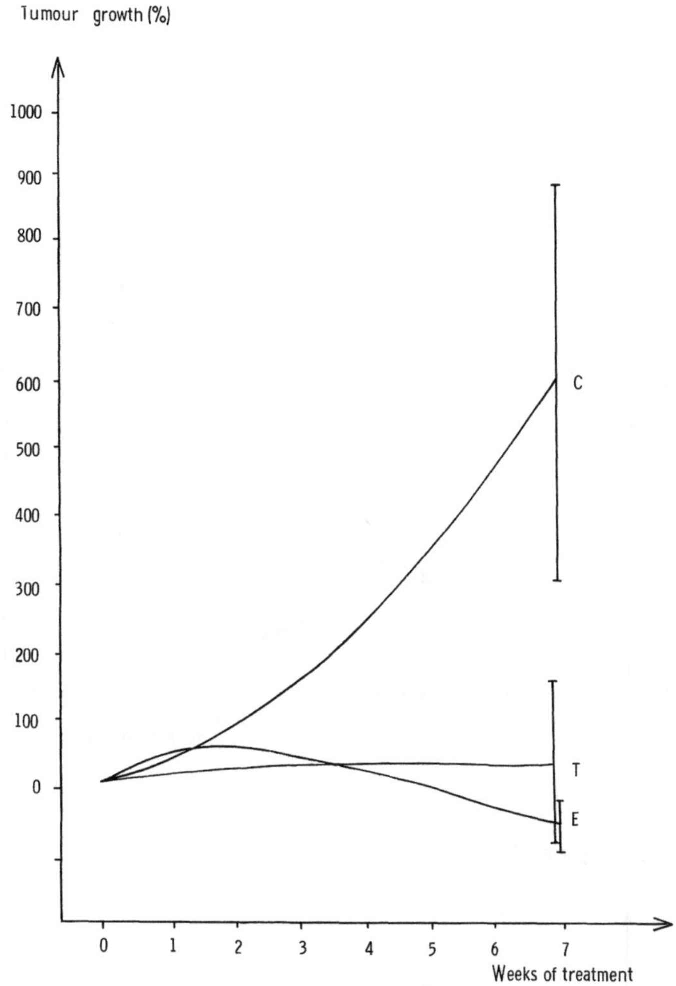

Fig. 7. Postmenopausal oestradiol receptor-positive and progesterone receptor-positive human breast cancer (CA) treated with tamoxifen (T: 14 animals) or oestradiol (E: 7 animals). The control group (C) contained 10 animals

The nude mouse model as presented here might have a further value for testing the individual reaction of a tumour to endocrine treatment. In comparison with clinical results there is not yet enough material to be published.

According to these data, in oestrogen receptor-positive and progesterone receptor-positive premenopausal women only major ablative therapy, including adrenalectomy, seems to yield adequate results. Additional antihormonal treatment can be of value. Antihormonal treatment with tamoxifen alone seems to be less effective, and tamoxifen in combination with ovariectomy seems not to be equal to ovariectomy plus adrenalectomy. In postmenopausal women with positive oestradiol and progesterone receptors, additional treatment with oestradiol or antihormonal treatment is beneficial. The application of testosterone seems either to be ineffective or to enhance tumour growth in animals.

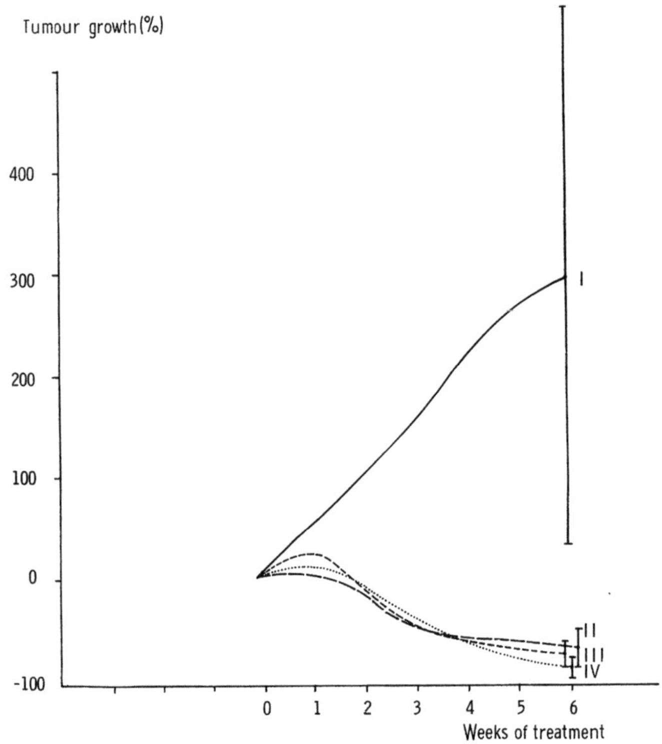

Fig. 8. Combined hormonal and cytotoxic treatment of a postmenopausal oestrogen receptor-positive, progesterone receptor-positive, and cyclophosphamide (Endoxan)-sensitive human breast cancer (KA). I, controls (14 animals); II, Endoxan + oestradiol (12 animals); III, Endoxan alone (10 animals); IV, Endoxan + tamoxifen (12 animals)

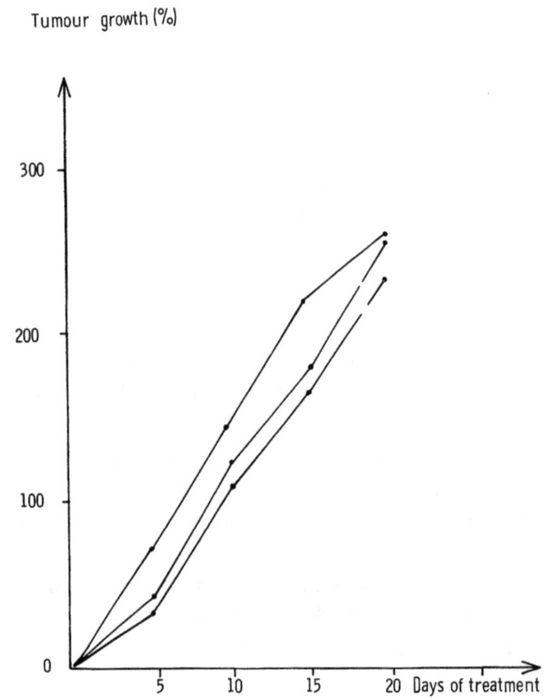

Fig. 9. Postmenopausal testosterone receptor-positive and oestrogen receptor-negative human breast cancer (LO) treated with testosterone (T) or oestradiol (E). C indicates the control results. The experiment involved 50 animals

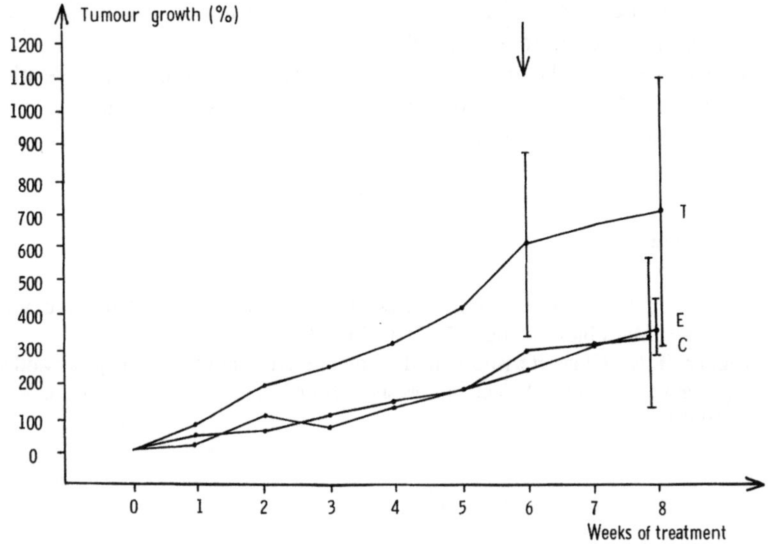

▲

Fig. 10. Postmenopausal testosterone receptor-positive human breast cancer (SI) treated with testosterone (T: 5 animals) or oestradiol (E: 5 animals). The control group (C) contained 12 animals. The *arrow* indicates the end of treatment

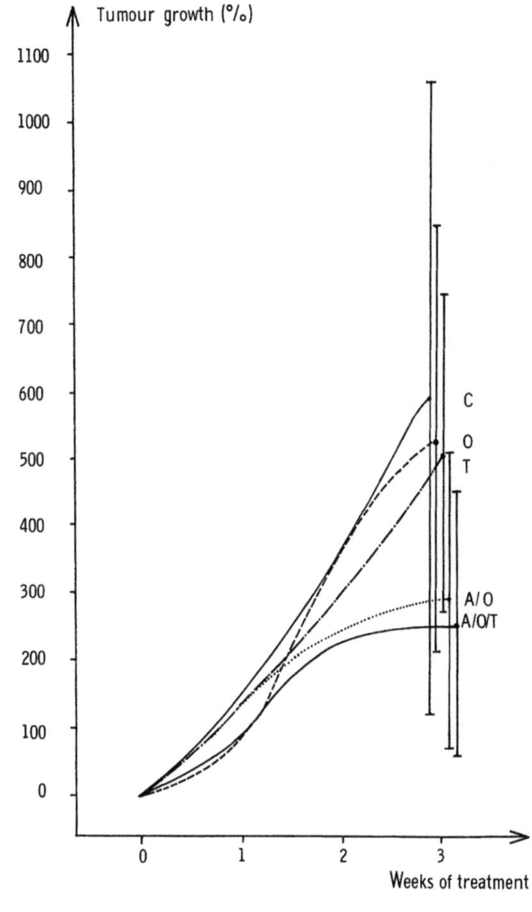

Fig. 11. Breast cancer of a fertile mouse (F1) treated with ovariectomy (O: 18 animals), tamoxifen (T: 16 animals), ovariectomy + adrenalectomy (A/O: 14 animals), or adrenalectomy + ovariectomy + tamoxifen (A/O/T: 10 animals). The control group (C) contained 16 animals

Combined endocrine and cytotoxic treatment in tumours sensitive to both had no better results than cytotoxic treatment alone.
Concerning steroid hormone receptors, cytotoxic treatment might result in a loss of specific binding sites. There seems to be some evidence for this in our material, and a study concerning this question is under way.

References

Rygaard, J., Povlsen, C. O.: Heterotransplantation of a human malignant tumor to "nude" mice. Acta Pathol. Microbiol. Scand. *77,* 758–760 (1969)

Wagner, R. K.: Characterisation and assay of steroid-hormone receptors and steroid-binding serum proteins by agargel-electrophoresis. Hoppe-Seylers Z. Physiol. Chem. *353,* 1235–1245 (1972)

10. A Hormone-Dependent Human Breast Cancer Cell Line Grown in Defined Medium[1]

M. E. Lippman, J. C. Allegra, and J. S. Strobl

Medicine Branch, National Cancer Institute, National Institutes of Health, Building 10, Room 6B02, Bethesda, MD 20014 (USA)

Introduction

It has long been appreciated that mammary cancer, in both humans and experimental animals, is frequently an endocrine-responsive illness. In fact, a large number of hormonal manipulations, including ablation of ovaries, adrenals, or pituitary or additive therapies such as estrogen, progestin, androgen, or glucocorticoid administration have all been shown occasionally to induce beneficial tumor regressions. The mechanisms by which these responses are induced are largely obscure. In part, this obscurity reflects the lack of suitable model systems in which hormonal effects can be studied. Experimental animal systems are enormously complex. It is impossible to administer a hormone to an experimental animal without altering the activities or concentrations of numerous other trophic substances. In addition, it is not safe to conclude that the effects of the hormone are due to direct interactions on the target cell, as opposed to indirect effects mediated by interactions of the hormone with the immune system or supporting stroma. Thus there is an extraordinary need for human mammary cell lines of undisputed pedigree that retain hormonal responses characteristic of in vivo tissues. In addition, systems need to be provided in which hormonal effects can be studied free from the presence of unknown factors present in serum supplements. In this report we review our studies with the ZR-75-1 cell line, which is derived from a human mammary cancer (Engel et al., 1978). This cell line can be propagated indefinitely in serum-free defined medium, and exhibits striking growth dependence on the presence of insulin, 17β-estradiol, transferrin, triiodothyronine, and dexamethasone.

Materials and Methods

Cells

ZR-75-1 cultures were derived from a malignant ascitic effusion in a 63-year-old white female who had undergone modified radical mastectomy 34 months previously for infiltrating duct carcinoma of the right breast.

1 We thank Le Esta Moran for invaluable help with manuscript preparation.

Establishment and characterization of the cell line has been described elsewhere and the reader is referred to the earlier publication for detailed methodology (ENGEL et al., 1978). Briefly, the salient features are as follows:

1) The morphology of the cells in culture is clearly epithelial, and is similar to that seen in biopsy material and in preparations of exfoliated cells from the original patient.
2) The cells exhibit ultrastructural features characteristic of breast carcinoma cells, such as desmosomes, tonofibrils, and intracytoplasmic ductlike vacuoles (BUEHRING and HACKETT, 1974).
3) The cells possess human chromosomes (model number 74—75), with markers different from those of HeLa cells by trypsin-Giemsa banding techniques, and distinct enzyme phenotypes, which further serve to assure their non-HeLa origin.
4) The cells possess specific receptors for glucocorticoids, estrogens, androgens, progestins, and insulin, and are responsive to a number of hormonal factors, which are discussed in this report.
5) These cells neither secrete nor synthesize significant amounts of the milk proteins casein and α-lactalbumin.

The line has been maintained in serial culture for 3 years through approximately 100 passages.

Hormone Receptors

The detailed methodology employed for steroid receptor analyses has already been published (LIPPMAN et al., 1976; 1977). Briefly, competition binding assays were performed on either cytoplasmic extracts or intact cells, multiple concentrations of radiolabeled ligand being used. Binding was examined by the Scatchard technique (SCATCHARD, 1949) to analyze data prepared by computer-assisted methods (AITKEN and LIPPMAN, 1977).

Medium and Hormones for Serum-Free Experiments

The cell line was initially established and maintained in RPMI 1640 medium supplemented with 25 n*M* Hepes (2-hydroxyethyl piperazine N-2-ethane sulfonic acid) buffer, 100 units penicillin/ml, 100 µg streptomycin/ml, 75 µg neomycin/ml, and fetal calf serum (FCS). Later any of several tissue culture median (Ham's F-10, IMEM, or MEM) supplemented as above proved equally satisfactory.

Improved Minimal Essential Medium (IMEM) (RICHTER et al., 1972) supplemented with L-glutamine (0.6 g/l), penicillin (62 mg/l), and streptomycin (135 mg/l), was the basic culture medium to which hormones and growth factors were added. Transferrin (Sigma, St. Louis, Mo.) was added at a final concentration of 1 µg/ml. L-Triiodothyronine (Sigma, St. Louis, Mo.) 10^{-5} *M* stock solution was prepared in 0.1 *N* NaOH and added to medium to yield a final concentration of 10^{-8} *M*. Insulin U-100 (Eli Lilly and Co., Indianapolis, Ind.) was added at a concentration of 5×10^{-7} *M*. 17β-Estradiol and dexamethasone (Sigma, St. Louis, Mo.) in benzene-ethanol were evaporated to dryness, dissolved in ethanol and stored at −20° C until use. Final concentrations in the medium were 10^{-8} *M* 17β-estradiol and 10^{-8} *M* dexamethasone. The final concentration of ethanol was 0.1%, and this concentration has no effect on the growth of the cells. Tamoxifen (TAM, ICI 46,474) was similarly prepared. Fibroblast growth factor (Collaborative Research, Waltham, Mass.) at a concentration of 0.025 µg/ml was added to the tissue culture flasks when the cells were subcultured in addition to nucleosides (10^{-8} *M* cytidine, uridine, thymidine, and adenine: Sigma, St. Louis, Mo.) and nonessential amino acids. Other factors tested for growth-promoting activity include epidermal growth factor (Collaborative Research, Waltham, Mass.), 5α-dihydrotestosterone (Steraloids Inc., Pawling, N.J.), vasopressin (Calbiochem, Gaithersburg, Md.), oxytocin (Sigma, St. Louis, Mo.), and human placental lactogen (Sigma, St. Louis, Mo.).

Cell Growth Experiments

Cells growing exponentially in MEM + 5% fetal calf serum were suspended with trypsin-EDTA (trypsin 0.05%; EDTA 0.02%) and replicately plated in MEM supplemented with 5% charcoal-treated calf serum (ARMELIN et al., 1974). The cells were plated into sterile six-well (35-mm) plastic tissue culture dishes (Linbro Scientific Inc., Hamden, Conn.). After sufficient time for the cells to become adherent (usually 12—16 h), the medium was changed for IMEM supplemented with estradiol, L-Triiodothyronine, insulin, dexamethasone, and transferrin (IMEM-HS) or to IMEM-HS minus a specific hormone. After 24 h the medium was replenished with fresh medium of identical composition. At various times, cells were collected by suspension in trypsin-EDTA and counted in a hemocytometer.

Cell Transfer

The serum-free cells were transferred by treating with 0.02% EDTA in saline A (0.35 g $NaHCO_3$/liter, 8.0 g NaCl/liter, 0.4 g KCl/liter, 1.0 g dextrose/liter, and 0.02 g phenol red/liter). The cell layer was rinsed with this solution and the excess removed. When the cells began to detach, the action of the EDTA was stopped by simple dilution in IMEM-HS. Cells were passed at a 1 : 2 dilution.

Plating efficiency experiments were performed by plating 25 000 cells in a 75-cm^2 tissue culture flask. After 7 days the cell colonies were counted. Plating efficiency is defined as the number of colonies formed multiplied by 100 and divided by the number of cells added to the tissue culture flask.

Precursor Incorporation

In order to assess the effect of TAM on thymidine incorporation in the ZR-75-1 breast cancer cells growing in IMEM-HS minus 17β-estradiol, radiolabeled thymidine (Amersham-Searle) diluted in Dulbecco's phosphate-buffered saline (PBC: pH 7.4) was added to each dish 1—2 h before the cells were harvested. Each dish usually contained 1 μCi tritium. Cells were harvested by washing the dishes once with PBS, suspending the cells in EDTA (0.02%), and collecting cell pellets by centrifugation. Cell pellets were suspended in water and sonically dispersed for 3s in a Branson sonicator (Branson Sonic Power Co., Danbury, Conn.) at the lowest setting. Aliquots were then used for the determination of protein by the method of LOWRY et al. (1951) or by thymidine incorporation by precipitation in 10% trichloroacetic acid. Acid-insoluble counts were collected and washed on a 0.45 μm-millipore filter. After drying, the filters were solubilized in Aquasol (New England Nuclear, Boston, Mass.) and counted in a Packard Scintillation Counter (Packard Instrument Co., Downers Grove, Ill.) (efficiency for tritium ~ 35%).

Results

Hormone Receptors

The cells were examined for the presence of specific steroid receptors. The results (Table 1) show that each cell contains cytoplasmic receptors for all four classes of steroid hormones. In

Table 1. Steroid hormone in the human breast cancer cell line ZR-75-1

Cell line	17-β Estradiol			5-α-Dihydrotestosterone		
	Receptor[a] concentr.	Binding[b] constant	Correl.[c] coeff.	Receptor concentr.	Binding constant	Correl. coeff.
ZR-75-1	29.0	1.3	0.982	34.0	0.53	0.911

Table 1. (continued)

Cell line	Glucocorticoid			Progesterone		
	Receptor concentr.	Binding constant	Correl. coeff.	Receptor concentr.	Binding constant	Correl. coeff.
74.0	–	–	43.0	3.7	0.964	

[a] fmol/mg cytoplasmic protein.
[b] Equilibrium dissociation constant (nM).
[c] Least squares.

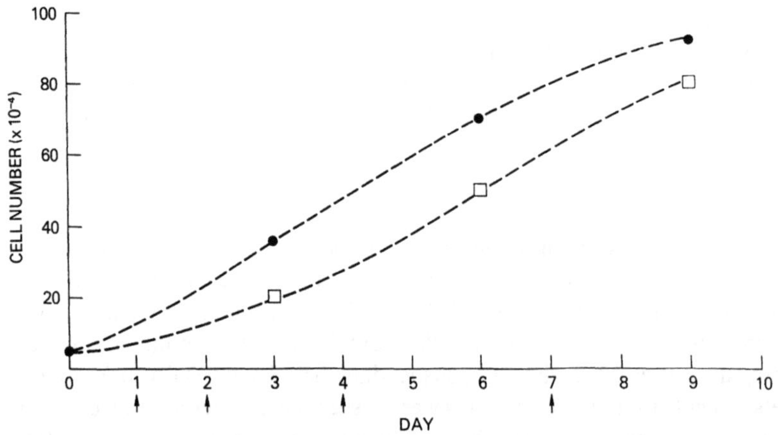

Fig. 1. Growth of the ZR-75-1 cell line in hormone-supplemented medium without serum. Cells were plated at a density of 50 000 cells/dish in MEM supplemented with 5% charcoal-treated calf serum. On day 1 medium was changed to IMEM-HS (●) and IMEM + 5% FCS (□). *Arrows* indicate days on which the cells were refed with fresh medium. Standard deviations of triplicate cell counts shown are generally less than 10%

terms of binding affinity and specificity these receptors appear entirely consistent with receptors described for other systems. In addition, these cells contain high-affinity receptors for insulin (OSBORNE et al., 1978). These receptors have features (affinity, specificity, negative cooperativity) of insulin receptors found in other target tissues. By inference, we assume that these cells also contain nuclear receptors for iodothyronines based on their hormonal responsiveness described below.

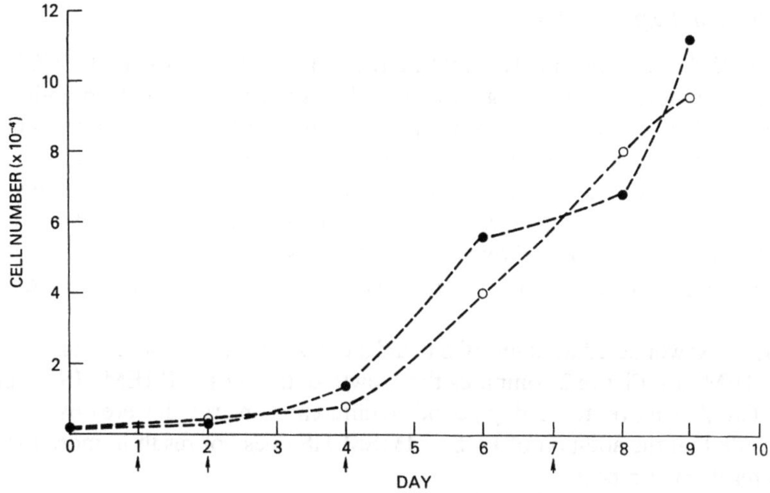

Fig. 2. Growth of the ZR-75-1 cell line in hormone supplemented medium without serum. Cells were plated at a density of 1000 cells/dish in MEM supplemented with 5% charcoal-treated calf serum. On day 1, the medium was changed to IMEM-HS (●) and IMEM-HS supplemented with 5% FCS (○). *Arrows* indicate days on which the cells were refed with fresh medium. Standard deviations of triplicate cell counts are generally less than 10%

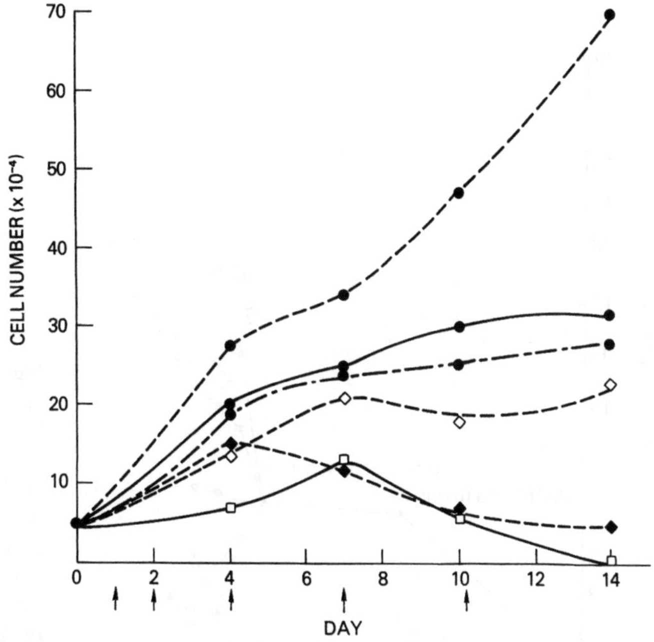

Fig. 3. Requirements for serum-free growth of ZR-75-1 human breast cancer cells. Cells were plated at a density of 50 000 cells/dish in MEM supplemented with 5% charcoal treated calf serum. On day 1, the medium was changed to IMEM-HS (– – ○ – –), IMEM-HS minus 17β-estradiol (——●), IMEM-HS minus insulin (– – – ●), IMEM-HS minus T_3 (– – ◇ – –), IMEM-HS minus transferrin (– – – ◆), IMEM (——□——). *Arrows* indicate days on which the cells were refed with fresh medium. Standard deviations of triplicate cell counts are generally less than 10%

Growth Experiments

ZR-75-1 cells grow rapidly in IMEM-HS. In Fig. 1, the growth of the ZR-75-1 cells in IMEM-HS is compared with their growth in IMEM supplemented with an optimal concentration of fetal calf serum. In this experiment the cells in IMEM-HS grew at a faster rate than those in FCS. In other experiments which are not shown, their growth rates are usually equal. The ZR-75-1 human breast cancer cell line grows rapidly in IMEM supplemented with hormones and the iron transport protein transferrin. The optimal concentration of 17β-estradiol in IMEM-HS has previously been shown to be 10^{-8} *M*. As described later, 5×10^{-7} *M* insulin, 10^{-8} *M* L-triiodothyronine, 10^{-8} *M* dexamethasone and 1 μg transferrin/ml are optimal for cell growth.

We next wondered whether FCS could increase the growth of cells already growing rapidly in IMEM-HS. Figure 2 compares the growth of the cells in IMEM-HS supplemented with 5% FCS. Again over this 9-day period no differences in growth were observed, and thus we conclude that the addition of FCS to IMEM-HS does not result in more rapid growth of these breast cancer cells.

The effects of each of the hormones and transferrin on growth is assessed in Fig. 3. As can be seen in this figure, the cells in IMEM-HS grow rapidly over the 14-day period. Control cells in IMEM alone remain viable for 4—7 days, as judged by attachment to the plastic tissue culture dishes, and then detach and die, as do the cells in IMEM-HS that lacks transferrin. Cells in IMEM-HS minus estradiol or insulin or L-triiodothyronine appear to grow progressively more slowly for approximately 7 days and then no net increment in cell number is seen,

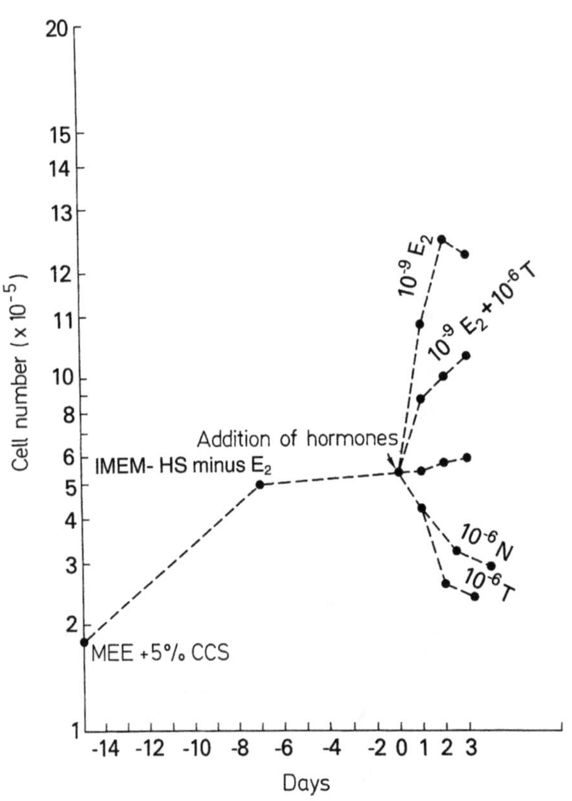

Fig. 4. Effects of estradiol or antiestrogen administration on ZR-75-1 cell growth. After 7 days (−14 to −7) in MEM plus charcoal-treated calf serum (CCS) cells were transferred to IMEM-HS minus 17β-estradiol (E_2) (from day −7 to day 0). On day 0, $10^{-9}M$ estradiol (E_2), 10^{-6} *M* TAM (T), or 10^{-6} *M* NAF (N) was added. Cells were harvested and counted on days shown. Medium was changed daily from day −14 to day 0

though viability is maintained for the 14-day period. The addition or subtraction of 10^{-8} *M* dexamethasone had no apparent effect on growth, but appeared to increase plating efficiency and was thus included in IMEM-HS. Higher concentrations of dexamethasone are growth-inhibitory.

The critical dependence of growth of these human mammary cancer cells on estradiol is illustrated in Fig. 4. As shown, the addition of a physiologically relevant concentration of 17β-estradiol (10^{-9} *M*) to cells in defined, serum-free medium results in rapid exponential growth. In this experiment, cells are initially plated on day −14 in MEM plus 5% charcoal-treated calf serum. This medium is changed daily. On day −7 the cells are transferred to IMEM-HS minus estradiol and this medium is changed daily. As seen, there is no further increase in cell number for the next 7 days. On day 0 either 10^{-9} *M* estradiol or one of the antiestrogens (tamoxifen: TAM, or nafoxidine: NAF) is added to the dish. Addition of estradiol results in a prompt resumption of exponential growth until the cells reach a maximum density of about 1.2×10^6 cells/well. Control cells show no net change in cell number. Cells treated with either antiestrogen are killed after an initial lag of 12–14 h. This killing is prevented by simultaneous administration of 1000fold less estradiol (Fig. 4). Thus these cells are exquisitely estrogen-dependent. While there is no net change in cell number in cells deprived of estradiol, this does not appear to be due simply to a cessation of growth. First, estradiol cells continue to incorporate thymidine, though at a lower rate than hormone-treated cells. Second, if the cells are prelabeled with thymidine there is loss of radioactivity into the medium in estrogen-deprived cells but not in estrogen-treated cells. Third, there is an obvious decrease in cell adhesiveness in estrogen-deprived cells, and detached cells are easily seen in the medium. Thus, it

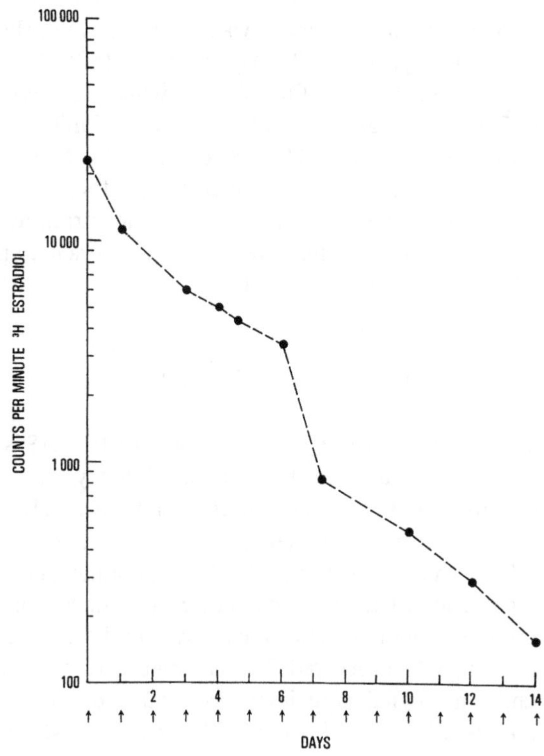

Fig. 5. Long-term retention of tritiated estradiol by ZR-75-1 cells. Subconfluent monolayers of ZR-75-1 cells in IMEM-HS minus E_2 were pulsed for 3 h with ^{3}H-17β-estradiol. At the end of the period, and daily thereafter, medium was exchanged for fresh serum-free IMEM-HS minus E_2 (*arrows*). Cells were harvested daily and radioactivity was assessed in the cell pellets

is likely that the ZR-75-1 cells are capable of a low rate of growth in estrogen-free medium, an effect masked by continued cell loss from the dish and replenishment. It is interesting to hypothesize that at least one estrogen-mediated effect is a modification of the cell surface resulting in an increased stickiness.

The long pretreatment with charcoal-treated calf serum and estradiol-free medium is required for complete removal of estradiol from these cells. An illustrative experiment is shown in Fig. 5. Cells are treated for 3 h with tritiated estradiol. Counts per minute in the cell pellet harvested each day are shown. The medium is exchanged daily (*arrows*) for fresh serum-free medium containing no estradiol. Fourteen days are required for a 2-log reduction in retained radioactivity. In experiments on another cell line, MCF 7, we have demonstrated that these retained counts are virtually all 17β-estradiol; they are specifically bound, and largely localized to the nuclear fraction. In addition, charcoal-treated serum or bovine serum albumin and antiestrogen or unlabeled estradiol addition can significantly accelerate the loss of nonspecifically and specifically retained estradiol.

Transferrin is mandatory for cell survival. As low a concentration as 0.25 μg/ml causes an increase in cell number after 4 days as compared with control cells. About 2–5 μg/ml is optimal.

Triiodothyronine is required for growth of the ZR-75-1 cells in defined medium. An effect on growth of L-triiodothyronine is observed at concentrations as low as 10^{-10} *M*, with maximal stimulatory effects on growth at 10^{-8} *M*. The effect on growth is diminished at higher concentrations, and 10^{-6}*M* and 10^{-5} *M* exhibit no growth-promoting activity.

Insulin is also required as a growth factor. An effect of insulin on growth is observed at concentrations as low as 10^{-11} *M*. The growth-promoting effect is maximal at 10^{-10} *M* and this maximal effect persists over a concentration range from 10^{-10} *M* to 10^{-6} *M*.

The effect of other factors on the growth of the ZR-75-1 cells was also investigated. No further growth-promoting activity was observed when the nucleosides, adenine (10^{-8} *M*), uridine (10^{-8} *M*), thymidine (10^{-8} *M*) or cytidine (10^{-8} *M*), nonessential amino acids, human placental lactogen (2 μg/ml), fibroblast growth factor (FGF) (0.025 μg/ml), epidermal growth factor (EGF) (0.01 μg/ml), vasopressin (1 milliunit/ml), oxytocin (1 milliunit/ml), or 5α-dihydrotestosterone (10^{-8} *M*) was added to IMEM-HS. The effects of growth factors, including FGF and EGF, were not determined either in the absence of insulin or at low (10^{-9} *M*) concentrations of insulin. At high concentrations insulin may interact with other growth peptide receptors. Thus, we cannot yet conclude positively that some growth response to EGF or FGF is not possible.

Cell Transfer and Long-Term Culture

The transfer of the ZR-75-1 cell line in IMEM-HS is difficult. Cells are passed at a dilution ratio of 1 : 2 because of a low plating efficiency. Table 2 lists the results of the plating efficiency experiments. The plating efficiency of the cells in IMEM-HS is approximately 1%. This can be improved to approximately 3%–4% by the addition of nonessential amino acids, nucleosides (10^{-8} *M* adenine, cytidine, thymidine, uridine) and 0.025 μg FGF/ml. We routinely add these factors at the time of subculture, and since none of these factors appears to have any growth-promoting activity in the ZR-75-1 cells, the flasks are refed with fresh IMEM-HS after plating has occurred. The plating efficiency of the cells in IMEM alone is less than 0.1% and is not significantly improved by the addition of bovine serum albumin (100 μg/ml). The plating efficiency of the ZR-75-1 cells in IMEM plus 5% FCS is greater than 50%.

Table 2. Effect of factors on plating efficiency of ZR-75-1 human breast cancer cells

Medium	Plating efficiency
IMEM	0.1%
IMEM plus bovine serum albumin	0.1%
IMEM-HS	1.2%
IMEM-HS plus bovine serum albumin	0.8%
IMEM-HS plus nucleosides	1.1%
IMEM-HS plus nonessential amino acids	1.0%
IMEM-HS plus FGF	1.8%
IMEM-HS plus nucleosides, nonessential amino acids, and FGF	3.4%
IMEM-HS plus nucleosides, nonessential amino acids, FGF, and conditioned medium	3.2%

We also attempted to improve plating efficiency by the addition of conditioned medium. We have preliminary data indicating that the ZR-75-1 cells condition their medium and that this conditioned medium, when added to the cells, leads to an increase in thymidine incorporation at 24 h and an increase in cell number at 48 h (ALLEGRA and LIPPMAN, unpublished data). As Table 2 shows, 50% (by volume) conditioned medium did not increase plating efficiency when added to IMEM-HS or IMEM-HS supplemented with nucleosides, nonessential amino acids, or FGF. Even under optimal conditions (in the presence of FCS) the ZR-75-1 require relatively large numbers of plated cells for satisfactory passage of the cells.

Discussion

The ZR-75-1 cell line has been characterized extensively and meets some criteria of inter- and intraspecies specificity and, most importantly, of organ specificity (ENGEL et al., 1978). The cells have a human karyotype. Allozyme phenotypes also show that the cell line is derived from a human donor and is distinct from HeLa. Finally, although lacking significant production of either casein or α-lactalbumin, its characteristic mammary epithelial morphology, including tonofibrils, desmosomes and intracytoplasmic vacuoles lined by microvilli, also supports its organ specificity (BUEHRING and HACKETT, 1974).

The adaptation of such a well-characterized human mammary cell line to serum-free growth has many potential benefits. Furthermore, it has receptors for estrogen, androgen, insulin, glucocorticoid, and progesterone, and responds to estrogen, androgen, insulin, and glucocorticoid. We felt that the establishment of the cell line in defined medium without the unknown effects of serum factors would equip investigators better to study the mechanisms of hormone interaction with breast cancer. Our preliminary data on the effect of the antiestrogen TAM are encouraging. In an environment totally devoid of estrogen (IMEM-HS minus 17β-estradiol), we are able to show a significant inhibition of cell growth and precursor incorporation, which suggests an effect of TAM that is totally independent of competition with estradiol. This system also allows the investigation of hormone stimulation in an environment in which the specific hormone studied can be eliminated for a fixed period of time. With this system, we are able to see pronounced stimulatory effects of 17β-estradiol and insulin, as measured by thymidine incorporation in cells grown for 7–10 days in IMEM-HS minus estradiol and insulin. The conversion of cells from a stable slow-growing state to exponential growth is a much closer approximation of hormone-dependent tissue than the relatively paltry stimulation usually observed in culture. The attainment of the effects of hormones of this magnitude and specificity may be important in allowing investigators to isolate specific cellular induced products.

Interestingly, none of these hormonal components, either alone or in any combination attempted by us, permits growth of another human breast cancer cell line (MCF-7).

Finally, the ZR-75-1 cell line growing in IMEM-HS may become a useful system for study of the effects of single drugs, drug combinations, and hormone and drug interactions in human breast cancer. It provides a growing cell system, free of serum contamination, for the study of drug interaction. It allows for the study of mechanisms of drug action without the presence of nucleosides, which are present in serum. The system may be easily modified by the addition of purines, pyrimidines, amino acids, and rescue agents such as folinic acid to allow evaluation of the mechanisms of drug action and drug toxicity. Furthermore, the growth rate of the system can be altered by the omission of a single hormone, allowing one to study the relationship of drug action and growth rate.

The major problem with the system, thus far, lies in the low plating efficiency. At present, the production of large quantities of cells is not practical; however, in studying hormone or drug interactions this is not a problem, since it is possible to plate the cells in charcoal-treated calf serum and change to IMEM-HS as soon as the cells become adherent. This low plating efficiency has also been noted in many of the other cell lines that have been adapted to defined medium. The HTC cells growing in IMEM-ZO reported by Thompson et al. (1975) have a plating efficiency of 0.1%–1%. The HTC cells were fastidious in their requirements for gentle handling and quality of medium. Burks and Peck (1978) also report a low plating efficiency for their primary bone cell cultures in serum-free medium. They found their plating efficiency to be density-dependent, with the cells exhibiting a low plating efficiency and a failure to proliferate at a low density.

In summary, the ability to grow the ZR-75-1 human breast cancer cell line in a defined serum-free medium supplemented with hormones and transferrin will be advantageous to the study of hormone interaction with human breast cancer.

References

Aitken, S. C., Lippman, M. E.: A simple computer program for quantification and Scatchard analysis of steroid receptor proteins. J. Steroid Biochem. *8*, 77 (1977)

Armelin, H. A., Wishikawa, K., Sato, G. H.: Control of mammalian cell growth in culture: The action of protein and steroid hormones as effector substances. In: Control of proliferation in animal cells. Clarkson, B., Baserga, R. (eds.), p. 97. Cold Spring Harbor, N.Y.: Cold Spring Harbor Lab. 1974

Buehring, G. C., Hackett, A. J.: Human breast tumor cell lines: Identity evaluation by ultrastructure. J. Nat. Cancer Inst. *53*, 621 (1974)

Burks, J. K., Peck, W. A.: Bone cells: A serum-free medium supports proliferation in primary culture. Science *199*, 542 (1978)

Engel, L. W., Young, N. A., Tralka, T. S., Lippman, M. E., O'Brien, S. J., Joyce, M. J.: Human breast carcinoma cells in continuous culture: Establishment and characteristics of three new cell lines. Cancer Res. *38*, 3352 (1978)

Lippman, M. E., Bolan, G., Huff, K.: The effects of androgens and antiandrogens on hormone-responsive human breast cancer in long-term tissue culture. Cancer Res. *36*, 4610 (1976)

Lippman, M. E., Huff, K., Bolan, G., Neifeld, J. P.: Interactions of R5020 with progesterone and glucocorticoid receptors in human breast cancer and peripheral blood lymphocytes in vitro. In: Progesterone receptors in normal and neoplastic tissues. McGuire, W. L. (ed.), p. 193. New York: Raven Press 1977

Lowry, O. H., Rosebrough, N. J., Farr, A. L., Randall, R. J.: Protein measurement with the folin phenol reagent. J. Biol. Chem. *193*, 265 (1951)

Monaco, M. E., Osborne, C. K., Lippman, M. E.: Insulin stimulation of fatty acid synthesis in human breast cancer cells: Brief communication. J. Nat. Cancer Inst. *58*, 1591 (1977)

O'Brien, S. J., Kleiner, G., Olson, R., Shannon, J. E.: Enzyme polymorphisms as genetic signatures in human cell cultures. Science *195*, 1345 (1977)

Osborne, C. K., Monaco, M. E., Lippman, M. E., Kahn, C. R.: Insulin receptors in human breast cancer cells in long term tissue culture: Correlation between insulin binding, degradation and biologic activity. Cancer Res. *38*, 94 (1978)

Richter, A., Sanford, K. K., Evans, V. J.: Influence of oxygen and culture medium on plating efficiency of some mammalian tissue cells. J. Nat. Cancer Inst. *49*, 1705 (1972)

Scatchard, G.: The attractions of proteins for small molecules and ions. Ann. N.Y. Acad. Sci. *51*, 660 (1949)

Thompson, E. B., Anderson, C. V., Lippman, M. E.: Serum-free growth of HTC cells containing glucocorticoid- and insulin-inducible tyrosine aminotransferase and cytoplasmic glucocorticoid receptors. J. Cell. Physiol. *86*, 403 (1975)

11. Endocrine and Cytostatic Treatment of Experimental Mammary Cancer

H. H. Fiebig and D. Schmähl

Abteilung für Innere Medizin, Klinikum der Albert-Ludwigs-Universität, Hugstetter Straße 55, D-7800 Freiburg (FRG)
Deutsches Krebsforschungszentrum, Institut für Toxikologie und Chemotherapie, Im Neuenheimer Feld 280, D-6900 Heidelberg 1 (FRG)

Introduction

Progress in clinical cancer chemotherapy is due mainly to the advent of controlled clinical trials. However, using experimentally transplanted tumours, investigators were able to identify all anticancer drugs that are effective in human cancer (GOLDIN et al., 1966). Nevertheless, no single transplantation tumour could simulate a specific human cancer.

Primary autochthonous tumours in animals resemble their human counterparts in biological behaviour. Experimental chemotherapy in autochthonous tumours appears to be more comparable to the human situation than do studies of transplantation tumours (SCHMÄHL, 1966, 1970).

Our first investigations into the treatment of autochthonous rat tumours such as hepatomas, subcutaneously growing sarcomas, cancers of the ear duct, breast, forestomach, bladder, and colon yielded, in part, a longer lifespan than in untreated rats (SCHMÄHL and SCHRICK, 1964; SCHMÄHL et al., 1963, 1966, 1968; FRETZ et al., 1969; HABS et al., 1977a; HABS et al., 1977b; SYCH et al., 1978).

In this paper, the effects of endocrine and cytostatic therapy on chemically induced autochthonous mammary carcinoma of the rat are presented. Carcinogenic aromatic hydrocarbons and nitrosoureas were used for induction of the tumours. Earlier therapeutic studies in this tumour model were carried out by HUGGINS et al. (1959), GRISWOLD et al. (1966), TELLER et al. (1966), SHIMKIN et al. (1967), and GROPPER and SHIMKIN (1967).

Biological Properties of the Tumour Model

For induction of primary mammary tumours we used the aromatic hydrocarbon 7,12-dimethylbenz[a]anthracene (DMBA), as first described by HUGGINS et al. (1959), and methylnitrosourea (MNU), following GULLINO et al. (1975).

Female Sprague-Dawley rats between 50 and 55 days old each received three i.v. injections of DMBA within 1 week, to a total dose of 4 mg. Tumours developed multicentrically along the milkline (Fig. 1). The rats were checked weekly for palpable tumours. Between 42 and 77 days (median 56 days) after the first DMBA injection, 85%–90% of the rats were randomly assigned to different therapy groups. At the beginning of treatment the mean

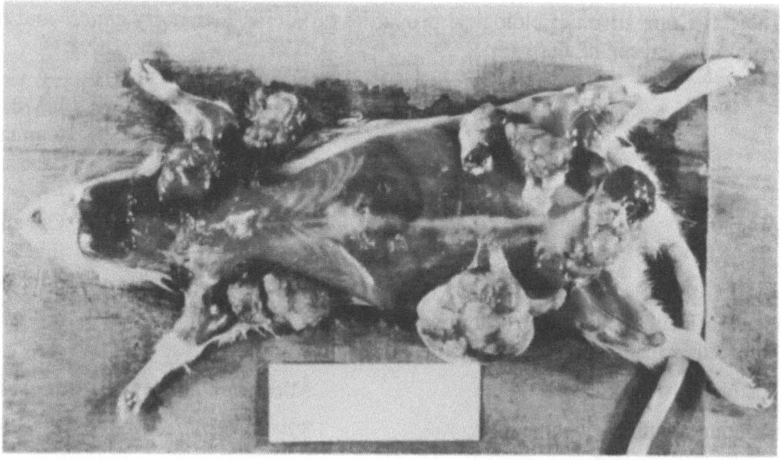

Fig. 1. DMBA-induced mammary cancer of the rat, developing multicentrically along the milk-line

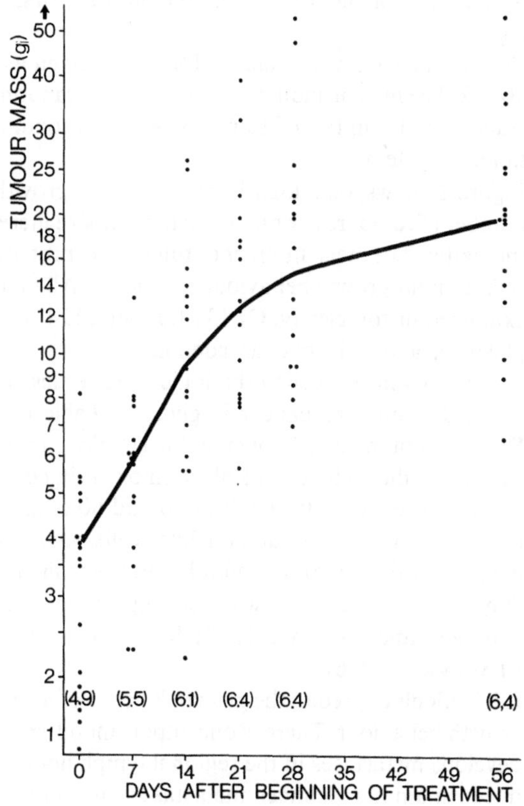

Fig. 2. Growth behaviour of total tumour size and mean number of tumours per rat (in parenthesis) in 16 untreated controls bearing DMBA-induced mammary cancer. Induction time ranged from 42 to 77 days

Table 1. Comparison of biological properties of human mammary cancer and the DMBA-induced mammary cancer of the rat

	Human mammary cancer	DMBA-induced mammary cancer of the rat
Aetiology	Chemical carcinogens? Hormones? Radiation? Nutrition? Virus?	Chemical carcinogens injected during adolescence
Genetic identitity between tumour and host cells except malignant transformation	+	+
Histology	Adenocarcinoma with subtypes	
Tumour volume doubling time	30–90 days	6.3–49 days
Variation in growth behaviour	+	+
Metastases	+	–
Effect of endocrine therapy	+	++
Effect of chemotherapy	++	+

number of tumours per rat was 4.8 ± 0.6 and the mean total tumour size, which was obtained by addition of the sizes of individual tumours, was 3.3 ± 0.5 g, usually between 2 and 6 g.

The second carcinogen used, MNU, was given as a single i.v. injection of 50 mg/kg on day 50 ± 2. The median induction period before randomisation for treatment was 77 days. The incidence and number of tumours were approximately the same as in the DMBA-induced tumour system.

Figure 2 shows, on a logarithmic scale, the growth curve of total tumour size and the mean number of tumours per rat. Total tumour size increased exponentially for 21 days and sloped thereafter. The mean number of tumours per rat increased from 4.9–6.4. A marked variability in tumour growth behaviour was noted. All mammary tumours from 18 control rats were examined histologically. Of 131 tumours, 124 were classified as carcinomas, five as preneoplasmas, and only two as adenomas.

A comparison between the biological properties of human mammary cancer and the DMBA-induced mammary cancer is given in Table 1.

Whereas not much is known on the aetiology of human mammary cancer, its counterpart in the rat is induced by chemical carcinogens injected during a critical phase of development of breast tissue, i.e., between days 50 and 60 of life. For both tumour types, there is a genetic identity between tumour and host cells, and histological examinations reveal adenocarcinomas with subtypes in addition to the malignant transformation. Tumour volume-doubling time is more than twice as long for human mammary cancer (RIGBY-JONES, 1962; PHILIPPE and LE GAL, 1968; KUSAMA et al., 1972; CHARLSON and FEINSTEIN, 1974; PEARLMAN, 1976).

It is difficult to predict the growth kinetics of a single tumour, since we find great variation in growth behaviour. There is one important difference, i.e., human mammary cancer normally develops metastases in the regional lymph nodes and distant organs, whereas in DMBA-induced mammary cancer metastases are only rarely seen.

Table 2. Effect of single agent chemotherapy in DMBA-induced mammary cancer of the rat

Drug	Dose (mg/kg day)	Schedule day	Application	TWI[b] (%) day 28	R+NC[a,b] % day 21 or 28	Change in body weight day 0–28 (%)	Mortality[c] day 56/ total day 0
ADR	1.2	1–3, 14–16	i.p.	45	31	0	2/16
Cyclophosphamide	20	1 × 4 weeks	i.p.	56	38	0	2/16
Vincristine	0.15	1 × 4 weeks	i.p.	48	12	+ 4	2/16
Prednisolone	10	1–21	p.o.	32	31	− 2	0/16
5-Fluorouracil	20	1–4, 14–17	i.p.	28	31	+ 9	1/16
Methotrexate	0.4	1–4, 15–18	i.p.	31	6	− 7	1/16
BCNU	6.0	1, 2	i.v.	39	19	− 6	5/16
Control M3					0	+ 5	0/16
Control M8M14					0	+ 7	0/18

[a] R + NC, total tumour size ≧ 150% of initial total tumour size.
[b] Rats dying of toxicity by day 56 were excluded.
[c] Due to toxicity.

In summary, the biological behaviour of human and DMBA-induced mammary cancers is markedly similar. However, before using the rat tumour model as a predictive system, we have to investigate whether there is a correlation in the results obtained from cytostatic and endocrine therapy.

Effect of Cytostatic Treatment

First we examined the effect of seven anticancer drugs that are effective in human mammary cancer (Table 2). The schedules were adopted from clinical experience, i.e., adriamycin (ADR) was given intermittently at 14-day intervals. The dosage was reduced for the next treatment cycle in rats showing a loss of body weight as a sign of toxicity. The selected doses resulted in a mortality rate due to toxicity around the LD_{10} level, except for treatment with BCNU, which was more toxic. For statistical evaluation, differences in tumour size were calculated by the Kruskal-Wallis test followed by multiple comparisons (Dunn, 1964), and the remission/no change rate with simultaneous tests by Gabriel (1966). Single-agent therapy effected remissions apparent in total tumour size in rare cases only; on the other hand, the total tumour size in 146 untreated rats did not show spontaneous remission or stationary growth behaviour in a single case, indicating that both remission and no change in total tumour size must be considered a treatment success. In terms of remission plus no change rate, ADR, cyclophosphamide (CY), vincristine, prednisolone, 5-fluorouracil (5-FU), and BCNU were effective (Table 2). Methotrexate was studied in four different dosages, three of which were toxic. At a dose of 0.4 mg/kg, given on days 1–4 and 15–18, methotrexate resulted in only one no change out of 16 treated rats. However, in terms of tumour weight inhibition (TWI) over untreated rats, calculated as control-test/control × 100 (TWI), methotrexate was active, effecting a TWI of 31%. The other drugs listed in Table 2 also showed a marked TWI

Table 3. Effect of single-agent chemotherapy in mammary cancer

Drug	Human mammary cancer Remission (%)	DMBA-induced mammary cancer of the rat: R + NC	
		Number/Total	%
Adriamycin	41[a]	21/63	33
Cyclophosphamide	34[b]	6/16	38
Methotrexate	34[b]	1/16	6
5-Fluorouracil	26[b]	5/16	31
BCNU	21[c]	3/16	19
Vincristine	20[b]	2/16	12
Prednisolone	18.5[d]	5/16	31
Chlorozotocin	NE[e]	8/16	50
$CH_3SO_2O(CH_2)_2$-CNU	NE	7/16	47
$H_2NC(O)CH_2$-CNU	NE	9/16	64

[a] Adriamycin (1975).
[b] CARTER (1976).
[c] CARTER et al. (1972).
[d] LIVINGSTONE and CARTER (1970).
[e] NE, not evaluated.

Table 4. Effect of ADR and nitrosoureas in DMBA-induced mammary cancer. Analysis of total tumour size per rat

Compound	Dose (mg/kg/ day, i.v.)	Schedule day	TWI (%) day 21	R + NC[a] (%) day 21 or 28	Change of body weight % day 0–21[b]	Mortality[b] day 56/ total day 0
$CH_3SO_2O(CH_2)_2$-CNU	8.0	1, 2	71[NS c]	47	− 2	2/15
	4.0	1, 2	8	0	+ 6	0/8
$H_2NC(O)CH_2$-CNU	7.5	1, 2	70[NS]	64	−13	1/14
	10.0	1, 2	Toxic			6/8
Chlorozotocin	10.0	1, 2	64[NS]	50	− 7	2/16
	20.0	1, 2	Toxic			7/17
BCNU	6.0	1, 2	56[NS]	19	− 2	5/16
ADR	3.0	1, 15	58	44	0	1/16
Control				0	+ 6	0/18

CNU = $NHCON(NO)CH_2CH_2CL$.
[a] R + NC, total tumour size ≥ 150% of initial total tumour size.
[b] Due to toxicity.
[c] NS, no significant difference from ADR.

Table 5. Effect of ADR and nitrosoureas in DMBA-induced mammary cancer. Analysis of individual tumours per rat

Compound	Numbers of tumours ≧ 0.6 g day 0	TWI (%) Median	TWI (%) 95% Confidence interval	R[b] day 21 %	R/total evaluable tumours[a]
$CH_3SO_2O(CH_2)_2$-CNU	32	78[NS c]	68–87	46[NS]	13/28
	17	5	0–41	0	0/17
$H_2NC(O)CH_2$-CNU	31	65[NS]	57–80	32[NS]	9/28
Chlorozotocin	28	65[NS]	41–79	26[NS]	6/23
BCNU	24	52	29–66	17	4/24
ADR	36	59	54–73	21	7/33
Control	32			3	1/32

[a] Tumours from rats dying of toxicity were excluded.
[b] R, remission; tumour size ≦ 50% of initial tumour size.
[c] NS, not significant vs ADR.

Table 6. Effect of combination chemotherapy in DMBA-induced mammary cancer of the rat

Combination	TWI[b] day 28 (%)	R + NC[a, b] day 21 or 28 (no.)	R + NC[a, b] day 21 or 28 (%)	Change in body weight day 0–28 (%)	Mortality[c] day 56/ total day 0
Control		0	0	+ 5	2/27
ADR alone[d]	52	11	30	0	3/37
ADR + 5-FU	73[e]	23	62[e]	+ 1	2/37
ADR + prednisolone	79[f]	30	81[f]	– 4	2/37
ADR + cyclophosphamide	81[g]	20	57	0	10/37

[a] R + NC, total tumour size ≥ 150% of initial tumour size.
[b] Rats dying of toxicity by day 56 were excluded.
[c] Due to toxicity.
[d] ADR 1.2 mg/kg/day, days 1–3, 14–16, i.p., for 16 animals; ADR 3.0 mg/kg/day, days 1, 15, i.v., for 21 animals. For dose reduction see text.
[e] P vs ADR alone < 0.05.
[f] $P < 0.01$.
[g] $P < 0.001$.

over untreated rats, ranging from 28%–56%. A slight decline in body weight was observed after treatment with prednisolone, methotrexate, and BCNU.

In Table 3 the effect of single-agent chemotherapy on remission rate in human mammary cancer is compared with the remission plus no change rate obtained in the DMBA-induced tumour system. We find a marked correlation for ADR, cyclophosphamide, 5-FU, BCNU, vincristine, and prednisolone. In terms of remission/no change rate, only methotrexate was less active in the rat model than in human breast cancer. It is possible that with another schedule, e.g., administration twice weekly, the effect of methotrexate could be improved. Our findings indicate that – in terms of total tumour size per rat – the DMDA-induced tumour model is less sensitive than human mammary cancer, but a remarkable correlation must be noted in the relative sensitivities.

Thus the DMBA-induced mammary cancer seems to be an excellent model for use in extended screening experiments to assess the antitumour activity of compounds effective in transplantation tumour systems.

We tested a number of new nitrosoureas synthesised by G. EISENBRAND, German Cancer Research Center, Heidelberg (EISENBRAND et al., 1976; FIEBIG et al., 1977). Three nitrosoureas had marked antitumour activity. The water-soluble 1-(2-chloroethyl)-1-nitroso-3-(methylene-carboxamido)-urea (CNMCU) and 2-[3-(2-chloroethyl)-3-nitrosoureido]ethyl-methansulphonate (CNUEMS) resulted in remission plus no change rates of 64% and 47% in total tumour size, respectively.

Chlorozotocin, a sugar derivative synthesised by the method of JOHNSTON et al. (1975), was also remarkably active, with a remission/no change rate of 50%. The three new nitrosoureas produced a more pronounced TWI, ranging from 71% to 64%, than did BCNU and adriamycin, with 56% and 58% (Table 4). However, the differences against ADR were not statistically significant, which may be due to the limited number of rats and the large 95% confidence interval for the results. Analysis of individual tumours per rat, which were at least 0.6 g at the beginning of treatment, revealed 23–32 evaluable tumours per test group (Table 5).

The methansulphonate derivative CNUEMS resulted in 13 remissions in 28 cases, the amino acid derivative CNMCU in 9 remissions in 28, and the sugar derivative chlorozotocin in 6 remissions in 23 treated rats. The remission rate was between 26% and 46%, as against 21% for treatment with adriamycin and 17% for treatment with BCNU. However, these differences were again not statistically significant. The evaluation of TWI showed the same results.

A higher TWI of between 65% and 78% was obtained with the new nitrosoureas, in comparison with 52% and 59% for treatment with BCNU and adriamycin, respectively.

The DMBA-induced tumour system allowed us to identify three nitrosoureas, two of which were first synthesised in our own institute, that showed at least the same and possibly a higher antitumour activity than adriamycin, clinically the most active anticancer agent in breast cancer.

In human mammary cancer, combination chemotherapy resulted in a higher remission rate than single-agent therapy. ADR was therefore given in combination with other active drugs. In 1975 we started combination chemotherapy in DMBA-induced mammary cancer of the rat. The effect of ADR in combination with six other drugs active in human mammary cancer was investigated. A schedule with simultaneous application of two drugs was chosen. The purpose of these studies was to find out which combination had a synergistic effect in tumour inhibition without increasing toxicity. The effects of three combinations producing statistically higher antitumour effects than ADR alone are shown in Table 6 (FIEBIG and SCHMÄHL, 1976). Each test group consisted of 37 rats. The remission/no change rate was 62% for ADR + 5-FU, 81% for ADR + prednisolone, and 57% for ADR + cyclophosphamide. ADR alone resulted in 30% remissions/no change. The three combinations yielded a TWI of between 73% and 81%. The differences in comparison with ADR alone were

Table 7. Effect of combination chemotherapy in DMBA-induced mammary cancer of the rat

Combination	Dose (mg/kg day)	Schedule day	Application	TWI[b] (%) day 28	R + NC[a, b] day 21 or 28 (%)	Change in body weight day 0–28 (%)	Mortality[c] day 56/ total day 0
ADR alone	1.2	1–3, 14–16	i.p.	45	31	0	2/16
ADR + vincristine	1.2 0.15	1–3, 14–16 1 × 4 weeks	i.p. i.p.	47[NS d]	38	+ 4	1/16
ADR alone	3.0	1, 15	i.v.	66	44	+ 1	1/16
ADR + methotrexate	3.0 0.4	1, 15 1–4, 15–18	i.v. i.p.	64	50	0	1/16
ADR + BCNU	2.5 4.0	1, 15 1, 2	i.v. i.v.	59	44	− 3	3/16
Control					0	+ 6	0/18

[a] R + NC, total tumour size ≥ 150% of initial total tumour size.
[b] Rats dying of toxicity by day 56 were excluded.
[c] Due to toxicity.
[d] NS, no significant vs ADR.

Table 8. Effect of combination chemotherapy on human breast cancer, DMBA-induced mammary cancer of the rat, and mouse leukaemia L 1210

Combination	Human breast cancer remission rate (%)	Mammary cancer of the rat	Leukaemia L 1210[a, b]
		Therapeutic synergism	
ADR alone	41[c]		
ADR + cyclophosphamide	80[d]	+	+
ADR + 5-FU	47–70[e] (+ CY)	+	−
ADR + methotrexate	42[e]	−	+
ADR + vincristine	45–48[e]	−	+
ADR + BCNU	NE[f]	−	±
ADR + prednisolone	NE[f]	+	NE

[a] GOLDIN and JOHNSON (1975).
[b] GOLDIN and JOHNSON (1975).
[c] Adriamycin (1975).
[d] JONES et al. (1975).
[e] TORMEY (1975).
[f] NE, not evaluated.

statistically significant at the levels listed in Table 6. In combination chemotherapy the same doses as in single-agent therapy could be given for the combinations ADR + 5-FU and ADR + prednisolone.

Only when the combination ADR + cyclophosphamide was used a reduction of dose was necessary for the second treatment cycle. However, an increase in toxicity was seen. Table 7 lists the results of three combinations that showed no synergistic effect. The combinations ADR + vincristine and, in further experiments, ADR + methotrexate and ADR + BCNU were no more effective than ADR alone.

A comparison of results obtained with combination chemotherapy in human mammary cancer, in the DMBA-induced tumour system, and in mouse leukaemia L 1210 is given in Table 8. In human mammary cancer, a higher remission rate was evident for the combinations ADR + CY and ADR + 5-FU. No synergistic or additive effect was demonstrable for ADR + methotrexate and ADR + vincristine (JONES et al., 1975; TORMEY, 1975). The combinations ADR + BCNU and ADR + prednisolone have not been tested clinically. Four combinations were evaluated in the three tumour systems. Leukaemia L 1210 predicted correctly that only the combination ADR + CY would be synergistic. The DMBA-induced rat mammary cancer showed the same findings as in clinical practice for all four combinations. In summary, a marked correlation is evident both for single-agent chemotherapy and for combination chemotherapy between the results of treatment in human breast cancer and in DMBA-induced mammary cancer of the rat.

Effect of Endocrine Therapy

In their early experiments, HUGGINS et al. (1959) showed that DMBA-induced mammary tumours are highly sensitive to ablative and additive endocrine therapy. Later on, specific oestrogen, progesterone, prolactin, androgen, insulin, and corticoid receptors were found in DMBA-induced mammary cancer (LECLERQ and HEUSON, 1973).

Present Studies

Purpose, Methods and Results

Our studies were carried out to investigate the effects of ovariectomy (OV), the anti-oestrogen tamoxifen (TAM), and the prolactin inhibitor ergocornine (EC), alone and in combination, on chemically induced mammary cancer. We were especially interested to ascertain whether TAM or EC could replace OV, and whether a combined endocrine therapy with OV could improve the effect of OV alone. Intact rats were used in an attempt to reflect the premenopausal hormonal situation.

Treatment with TAM (tamoxifen citrate) and EC was given at a dose level of 2.0 mg/kg body weight, corresponding to 14 mg/m² (FREIREICH et al., 1966), daily until the tumour size was greater than 150% of the initial tumour size and for at least 21 days. TAM was administered as a solution in oil through a stomach tube, and EC, which is soluble in 3% ethanol, was injected s.c. The effectiveness of TAM in DMBA-induced breast cancer has been described by JORDAN and KOERNER (1976), and the efficacy of EC by CASSEL et al. (1971).

In premenopausal women with advanced oestradiol-receptor (ER)-rich breast cancer, OV is the treatment of choice. The anti-oestrogen TAM also displayed some activity, producing 36

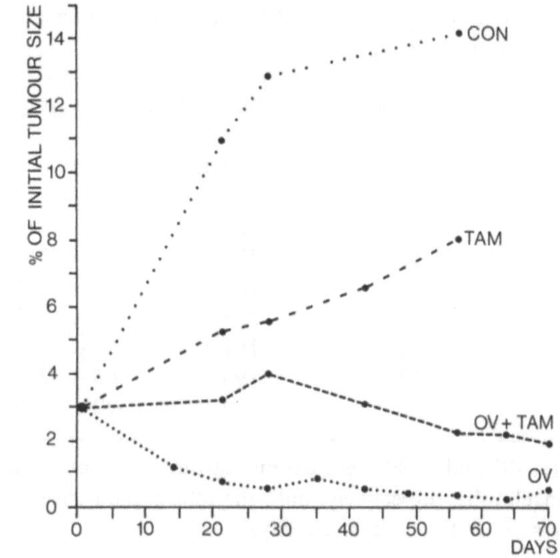

Fig. 3. Effect of OV and TAM, alone and in combination, on DMBA-induced mammary cancer of the rat. Difference in results between OV + TAM and OV alone is statistically significant ($P < 0.001$)

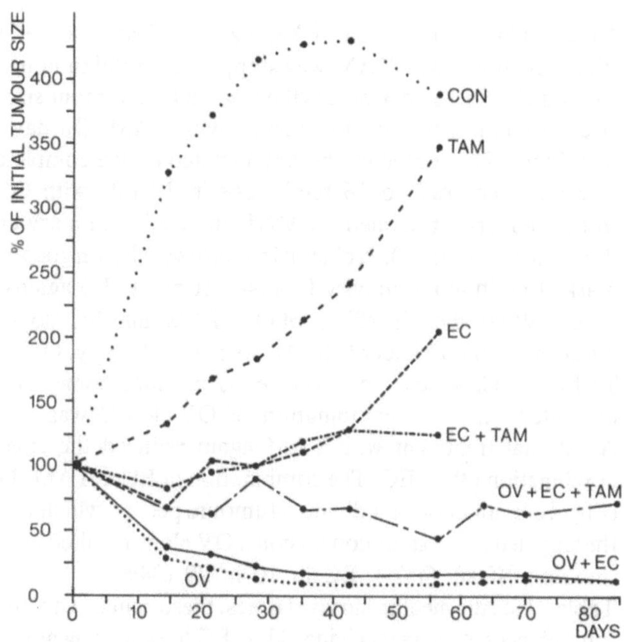

Fig. 4. Effect of OV, EC, and TAM, alone and in combination, on MNU-induced mammary cancer of the rat. Difference in results between OV alone and OV + EC + TAM is statistically significant ($P < 0.001$)

remissions in 141 patients (25%) treated at different institutes (PATTERSON, personal communication). Clinical trials comparing OV and TAM are in progress.

In DMBA-induced mammary cancer, we compared OV with TAM and combination chemotherapy with ADR + 5-FU. OV was significantly more effective than TAM and ADR + 5-FU (FIEBIG and SCHMÄHL, 1977).

In accordance with the hypothesis that the competitive blocking of oestrogens synthesised by the adrenal glands after OV could yield an additional effect, we compared OV alone with OV + TAM (Fig. 3).

Table 9. Effect of OV, TAM[a], and EC[a] alone and in combination on survival time in MNU-induced mammary cancer of the rat

Treatment	Number of rats	Survival time (days)		Increase in lifespan over controls (%)
		Median	Range	
OV	11	223	180– 310	77
OV + EC	12	220	136–> 347	75
OV + EC + TAM	11	183	76–> 394	45
EC	12	127	41– 267	1
TAM	12	181.5	82– 283	44
EC + TAM	12	195	65– 275	55
Control	12	126	22– 215	

[a] Doses for EC and TAM were 2.0 mg/kg/day, corresponding to 14 mg/m^2, administered s.c. and by stomach tube, respectively, until the total tumour size was greater than 150% of initial total tumour size, or for at least 21 days.

The combination of OV and TAM was significantly less effective than OV alone ($P < 0.001$). When treatment with TAM was stopped, the total tumour size of rats receiving TAM alone continued to increase, whereas the median total tumour size of ovariectomised rats decreased after discontinuation of the therapy with TAM. On day 70 the difference was no longer significant. The combined therapy resulted in one complete and one (?) partial remission in 17 rats, in contrast to 16 remissions in 18 rats with OV alone.

In the endocrine treatment of MNU-induced mammary cancer, only OV has been studied (Gullino et al., 1975). Prolactin inhibitors such as ergocornine (EC) and ergocryptin showed marked antitumour activity (Cassel et al., 1971) against DMBA-induced mammary tumours. We studied the effects of OV, TAM, and EC alone and in combination on MNU-induced mammary cancer (Fig. 4). As single therapy, OV was markedly more effective than TAM + EC, which did nevertheless produce some tumour inhibition in comparison to untreated rats. The combination of OV + EC was no more effective than OV alone. Additional treatment with TAM again reduced the effect of both OV alone and of the combination OV + EC. The combination of EC + TAM showed the same effect as EC alone (Fig. 4). Evaluation of individual tumours per rat, which were at least 0.6 g at the beginning of therapy, led to the same conclusions. OV alone resulted in 12 complete remissions in 30 single tumours (40%), OV + EC in 10 in 29 (34%).

Table 9 lists the median survival times, these being a valuable parameter in the MNU-induced tumour system. Rats receiving OV + EC lived as long as rats subjected to ovariectomy alone. The addition of TAM produced a decrease in the survival time. Therapy with TAM alone resulted in a markedly longer survival time than in the untreated rats, whereas rats receiving EC alone lived no longer than untreated controls. The combination TAM + EC did not increase the survival time over that obtained with TAM alone.

Conclusion

The purpose of these experiments was to study whether the effect of OV could be enhanced by simultaneous combination with TAM and/or EC in chemically induced mammary cancer of intact rats. TAM was given at the dose level of 14 mg/m^2, the same as is used in women.

The results of our studies were negative. In this experimental model OV was significantly more effective than TAM. The combination of TAM + OV significantly reduced the effect of OV alone, and suggests caution in any clinical trial of the combined therapies.

While the prolactin inhibitor ergocryptin showed no effect in mammary cancer of postmenopausal women (EORTC, 1972), EC had a marked antitumour activity in chemically induced mammary cancer of intact rats. The possible therapeutic value of prolactin inhibitors in breast cancer of premenopausal women has not yet been studied.

In the DMBA-induced tumour system, the mechanism of action of oestrogen removal produced by OV is probably via a direct effect on tumour cells. However, OV produced a simultaneous decrease in the prolactin level, which could contribute to the tumour regression (JORDAN, 1976). In our experiments, the combination OV + EC was no more effective than OV alone. Thus, further blocking of the reduced prolactin level following OV had no more pronounced antitumour effect.

Discussion

To determine whether the chemically induced mammary cancer of the rat is a suitable model for human breast cancer we have to compare the effect of established therapeutic measures in both tumour types.

Cytostatic treatment was effective in DMBA-induced mammary cancer, but to a lesser degree than in human breast cancer. However, there was a marked correlation between the remission/no change rate in total tumour size and the remission rate obtained in clinical practice (Table 3). In the DMBA-induced model no change must be considered as successful treatment, since in 146 control rats in different experiments no spontaneous remission or stationary growth behaviour of total tumour size was observed. As in the clinical situation, combination cytostatic treatment was more effective than single-agent chemotherapy (Table 6).

Four cytostatic combinations were evaluated in human breast cancer, in experimentally induced mammary cancer, and in the widely used mouse leukaemia L 1210 (Table 8). DMBA-induced mammary cancer gave a correct prediction for all four combinations, whereas L 1210 only predicted correctly that the combination ADR + cyclophosphamide would be synergistic.

The comparable relative efficacy of single-agent and combination therapy suggests that the results of cytostatic treatment of DMBA-induced mammary cancer can be extrapolated to human breast cancer. However, in evaluating cytostatic treatment, it must be kept in mind that anticancer drugs influence the endocrine situation and that they might act via a chemical castration, besides having a direct effect on tumour cells.

Furthermore, the dose of cytostatic drugs must be limited to a level where any loss of body weight can be avoided. In 1967 GROPPER and SHIMKIS demonstrated that a loss of body weight displayed in itself a marked antitumour effect in hormone-sensitive mammary cancer of the rat. This finding is probably due to a disturbance of the endocrine situation of the female rat produced by a reduced food intake (GREENSTEIN, 1954).

The endocrine therapy effected a higher remission rate in the experimental mammary cancer than in human breast cancer. In DMBA-induced mammary cancer OV resulted in remissions of 86% and 89% in two different experiments. MNU-induced mammary cancer is even more susceptible to OV, which yields a remission rate of 95%. Breast cancer in premenopausal women is less sensitive to castration, the remission rate with this procedure being about 30%. These findings can be explained by the different ER concentrations. DMBA-induced tumours are ER-rich in 90% of cases, in contrast to 60% or less of cases of human breast cancer tissue.

In the DMBA- and MNU-induced tumour models, OV was markedly more effective than TAM, which was given at the same dose level as in humans, based on body area. Clinical trials comparing OV and TAM in premenopausal women with breast cancer are in progress. EC, which was active in MNU-induced tumours, has not been investigated in premenopausal women.

The combination of OV and TAM produced an antagonistic effect, reducing the effect of OV alone. This finding can be explained by the fact that TAM has intrinsic weak oestrogenic properties, stimulating, for example, the growth of the uterus in adolescent female rats (JORDAN, 1976).

Our experimental findings suggest a cautious approach to any clinical trial combining OV with TAM in mammary cancer of premenopausal women. However, our experiments do not answer the question as to whether the duration of a remission or no change could be increased by subsequent treatment with TAM given when new signs of tumour activity become evident or when the level of oestradiol synthesised in the adrenal glands increases.

Summary

DMBA-induced mammary cancer of the rat shares a number of characteristics with human breast cancer, but there are also differences, the main one being that metastases are rarely observed. A marked similarity was demonstrable in the relative sensitivity to cytostatic and endocrine treatment. In single-agent chemotherapy six of seven drugs that are active in man were also active in DMBA-induced mammary cancer, although to a lesser extent than in man. Of a number of new compounds tested, three new anticancer agents of the nitrosourea class could be identified that displayed a higher antitumour activity than BCNU and an effect at least equal to, and probably more pronounced, than that of adriamycin (ADR). Among the new compounds the water-soluble amino acid derivative 1-[2-(chloroethyl)-1-(nitroso-3) methylenecarboxamido]-urea (CNMCU) and the sulphonic acid ester 2-[3-(2-chloroethyl)-3-nitrosoureido]ethylmethansulphonate (CNUEMS) were first synthesised in our own institute by EISENBRAND. Chlorozotocin, a sugar derivative, was also remarkably active.

In combination chemotherapy, a marked agreement with clinical results is evident. The combinations ADR + cyclophosphamide, ADR + 5-FU and ADR + prednisolone demonstrated a therapeutic synergism, whereas methotrexate, vincristine, and BCNU yielded no additional effect. In the four combinations investigated clinically, the DMBA-induced mammary cancer showed identical findings for all combinations, in contrast to the mouse leukaemia L 1210, which gave a false result for three of four combinations. The encouraging results of the combination ADR + prednisolone, which has not been tested in human mammary cancer, should stimulate a clinical trial.

In the endocrine therapy of induced mammary cancer in intact rats, OV alone remains the most effective treatment. As a single therapy, OV was significantly more effective than the prolactin inhibitor ergocornine (EC) or the anti-oestrogen tamoxifen (TAM). At the doses given the combination of OV + EC produced no added effect. Additional treatment with TAM

weakened the effect of OV alone and of the combination OV and EC. These findings suggest caution in clinical testing of OV and simultaneous therapy with TAM.
The common characteristics in biological behaviour and the comparable relative sensitivity to cytostatic and endocrine treatment make chemically induced mammary cancer of the rat an excellent experimental model for human breast cancer.

Acknowledgements

We gratefully acknowledge the technical assistance of Mrs. Maria Zimmermann, Mrs. Karin Hannen, and Miss Andrea Pohl.
Dr. P. Schurr, Upjohn Company, Kalamazoo, Michigan, USA, is thanked for the supply of DMBA.
We are indebted to Prof. Dr. K. Goerttler and Doz. Dr. D. Komitowsky for carrying out the histological examinations.

References

Adriamycin: Adria Laboratories Inc., Delaware. Current Clinical Experience (1975)

Carter, S. K.: Integration of chemotherapy into combined modality treatment of solid tumors. VII. Adenocarcinoma of the breast. Cancer Treat. Rep. *3*, 141–174 (1976)

Carter, S. K., Schabel, F. M., Jr., Broder, L. E., Johnston, T. P.: 1,3-bis(2-Chloroethyl)-1-nitrosourea (BCNU) and other nitrosoureas in cancer treatment: A review. Adv. Cancer Res. *16*, 237–237 (1972)

Cassel, E. E., Meites, J., Welsch, C. W.: Effects of ergocornine and ergocryptine on growth of 7,12-dimethylbenzanthracene-induced mammary tumors in rats. Cancer Res. *31*, 1051–1053 (1971)

Charlson, M. E., Feinstein, A. R.: The auxometric dimension. A new method for using rate of growth in prognostic stage of breast cancer. JAMA *228*, 180–185 (1974)

Dunn, O. J.: Multiple comparison using rank sums. Technometrics *6*, 241–252 (1964)

Eisenbrand, G., Fiebig, H. H., Zeller, W. J.: Some new congeners of the anticancer agent 1,3-bis (2-chloroethyl)-1-nitrosourea (BCNU). Synthesis of bifunctional analogs and water soluble derivatives and preliminary evaluation of their chemotherapeutic potential. Z. Krebsforsch. *86*, 279–286 (1976)

E.O.R.T.C. Breast Cancer Group: Clinical trial of 2-bromo-ergocryptine (CB 154) in advanced breast cancer. Eur. J. Cancer *8*, 155–156 (1972)

Fiebig, H. H., Schmähl, D.: Synergismus von Adriamycin mit 5-Fluoruracil mit Prednisolon und mit Cyclophosphamide. Klin. Wochenschr. *18*, 710–716 (1976)

Fiebig, H. H., Eisenbrand, G., Zeller, W. J., Deutsch-Wenzel, T.: Water soluble derivatives and bifunctional analogs of the anticancer agent 1,3-bis(2-chloroethyl)-1-nitrosourea (BCNU). Eur. J. Cancer *13*, 937–945 (1977)

Freireich, E. J., Gehan, E. A., Rall, D. P., Schmidt, L. H., Skipper, H. E.: Quantitative comparison of toxicity of anticancer agents in mouse, rat, hamster, dog, monkey and man. Cancer Chemother. Rep. *50*, 219–244 (1966)

Fretz, J., Rohde, W., Schmähl, D., Thomas, C.: Therapieversuche am autochthonen Mammacarcinom der Ratte. Arzneim.-Forsch. *19*, 1291–1295 (1969)

Gabriel, K. R.: Simultaneous test procedures for multiple comparisons on categorical data. JASA *61*, 1081–1096 (1966)

Goldin, A., Johnson, R. K.: Experimental tumor activity of Adriamycin (NSC-12 3127). Cancer Chemother. Rep. *6*, 137–147 (1975)

Goldin, A., Johnson, R. K.: Antitumor effects of Adriamycin in comparison with related drugs, and in combination with chemotherapy. In: Adriamycin review. Staguet, M., Tagnon, H., Kenis, Y. (eds.), pp. 37–54. Gent: European Press Medikon 1977

Goldin, A., Serpich, A. A., Mantel, N.: A comentary-experimental screening procedures and clinical predictability value. Cancer Chemother. Rep. *50,* 173–218 (1966)

Greenstein, J. P.: Biochemistry of cancer. 2nd Edit. p. 237. New York: Academic Press Inc. 1954

Griswold, D. P., Skipper, H. E., Laster, W. R., Jr., Wilcox, W. S., Schabel, F. M., Jr.: Induced mammary carcinoma in the female rat as a drug evaluation system. Cancer Res. *26,* 2169–2180 (1966)

Gropper, L., Shimkin, M. B.: Combination therapy of 3-Methylcholantrene-induced mammary carcinoma in rats: Effect of chemotherapy, ovariectomy and food restriction. Cancer Res. *27,* 26–32 (1967)

Gullino, P. M., Pettigrew, H. M., Grantham, F. H.: N-Nitrosomethylurea as mammary gland carcinogen in rats. J. Natl. Cancer Inst. *54,* 401–414 (1975)

Habs, M., Aug, J., Schmähl, D.: Chemotherapy studies in autochthonous rat tumors. Forestomach and bladder cancer. Z. Krebsforsch. *89,* 119–136 (1977a)

Habs, M., Habs, E., Schmähl, D.: Chemotherapy studies in autochthonous rat tumors. Hepatomas. Z. Krebsforsch. *90,* 167–173 (1977b)

Huggins, C., Briziavelli, G., Sutton, H.: Rapid induction of mammary carcinoma in the rat and the influence of hormones on the tumor. J. Exp. Med. *109,* 25–41 (1959)

Johnston, T. P., McCaleb, E. S., Montgomery, J. A.: Synthesis of chlorozotocin, the 2-chloroethyl analog of the anticancer antibiotic streptozotocin. J. Med. Chem. *18,* 104–106 (1975)

Jones, E. S., Durie, B. G. M., Salmon, S. E.: Combination chemotherapy with adriamycin and cyclophosphamide for advanced breast cancer. Cancer *36,* 90–97 (1975)

Jordan, V. C., Koerner, S.: Tamoxifen as an anti-tumor agent. J. Endocrinol. *68,* 305–311 (1976)

Jordan, V. C.: Antiestrogenic and antitumor properties of tamoxifen in laboratory animals. Cancer Treat. Rep. *60,* 1409–1419 (1976)

Kusama, S., Spartt, J. S., Donegan, W. L., Watson, F. R., Cunningham, C.: The gross rates of growth of mammary carcinoma. Cancer *30,* 594 (1972)

Leclerq, G., Heuson, J. C.: Specific estrogen receptor of the DMBA-induced mammary carcinoma of the rat and its estrogen-requiring molecular transformation. Eur. J. Cancer *9,* 675–685 (1973)

Livingstone, R., Carter, S. K.: Single agents in cancer chemotherapy. New York: Plenum Press 1970

Pearlman, A. W.: Breast cancer-influence of growth rate on prognosis and treatment evaluation. Cancer *38,* 1826–1833 (1976)

Philippe, E., Le Gal, Y.: Growth of 78 recurrent mammary cancers. Cancer *21,* 461–467 (1968)

Rigby-Jones, P.: Prognosis of malignant tumors of the breast in relation to rate of growth and axillary lymph nodes observed clinically. Acta UICC *18,* 815 (1962)

Schimkin, M. B., Gropper, L., Thatcher, D., Gruenstein, M.: Hormonal treatment of mammary tumors in rats induced by 3-Methylcholanthrene (NSC-21970) and 7,12-Dimethylbenz(a)anthracene (NSC-408823). Cancer Res. *27,* 1284–1288 (1967)

Schmähl, D.: Die heutige Situation in der experimentellen Chemotherapie von Tumoren. Dtsch. Med. Wochenschr. *91,* 2132–2135 (1966)

Schmähl, D.: Entstehung, Wachstum und Chemotherapie maligner Tumoren. 2. Aufl. Aulendorf: Editio Cantor 1970

Schmähl, D., Schrick, G.: Chemotherapieversuche an autochthonen Gehörgangscarcinomen bei Ratten. Arzneim.-Forsch. *14,* 72–73 (1964)

Schmähl, D., Schrick, G., König, K.: Chemotherapieversuche an Hepatomen. Arzneim.-Forsch. *13,* 370–371 (1963)

Schmähl, D., Osswald, H., Brune, H.: Chemotherapieversuche mit Endoxan an autochthonen Benzpyren-Sarkomen bei Ratten und Mäusen. Z. Krebsforsch. *68,* 293–302 (1966)

Schmähl, D., Osswald, H., Brune, H.: Einfluß von Dosis und Tumorgröße für das Ansprechen autochthoner Benzpyren-Sarkome bei Ratten und Mäusen auf chemotherapeutische Behandlung mit Endoxan. Z. Krebsforsch. *70,* 246–251 (1968)

Sych, F., Habs, M., Schmähl, D.: Chemotherapy studies in autochthonous rat tumors. Intestinal Cancer. Z. Krebsforsch. *92,* 105–117 (1978)

Teller, M. N., Stock, C. C., Stohr, P. C., Merker, P. C., Kaufman, R. J., Escher, G. C., Bowie, M.: Biologic characteristics and chemotherapy of 7,12-dimethylbenz(a)anthracene-induced tumors in rats. Cancer Res. *26,* 245–252 (1966)

Tormey, C. C.: Adriamycin (NSC-123127) in breast cancer: An overview of studies. Cancer Chemother. Rep. *6,* 319–328 (1975)

12. The Direct Inhibition of Prostaglandin Synthetase of Human Breast Cancer Tumour Tissue by Tamoxifen[1]

G. A. F. Ritchie

Imperial Chemical Industries Ltd., Biochemistry Department, Mereside Alderley Park, Macclesfield, Cheshire SK10 4TG (U.K.)

Introduction

Patients with breast cancer in the early clinical stages often complain of bone pain although they may not have radiologically apparent bone metastases and indeed clinical tests may reveal evidence of hypercalcaemia. There is a high incidence of bone metastases in advanced breast cancer and a well-correlated increase in the incidence of hypercalcuria and hypercalcaemia. It is also known that bone pain can increase dramatically whenever hypercalcaemia develops. We have been impressed by the clinical effects of tamoxifen, which in addition to its anti-oestrogenic properties causing tumour regression has been observed to relieve bone pain in many other patients in the absence of measurable tumour regression and in the absence of recalcification of bone metastases.

In a study involving 127 patients with advanced breast cancer, GALASKO and BURN (1971) diagnosed some abnormality of calcium balance in 63 patients (50%), and most patients in the survey had radiologically apparent bone metastases. Of 18 patients who did develop pronounced hypercalcaemia with acute bone pain, 17 had bone metastases. In two clinical trials of tamoxifen as a palliative therapy in advanced breast cancer, significant numbers of patients experienced relief of bone pain. In the trial of BRULE (1976), 54 of 84 patients with bone pain obtained relief during 2 months of therapy with tamoxifen (20 mg b.i.d.). In the study of RIBEIRO (1977), 32 of 111 patients responded objectively to tamoxifen as the first endocrine agent (10 mg b.i.d.) and a further 12 patients with bone metastases who did not respond objectively to tamoxifen obtained complete symptomatic relief for approximately 6 months without concomitant radiotherapy. Osteolysis of bone by primary or secondary tumours, whether or not accompanied by overt hypercalcaemia, is the result of aberrant mobilisation of bone calcium triggered by local or humoral stimuli.

In most cases of hypercalcaemia associated with carcinoma it appears that levels of parathyroid hormone (PTH) and related polypeptides are not abnormal in either plasma or tumour tissue. Therefore other osteolytic substances seem to be implicated.

The prostaglandins comprise a group of potential mediators of bone pain, and there are two sources of support for this statement. First, prostaglandins of the "E" series are potent bone

1 The author wishes to thank Mr. D. GEORGE and Mr. J. HOWAT of the Withington Hospital, Manchester, for kindly helping to provide samples, and Mr. L. SKINNER of the Christie Hospital, Manchester, for the receptor measurements.

resorption stimulators in cultures of foetal bone. Second, prostaglandin E_2 is probably responsible for the hypercalcaemia seen in transplantable tumours in animals.
The prostaglandins are generally accepted to be synthesised by all mammalian cells and to act as local hormones mediating biological control mechanisms within the tissues. Although there are now nine known classes of prostaglandins, those of interest in this context are PGE_2 and $PGF_{2\alpha}$. Both these prostaglandins are derived from the essential unsaturated fatty acid, arachidonic acid, by incorporation of two moles of oxygen catalyzed by the cyclo-oxygenase enzyme, a component of the prostaglandin synthetase complex.
The enzymic product is an unstable hydroperoxy acid (PGG_2), which is converted to the equally unstable PGH_2 by loss of an oxygen atom at C_{15}. PGH_2 is then converted to one or more prostaglandins, including PGE_2 and $PGF_{2\alpha}$, by enzymes present in a membrane-bound complex.
The biological properties of these two prostaglandins are diverse and often produce opposing effects in pharmacological preparations. Furthermore, it is likely that the prostaglandins synthesised by a particular cell type are in a fixed ratio under normal physiological conditions. This ratio may be changed under pathological conditions.

In Vitro Studies

Since the prostaglandins are potential mediators it was postulated that the relief of bone pain by tamoxifen might be due to an effect on prostaglandin biosynthesis in breast tumour tissue. Preliminary investigations indicated that tamoxifen is a potent inhibitor of prostaglandin synthetase activity in ram seminal vesicles. Tamoxifen was therefore investigated as an inhibitor of this enzyme in human breast tumour tissue.
Malignant breast tumour samples were obtained from patients in clinical stages I—II and used within 2 h of surgery. The sample of breast tumour tissue (0.25—2.0 g) was chopped and mixed with a buffer solution (Tris/sucrose/EDTA; pH 7.4), rapidly homogenised (15 s) and briefly centrifuged. From this a cell-free extract containing the enzyme was obtained, which was immediately used for assay. The enzyme was preincubated in Tris-HCl buffer (pH 7.9) with or without inhibitor (acetylsalicylic acid, indomethacin, or tamoxifen) in ethanol at a 1% final concentration. The co-factors, adrenaline and substrate, arachidonic acid or ^{14}C-arachidonic acid, were added to give a final volume of 0.1 ml. After incubation for 30 min at 30° C the solutions were acidified to stop the reaction.
The prostaglandins synthesised during the incubation process were determined by one of the following three procedures:

1) *Silicic acid microcolumn chromatography.* Total synthesis of a prostaglandin-like material was measured. Oxygenated products from arachidonic acid are more polar, so arachidonic acid was separated from these products and the total conversion measured.
2) *Radio thin-layer chromatography.* The prostaglandins were extracted from the incubation mixture and chromatographed on thin-layer plastic-backed plates. These were then cut up and the areas corresponding to authentic prostaglandins E and F were counted.
3) *PGE determination by radioimmune assay.* In this procedure the cold synthesised prostaglandin E is determined after extraction with a rabbit antiserum of high specificity. The sensitivity of this assay is such that 20 pg PGE in a sample can be measured and the cross-reaction with PGF is less than 0.01%.

Results

The results of silicic acid chromatography on microcolumns are shown in Table 1. Conversion of substrate in these experiments is about 1%. Indomethacin at a high concentration completely inhibits the enzyme. Tamoxifen at high concentrations produces variable, but potent inhibition. The *cis*-isomer of tamoxifen (ICI 47,699), which has little anti-oestrogen activity, shows some inhibitory activity but it is not dose-dependent. The thin-layer radio chromatogram method yielded prostaglandins E and F in roughly equal amounts (Fig. 1).

Table 1. Inhibition of malignant breast tissue PGS activity by tamoxifen, ICI 47,699, and indomethacin (radioassay and microcolumns separation method)

	Inhibition (*M*)	Total ^{14}C-prostaglandin (cpm)	Inhibition of PGS (%)
	None	1279	–
Tamoxifen	2×10^{-3}	178	86
	1×10^{-3}	0	100
	5×10^{-4}	149	88
	1×10^{-4}	936	65
ICI 47,699	2×10^{-3}	1215	2
	1×10^{-3}	884	28
	5×10^{-4}	672	46
	1×10^{-4}	1235	0
Indomethacin	1×10^{-4}	0	100
	1×10^{-5}	0	100

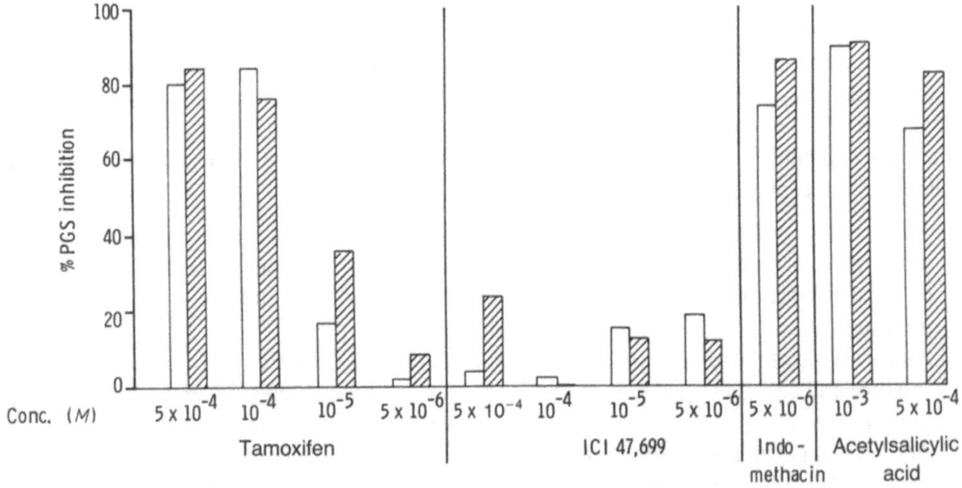

Fig. 1. Inhibition of malignant breast tissue prostaglandin synthetase (radioassay and thin-layer chromatographic separation of prostaglandins). □, PGE; ▨, PGF. Ratio, PGE : PGF = 0.82

Table 2. Receptor levels, PGE-synthesising capacity, and its inhibition by tamoxifen in malignant breast tumour

Patient	% Inhibition of PGE synthesis by		Net PGE synthesis (ng PGE/g wet tissue)	Receptor level[a]	
	Indomethacin (10^{-5} *M*)	Tamoxifen (5×10^{-5} *M*)		ER	PgR
1	44	0	125	5	15
2	100	29	138	5	818
3	99	33	661	5	1000
4	90	55	471	145	472
5	97	60	796	400	15
6	97	66	957	57	15
7	100	69	248	795	15
8	99	69	381	48	68

[a] fmol/mg cytosol protein.

Tamoxifen produced a high dose-dependent inhibition of prostaglandin synthetase activity, whereas ICI 47,699 dit not. Prostaglandin E and F were equally affected by the inhibitors. The main reason for using the radioimmune assay is because PGE is implicated as a mediator of calcium release. PGE synthesis has been measured after incubation with a cell-free extract. The results confirm that tamoxifen produces at least 50% inhibition of PGE synthesis at concentrations as low as 10^{-6} *M*.

These results with cell-free extracts have shown that malignant breast tumour tissue contains significant prostaglandin synthetase activity and produces prostaglandins of the E and F series. It has also been shown that tamoxifen directly inhibits the cyclo-oxygenase reaction of prostaglandin synthetase in a dose-dependent manner, and that the *cis*-isomer does not. Further investigations of this property have been carried out in a number of breast tumours and a comparison made of total prostaglandin synthesis and the extent of inhibition by tamoxifen. Data were also collected on oestrogen and progesterone receptors.

The actual process of homogenising a tissue releases arachidonic acid and permits a very rapid burst of synthetase activity. This activity is itself inactivated by the formation of excess intermediate endoperoxide, and this means that in cell-free extracts the prostaglandin synthetase activity underestimates the true prostaglandin-synthesising capacity of that tissue. Consequently, the following procedure was adopted to estimate prostaglandin synthetase.

Weighed samples (50 mg wet wt.) of malignant or nonmalignant breast tissue were added to acidified ethanolic Krebs' solution, which inactivates the enzyme during homogenisation; this will thus be a measure of the content of preformed (basal) prostaglandin in that tissue. A second sample was homogenised in Krebs' solution for 10 s to provide a measure of the total prostaglandin-synthesising capacity. The inhibitor was added before the samples were homogenised. After a brief incubation (15 min at 37° C), the prostaglandins were extracted and PGE was determined by radioimmune assay. In nonmalignant tissues the basal levels were not detectable by the assay method, but the synthesising capacity of nonmalignant tissue is about 7 ng PGE/g tissue (wet wt.); in malignant tissues the amount preformed in the tissue is similar to that synthesised in nonmalignant tissue (5.5 ng/g wet wt.), but the synthesising capacity is very much greater, giving a median of 310 ng PGE/g wet wt. This represents 40 fold PGE synthesis in malignant tissues compared with nonmalignant tissue. These values are similar to those reported by BENNETT et al. (1975) in a survey of breast tumour tissue in which he measured prostaglandins by bioassay.

The effectiveness of indomethacin and tamoxifen under these incubation conditions has been determined in a number of malignant tissue samples, most of which have been taken from infiltrating duct carcinomas. The data are shown in Table 2.

In eight tumour samples, indomethacin was almost completely inhibitory at 10^{-5} *M* in all cases but one; tamoxifen produced significant prostaglandin synthetase inhibition in seven of eight tumours at 5×10^{-5} *M*. The individual values for the net prostaglandin E synthesised by these samples of malignant breast tissue vary from 100 to 1000 ng/g wet wt. Not all the tumours were equally inhibited by the dose of tamoxifen used, nor did the extent of inhibition appear, to correlate with the net PGE synthesis by that tumour. The *cis*-isomer (ICI 47,699) at the same concentration as tamoxifen failed to inhibit the enzyme activity in four of six malignant tumours.

Discussion

The number of experiments is insufficient to predict any correlation of receptor levels, but there is unlikely to be a correlation with progesterone receptor levels. It will be of interest to continue to monitor oestrogen receptor levels and compare them with the effect of tamoxifen under these conditions. The dose-response curve for tamoxifen has been determined in two malignant tumours; the inhibitory concentrations giving 50% inhibition in these two tumours are in the range between 10^{-7} and 10^{-6} *M*. These results provide conclusive evidence that tamoxifen is an effective inhibitor of human breast tumour prostaglandin synthetase in vitro.

The properties of tamoxifen described here may not be attributable to its potency as an antioestrogen, since oestradiol has no direct stimulatory effect upon prostaglandin synthetase

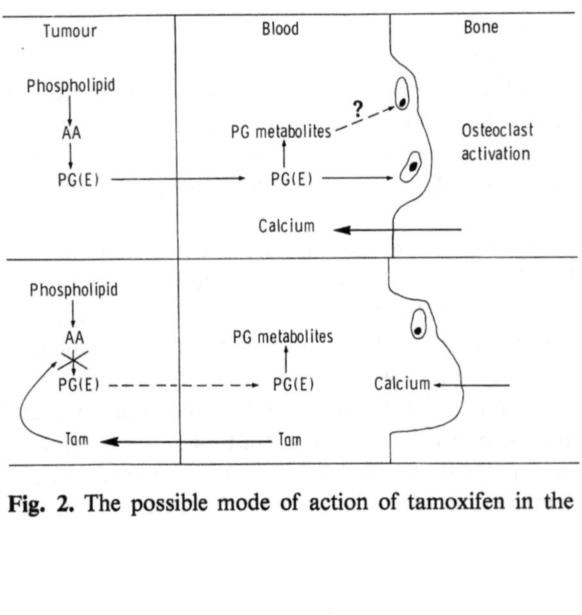

Fig. 2. The possible mode of action of tamoxifen in the relief of bone pain in breast cancer

and does not antagonise the inhibition caused by tamoxifen. It is interesting that high concentrations of stilboestrol also inhibit prostaglandin synthetase in vitro.

The role of prostaglandins as mediators of bone resorption in breast cancer is supported by the data of POWLES et al. (1976), who found a high incidence of in vitro osteolytic activity was produced by samples of human breast tumour incubated in tissue culture. All the samples from patients with bone metastases produced osteolysis, and eight of nine osteolytically active tumours showed reduced in vitro osteolysis when incubated with acetylsalicylic acid, a prostaglandin synthetase inhibitor. These results suggest that a prostaglandin-like material is produced by the tumours and may be one of the causative agents of bone resorption. If these results are substantiated, and if supportive evidence obtained from various model systems is applicable to all stages of breast cancer, then an anti-oestrogen possessing significant prostaglandin synthetase inhibitory activity may have advantages in therapy.

These results suggest an hypothesis that may account for the clinical observation of bone pain relief (Fig. 2). In tumour tissue arachidonic acid is released from phospholipids and converted to prostaglandins, which pass systemically to the bones where they may activate osteoclasts. There is evidence from model systems in support of this suggestion. When osteoclasts are activated calcium is released from the bone matrix with concomitant pain, caused by a combination of increased bone stress and made worse by the peripheral hyperalgesic action of prostaglandins at sites of inflammation.

It is suggested that tamoxifen may be preferentially taken up into tumour tissue, whereby it is able to effect inhibition of prostaglandin synthetase so reducing prostaglandin output and the resorption of bone calcium. Tamoxifen is known to be concentrated in certain tissues; the concentration in the human endometrium is three times that in serum (FROMSON and SHARP, 1974), and the concentration in hypertrophied human prostate is ten times the serum concentration (PATTERSON, unpublished data).

Such an hypothesis may be tenable for metastasised bone, since prostaglandins could reach their sites of action within their short half-lives. It is interesting to speculate whether prostaglandin output may be moderated in the primary tumour itself to influence calcium resorption either directly or indirectly.

References

Bennett, A., McDonald, A. M., Simpson, J. S., Stamford, I. F.: Breast cancer, prostaglandins, and bone metastases. Lancet *1975 I*, 1218–1220

Brule, G.: Co-operative clinical study of 178 patients treated with "Nolvadex". In: Proceedings of the Symposium 'Hormonal Control of Breast Cancer', Manchester 1976. Alderley Park: I.C.I. Ltd. Pharmaceuticals Division

Fromson, J. M., Sharp, D. S.: The selective uptake of tamoxifen by human uterine tissue. J. Obstet. Gynaecol. Br. Cwlth. *81*, 321–323 (1974)

Galasko, C. B. S., Burn, J. T.: Hypercalcaemia in patients with advanced mammary cancer. Br. Med. J. *1971 III*, 573–577

Powles, T. J., Dowsett, M., Easty, D. M., Easty, G. C., Neville, A. M.: Breast cancer osteolysis, bone metastases, and anti-osteolytic effect of aspirin. Lancet *1976 I*, 608–610

Ribeiro, G.: Advanced carcinoma of the breast treated with tamoxifen: a review of 141 patients. Proceedings of a Symposium 'Hormonal Aspects of Breast Cancer Therapy', pp. 24–31. Tel Aviv: ABIC Ltd. 1977

III. Endocrine Treatment of Advanced Breast Cancer

13. Endocrine Treatment of Advanced Breast Cancer

H. Maass and W. Jonat

Kliniken der Freien Hansestadt Bremen, Zentralkrankenhaus St. Jürgen-Straße, Frauenklinik, Abteilung II, St. Jürgen-Straße, D-2800 Bremen 1 (FRG)

The cure rates of breast cancer have not actually changed in recent decades, although many treatment procedures have been proposed. Although we can cure a lot of patients, we are confronted with the problem that the majority of them will develop metastases. Thus more patients have to be treated by systemic therapy than we can treat by surgery and radiotherapy. Probably the size of this group of patients is increasing because of adjuvant treatment modalities.

We all know that after metastases have developed the fate of the patient is decided, but prolongation of life can be achieved with systemic therapy. Thus patients with metastatic breast cancer are incurable but treatable. Endocrine treatment was the first, and for a long time the only method of treating cancer patients with metastases.

In the treatment of breast cancer there have been at least two landmarks, both at the end of the last century: the introduction of radical mastectomy by HALSTED (1890/91) in the United States and ROTTER (1899) in Germany, and the discovery by BEATSON (1896) in Scotland and SCHINZINGER (1889) in Germany that ovariectomy leads to regression of the tumour. Due to the disappointing results of prophylactic endocrine measures, e.g., ovariectomy and/or androgens and other measures, the main field of application is the advanced stage (HORSLEY and HORSLEY, 1962; KENNEDY et al., 1964; NISSEN-MEYER, 1967; TAYLOR, 1939).

When encouraging results were obtained with polychemotherapy, endocrine treatment fell into the background.

However, there is no doubt the lives of responding patients can be extended for some years, with an improved quality of life. This is one advantage of endocrine measures. Moreover, they are less expensive and easier to handle by the doctor. The disadvantage vis-à-vis polychemotherapy is the lower remission rate in unselected patients.

The overall remission rates are about 30%, ranging from 20% for androgens to 40%–45% after hypophysectomy. According to STOLL (1977), a 50% reduction in tumour size means a 99% tumour cell kill. Thus the arrest of a progressive disease can be an especially favourable response for the patient, because this arrest is often accompanied by increased well-being and relief of pain.

It is difficult to view these subjective remissions objectively. They are more frequent after ablative procedures and in the case of bone metastases. STOLL (1970) estimates the proportion of patients who experience this type of favourable treatment effect at about 50%.

Table 1. Incidence of regression after hormone ablative treatment, according to the dominant site of metastases. (FRACCIA et al., 1969; TAYLOR, 1966)

Location of metastases	Oophorectomy (premenopausal patients)		Adrenalectomy +/− oophorectomy		Hypophysectomy	
	No. of pts.	Regression (%)	No. of pts.	Regression (%)	No. of pts	Regression (%)
Soft tissue	103	35	425	35	148	30
Viscera	71	29	576	18	202	25
Bone	81	42	743	35	325	35
Total	225	35	1744	30	675	31

Table 2. Objective remission from oestrogen therapy according to site of involvement (Adapted from HEUSON, 1974)

Dominant lesion	A.M.A. (1960)	C.B.C.G. (1964)	KENNEDY (1965)	STOLL (1973)
Soft tissue	41%	32%	38%	29%
Bone	30%	12%	25%	5%
Visceral	32%	13%	26%	17%

Table 3. Influence of interval between menopause and beginning of hormone therapy (Adapted from HEUSON, 1974)

	A.M.A. (1960)	C.B.C.G. (1964)	STOLL (1973)
Interval (years)	Remissions (%)	Remissions (%)	Remissions (%)
0–4	12	7	7
5–9	38	29	23
> 9	37	20	26

The response to any kind of endocrine therapy depends on some clinical parameters. First, the site of the metastatic lesion is crucial. In general, visceral metastases show poor responses. Based on retrospective evaluations by TAYLOR (1966) and FRACCHIA et al. (1971), Table 1 illustrates the poor response of visceral metastases to ablative surgery. But the observed response rates related to the sites of the lesions vary widely in the various published series. Re-

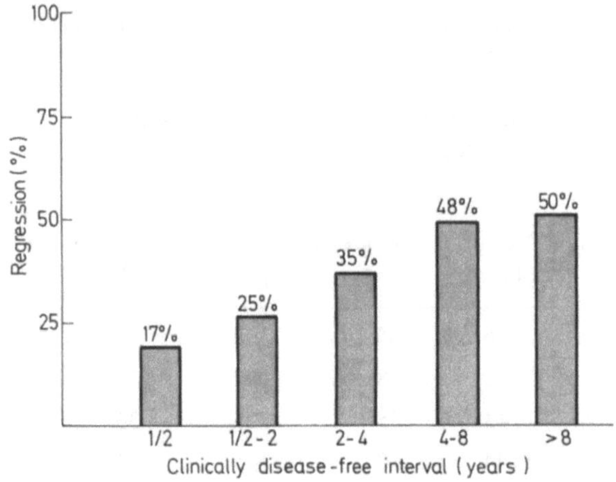

Fig. 1. Clinically disease-free interval in breast cancer, correlated with response to hypophysectomy. (Adapted from FRACCHIA et al., 1971)

cently VAN GILDER and GOLDENBERG (1975) reported remissions in 83% of patients with osseous metastases after trans-sphenoidal hypophysectomy. Similar deviations were reported in the effect of additive hormone therapy, e.g., oestrogen therapy (Table 2).

A more reliable clinical index is found in the duration of the menopause, especially for additive procedures. Table 3 shows that patients in the early menopause have little chance of responding. There is a tendency for results to improve with advancing age.

The third well-known observation is the negative correlation between a short disease-free interval after primary treatment and response to endocrine measures. As an example, Fig. 1 shows the response rate after hypophysectomy as a function of the disease-free interval. This observation was not confirmed by STOLL (1970).

Thus, there is a possibility of selecting patients with advanced cancer by clinical parameters. But the differences are not clear-cut and their predictive value is limited. Therefore the response after the first endocrine treatment was found to be the only reliable indicator as to whether the tumor was hormone-responsive or not. This led to the recommendation that patients be treated first by endocrine measures. Since polychemotherapeutic regimens have shown a higher efficacy independent of the site of lesion, the menopausal status, and the disease-free interval this is no longer thought advisable. However, the results of the various chemotherapeutic combinations are not so convincing that it is ethically justifiable to treat every patient with cytotoxic drug combinations. If we look at the data collected in controlled studies, more than half the patients have received aggressive and expensive treatments with many side effects and no beneficial effect (CARBONE et al., 1977). From the point of view of side effects and costs endocrine treatment is preferable, but it is of course not free of side effects. Major endocrine-ablative surgery is not acceptable unless there is a reasonable chance that the patient will benefit from this kind of treatment.

As more therapeutic alternatives are now available pretherapeutic prediction is more urgently needed than before.

The introduction of anti-oestrogens has been a substantial advance. Several controlled trials have shown that anti-oestrogens are at least as effective as conventional treatment procedures, and may have results comparable to those of major ablative surgery, e.g., adrenalec-

Table 4. Objective remission with tamoxifen. (MORIDSEN et al. 1978)

N	CR	PR	NC	PROG	CR + PR
1173	73	299	234	577	372/1173 = 31.7%

N, number of patients; CR, complete response; PR, partial response; NC, no change; PROG, progression.

Table 5. Clinical course after endocrine treatment of oestrogen receptor-positive vs -negative patients

	No. of patients	Objective remission	No change, partial remission, or R of another lesion	Previous remission	No effect
ER+	53	34 = 64%	5	7	7 = 13%
ER–	52	3	4	2	43 = 83%

tomy (COLE et al., 1972; HENNINGSEN and AMBERGER, 1977; TAGNON, 1977). Due to the photosensitising effect of nafoxidine, tamoxifen is now the compound of choice.

The data presented by PATTERSON (1977) are given in Table 4. The overall objective response rate is within the range for other procedures. An additional 20% of the patients showed an arrest of the disease. The observation time is still too short to permit any definitive statement, but the average duration of response seems to be quite long. Obviously tamoxifen is suitable as the first step of treatment, but it is also effective as a subsequent therapy after preceding treatments.

It is remarkable that patients who did not respond to a previous endocrine therapy have a good chance of achieving remission with tamoxifen. The number of cases in this group – 10 out of 17 – is still too low for definitive conclusions. Otherwise this observation would be of great clinical and biological importance. In any case, an attempt at treatment with tamoxifen after endocrine and chemotherapy seems to be justified. The dependence of the effects of anti-oestrogens on metastatic site, age, and disease-free interval is comparable to that seen with other endocrine measures. Soft tissue metastases show the best response. According to the data of HENNINGSEN and AMBERGER (1977), lung and pleural metastases, in particular, respond quite well, whereas in this study and that of FIRUSIAN and SCHMIDT (1977), bone lesions were poor responders. Side effects were rare and did not cause much stress on the patients.

As mentioned above, the predictive value of the clinical parameters is limited for practical use. An experienced oncologist may be able to achieve a rough selection. The choice of individualised therapy has been greatly facilitated by the introduction of receptor determinations as predictive tests by JENSEN et al. (1971). It is now a well-established fact that the presence of specific steroid hormone-binding proteins in target cells is a necessary condition for hormonal action.

However, cells lacking these receptors do not have any means of recognising the hormonal signal. This was confirmed by early clinical data indicating that patients lacking oestrogen receptors do not respond to endocrine treatment (ENGELSMAN et al., 1973; JENSEN et al., 1971;

Table 6. Objective breast tumour regression according to the site biopsied for ER assay. (McGuire et al., 1974, Leung et al., 1974; Singhakowinta et al., 1974)

Site of biopsy	ER+	ER−
Soft tissue	9/13	0/9
Visceral	14/23	2/14
Bone	2/3	1/3
Liver	5/12	0/1

Table 7. Receptor status and objective remission in advanced breast cancer

Receptor	Rate of remission			Author
	(No.)	(%)	mean, %	
ER+	> 1000	55–65	60	McGuire et al., 1974a
ER+ DHTR+	18	67–75	72	Persijn et al., 1975 Trams and Maass, 1977 McGuire et al., 1978
ER+ PR+	59	(57)–88	80	Bloom et al., 1977
ER+ CR+	53	90	90	Allegra et al., 1978

Maass et al., 1972; McGuire et al., 1974). In the meantime it has become widely known that the situation in the so-called receptor-positive group (ER^+) is less satisfactorily defined. The reason for this has often been discussed. In this paper we would like to indicate some clinical points.

The first point entering into the discussion was the discrepancy between the rate of ER^+ patients and the known remission rates after endocrine treatment without selection.

The application of more refined techniques has led to an increasing proportion of ER^+ patients. This led Leclerq and Heuson (1977) to assume that all tumours probably have receptor-containing cells and are consequently hormone-sensitive to some degree. This assumption might be supported by data shown in Table 5. In our material the percentage of ER^+ patients with general progression of their disease is only 13%. In the rest there is thus some kind of hormonal effect, but the number of complete treatment failures is much higher in the ER^- group. This means a clear distinction by clinical observation. On the basis of Heuson's hypothesis, a simultaneous combined endocrine and cytotoxic treatment was proposed for all cases. A preliminary indication as to the validity of this approach is given by the results of a trial performed by the Swiss Group for Clinical Cancer Research, in which no statistical differences between the two modalities – endocrine plus polychemotherapy and polychemotherapy alone have so far been demonstrated.

At present there is no evidence that combined endocrine and cytotoxic treatment is superior to sequential application of the two modalities. As far as we know there are no hard data providing information on what kind of sequence might yield the best survival time after manifestation of metastases.

Besides the negative results of trials with unselected patients the proposal of the Brussels Group is not convincing, as we know from the data on several hundred patients with no or only a low receptor content in their tumour tissue who are not responsive to ablative and additive endocrine treatment. In this context the problem of the too high rate of the ER^+ patients could be solved by quantification of the receptor findings. In our data there is no convincing correlation between the quantitative amount of oestrogen receptors and the response rate; we have patients with quite high numbers of ER who failed to respond, but nevertheless, the group with very low receptor contents did not respond. We therefore support the definition of JENSEN, who refers to receptor-poor or receptor-rich tumour specimens rather than ER^- and ER^+ ones.

Another possible way of achieving better response rates in receptor-rich patients is the additional consideration of clinical parameters in selection of the patients. Table 6 shows, as expected, that the response rate of patients with ER-containing visceral metastases is low, but higher than that in an unselected group of patients. Therefore the poor prognosis of patients with visceral, especially liver, metastases is not due solely to the biochemical attributes of the tumour cell.

It has been observed that non-responding ER^+ patients have a shorter disease-free interval on average (JENSEN, 1978; KNIGHT et al., 1977).

The introduction of clinical parameters must lead to higher response rates. Our data indicate that over 75% remissions can be achieved when clinical features and ER status are both used in patient selection.

In the last few years attempts had been made at better characterisation of the tumour by determination of other hormone receptors. The published data on steroid hormone receptors are summarised in Table 7. No clinical data are available on determinations of membrane-linked protein hormone receptors, especially the prolactin receptor.

Patients respond much better if more than one receptor is present in the tumour cell. The progesterone receptor is of special interest, because its synthesis and thus its presence is dependent on the whole biochemical reaction chain of oestrogen action (HORWITZ et al., 1975; HORWITZ and MCGUIRE, 1975). Further data will have to show whether the determination of the progesterone receptor alone is sufficient for characterisation of the tumour.

At present attempts are in progress in most laboratories to find more biochemical markers. In the receptor field early clinical observations indicate that the estimation of the nuclear oestrogen receptor shows better results. It is of biological interest that there are human breast tumours that have cytoplasmic but no nuclear receptors (FAZEKAS and MCFARLANE, 1978; LAING et al., 1977).

In conclusion, there is no doubt that receptor determinations together with some morphological and clinical parameters provide the best possibility that such a selected group of patients will benefit from endocrine treatment modalities. In this group, remission rates at least as high as those obtained with polychemotherapeutic regimens can be achieved, with the substantial advantages of a better quality of remission with the chance of attaining further responses and reserving polychemotherapy for later use, and of a therapy that is much easier for the doctor to handle and is less costly. These last two points are extremely important.

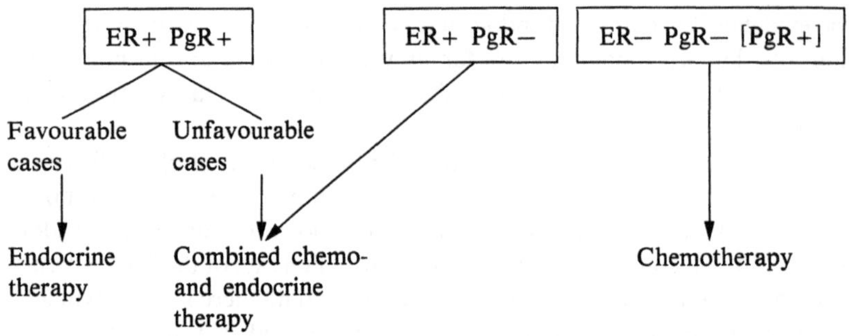

Fig. 2. Treatment of advanced breast cancer. ER, oestrogen receptor; PgR, progesterone receptor

At the present state of our knowledge we propose the following schematic procedure in the treatment of patients with metastatic breast cancer (Fig. 2). This will probably be changed if more facts about the predictive value of more receptor data or other biochemical markers become available. Patients with oestrogen and progesterone receptors in their tumour can be divided into two groups:

1) Clinically unfavourable cases. These are patients with rapidly growing, poorly differentiated tumours, who need a rapid therapy effect. Patients with extensive visceral metastases should also be treated by combined chemo- and endocrine therapy as the first step.
2) The remaining receptor-positive, clinically favourable group of patients should be treated with endocrine measures alone first, and if this is effective, also in later courses of treatment.
   Data on clinical experience with ER^+ and progesterone receptor-negative (PgR−) cases are rare. At the present state of our knowledge combined treatment procedures are therefore recommended. Patients lacking both types of receptor are candidates for cytotoxic polychemotherapy. Ablative endocrine procedures or an additive hormonal therapy with side effects are not acceptable in this group.

In our opinion this is a reasonable and practicable compromise at the moment. In this context receptor determination is a necessary step in the process of clinical decision.
This scheme (Fig. 2) refers to our clinical knowledge. The process of selecting the first endocrine measure is not essentially different from the well-known procedure recommended in the past. Unless reliable data showing that tamoxifen can be used instead of castration in premenopausal women become available, ovariectomy should be the first step.
In postmenopausal women tamoxifen can probably be given instead of oestrogens in high doses. The further treatment phases depend on whether the patients respond or not. Pre- and postmenopausal responders can be treated with tamoxifen if the latter have previously been treated with oestrogens. Major ablative procedures might be reserved for further steps.
A question that will have to be studied in the near future is the introduction of endocrine measures into adjuvant treatment procedures in primary breast cancer patients, based on receptor findings in the primary tumour.
The present state of the Bonadonna et al. (1978) trial shows that CMF treatment for 1 year after radical mastectomy has only been effective in premenopausal women. It is not yet clear

whether this effect will prolong survival or means "only" a prolongation of the disease-free interval. A similar dependence of the therapeutic effect on the menopausal status was observed in the Mayo Clinic Trial (AHMANN et al., 1978).

It is remarkable that in the group of patients who developed amenorrhoea during treatment there was a low but perceptible failure rate. The differences are not yet significant but might show a trend.

The reason for these observations is not clear. An indirect, cytotoxic castration effect may be involved, but is probably not the only causal factor.

Another finding is of importance in the discussion of adjuvant therapy schedules in breast cancer. LIPPMAN et al. (1978) showed that the response to chemotherapeutic treatment in advanced breast cancer is much better in receptor-negative than in receptor-positive patients. KING's (1978) and our own data show a similar trend (JONAT and MAASS, 1978). If this is true patients with receptors in their primary tumour are not suitable for an adjuvant cytotoxic therapy.

The data from the Milan trial and the Mayo Clinic Trial, and the possibility of selecting patients by receptor determinations, have stimulated discussion on adjuvant endocrine procedures.

In summary it can be stated that endocrine treatment retains an important role in the treatment of breast cancer patients. Better selection of patients by means of receptor determinations and the availability of effective compounds with low side effects, such as tamoxifen, lead to higher remission rates accompanied by an improvement in the quality of life for survivors.

References

Ahmann, O. L., Payne, W. S., Scanlon, P. W.: Repeated adjuvant chemotherapy with phenylalanine mustard or 5-fluorouracil, cyclophosphamide, and prednisone with or without radiation, after mastectomy for breast cancer. Lancet *1978 I,* 893–896

Allegra, J. C., Lippman, M. E., Thompson, E. B., Simon, R., Barlock, A., Green, L., Huff, K., Aitken, S., Do, M., Warren, R.: Steroid hormone receptors in human breast cancer. AACR abstract, 1978; Cancer Res. *19,* 336 (1978)

Beatson, G. T.: On the treatment of inoperable cases of carcinoma of the mamma. Suggestion for a new method of treatment with illustrative cases. Lancet *1896 II,* 104

Bloom, N., Tobin, E., Degenshein, G. A.: Clinical correlation of endocrine ablation with estrogen and progesterone receptors in advanced breast cancer. In: Progesterone receptors in normal and neoplastic tissue. McGuire, W. L., Raynaud, J. P., Baulien, E. E. (eds.), pp. 125–139. New York: Raven Press 1977

Bonadonna, G., Valagussa, P., Rossi, A., Zucali, R., Tancini, G., Bajetta, E., Brambilla, C., De Lena, M., Di Fronzo, G., Banfi, A., Rilke, F., Veronesi, U.: Are surgical adjuvant trials altering the course of breast cancer? Semin. Oncol. *5,* 450–464 (1978)

Carbone, P. P., Bauer, M., Band, P., Tormey, D.: Chemotherapy of disseminated breast cancer. Cancer *39,* 2916–2922 (1977)

Cole, M. P., Jones, C. T. A., Todd, I. D. H.: The treatment of advanced carcinoma of the breast with the antiestrogenic agent tamoxifen (ICI 46,474). A series of 96 patients. Adv. Antimicrob. Antineopl. Chem. *2,* 529 (1972)

Cooperative Breast Cancer Group: Progress report: Results of studies of the Cooperative Breast Cancer Group 1961–1963. Cancer Chemother. Rep. *41,* 1 (1964)

Council on Drugs: Androgens and estrogens in the treatment of disseminated mammary carcinoma. Retrospective study of nine hundred forty-four patients. Report to the Council. JAMA *172,* 1271 (1960)

Engelsman, E., Persijn, J. P., Korsten, C. B., Cleton, F. J.: Oestrogen receptor in human breast cancer tissue and response to endocrine therapy. Br. Med. J. *1973 II,* 750–752

Fazekas, A. G., McFarlane, J. K.: Nuclear estradiol receptors in human breast cancer tissue. AACR abstracts 1978; Cancer Res. *19,* 216 (1978)

Firusian, N., Schmidt, C. G.: Ergebnisse der Antiöstrogen-Therapie bei metastasierendem Mammakarzinom. Med. Welt *28,* 2035–2039, 2065–2067 (1977)

Fracchia, A. A., Murray, D. R., Farrow, J. H., Balachandra, V. K.: Comparison of prophylactic and therapeutic castration in breast carcinoma. Surg. Gynecol. Obstet. *128,* 270–276 (1969)

Fracchia, A. A., Farrow, J. H., Miller, T. R., Tollefsen, R. H., Greenberg, E. J., Knapper, W. H.: Hypophysectomy as compared with adrenalectomy in the treatment of advanced carcinoma of the breast. Surg. Gynecol. Obstet. *133,* 241–246 (1971)

Halsted, W. S.: Johns Hopkins Hosp. Rep. *2,* 255 (1890–1891)

Henningsen, B., Amberger, H.: Antiöstrogene Therapie des metastasierenden Mammakarzinoms. Dtsch. Med. Wochenschr. *102,* 713–716 (1977)

Heuson, J. C.: Hormones by administration. In: The treatment of breast cancer. Atkins, H. (ed.), pp. 113–163. St. Leonardgate: MTP Medical and Technical Publ. 1974

Horsley, J. S., III, Horsley, G. W.: Twenty years' experience with prophylactic bilateral oophorectomy in the treatment of carcinoma of the breast. Am. Surg. *155,* 935 (1962)

Horwitz, K. B., McGuire, W. L.: Specific progesterone receptors in human breast cancer. Steroids *25,* 497 (1975)

Horwitz, K. B., McGuire, W. L., Pearson, O. H., Segaloff, A.: Predicting response to endocrine therapy in human breast cancer: an hypothesis. Science *189,* 726 (1975)

Jensen, E. V.: Presented at the First Innsbruck Winter Conference on Biochemistry in Clinical Medicine. Jan. 1978, Innsbruck, Austria (in press)

Jensen, E. V., Block, G. E., Smith, S., Kyser, K., DeSombre, E. R.: Estrogen receptors and breast cancer response to adrenalectomy. Natl. Cancer Inst. Monogr. *34,* 55–70 (1971)

Jonat, W., Maass, H.: Some comments on the necessity of receptor determination in human breast cancer. Cancer Res. *38,* 4305–4306 (1978)

Kennedy, B. J.: Diethylstilboestrol versus testosterone propionate therapy in advanced breast cancer. Surg. Gynecol. Obstet. *120,* 1246 (1965)

Kennedy, B. J., Mielke, P. W., Fortuny, I. E.: Theapeutic castration versus prophylactic castration in breast cancer. Surg. Gynecol. Obstet. *118,* 524–540 (1964)

King, R.: Presented at the First Innsbruck Winter Conference on Biochemistry in Clinical Medicine. Jan. 1978, Innsbruck, Austria (in press)

Knight, III, W. A., Livingston, R. B., Gregory, E. J., McGuire, W. L.: Estrogen receptor as an independent prognostic factor for early recurrence in breast cancer. Cancer Res. *37,* 4669–4671 (1977)

Laing, L., Smith, M. G., Calman, K. C., Smith, D. L., Leake, R. E.: Nuclear estrogen receptors and treatment of breast cancer. Lancet *1977 II,* 168–169

Leclerq, G., Heuson, J. C.: Therapeutic significance of sex-steroid hormone receptors in the treatment of breast cancer. Eur. J. Cancer *13,* 1205–1215 (1977)

Leung, B. S., Fletcher, W. S., Lindell, T. D., Wood, D. L., Krippaehne, W. W.: Predictability of response to endocrine ablation in advanced breast carcinoma. Arch. Surg. *106,* 515–519 (1973)

Leung, B. S., Moseley, H. S., Davenport, C. E., Krippaehne, W. W., Fletcher, W. S.: Estrogen receptor in prediction of clinical responses to endocrine ablation. In: Estrogen receptors in human breast cancer. McGuire, W. L., Carbone, P. P., Vollmer, E. P. (eds.), pp. 93–105. New York: Raven Press 1974

Lippman, M. E., Allegra, J. C., Thompson, E. B., Simon, R., Barlock, A., Green, R. N. L., Huff, K. K., Do, H. M. T., Aitken, S. C., Warren, R.: The relation between estrogen receptors and response rate to cytotoxic chemotherapy in metastatic breast cancer. N. Engl. J. Med. *298,* 1223–1228 (1978)

Maass, H., Engel, B., Hohmeister, H., Lehmann, F., Trams, G.: Estrogen receptors in human breast cancer tissue. Am. J. Obstet. Gynecol. *113,* 377–382 (1972)

McGuire, W. L., Carbone, P. P., Vollmer, E. P. (eds.): Estrogen receptors in human breast cancer. New York: Raven Press 1974a

McGuire, W. L., Pearson, O. H., Segaloff, A.: Predicting hormone responsiveness in human breast cancer. In: Estrogen receptors in human breast cancer. McGuire, W. L., Carbone, P. P., Vollmer, E. P. (eds.), pp. 17–30. New York: Raven Press 1974

McGuire, W. L., Horwitz, K. B., Zava, D. T., Garola, R. E., Chamness, G. C.: Progress in endocrinology and metabolism. Hormones in breast cancer: Update 1978. Metabolism *27,* 487–501 (1978)

Mouridsen, H. T., Palshof, T., Patterson, J., Battersby, L.: Tamoxifen in advanced breast cancer. Cancer Treat. Rev. *5,* 131–141 (1978)

Nissen-Meyer, R.: The role of prophylactic castration in the therapy of human mammary cancer. Eur. J. Cancer *3,* 395–403 (1967)

Persijn, J. P., Korsten, C. B., Engelsman, E.: Oestrogen and androgen receptors in breast cancer and response to endocrine therapy. Br. Med. J. *1975 IV,* 503

Ravdin, R. G., Lewison, E. F., Slack, N. H., Gardner, B., State, D., Fisher, B.: Results of a clinical trial concerning the worth of prophylactic oophorectomy for breast carcinoma. Surg. Gynecol. Obstet. *129,* 1055–1064 (1970)

Rotter, J.: Zur Topographie des Mammacarcinoms. Arch. Klin. Chir. *58,* 346 (1899)

Schinzinger, A.: Über carcinoma mammae. Zentralbl. Chir. *16* (Suppl. 29), 55–56 (1889)

Singhakowinta, A., Mohindra, R., Brooks, S. C., Vaitkevivins, V. K., Brennan, M. J.: Clinical correlation of endocrine therapy and estrogen receptor. In: Estrogen receptors in human breast cancer. McGuire, W. L., Carbone, P. P., Vollmer, E. P. (eds.), pp. 131–155. New York: Raven Press 1974

Stoll, B. A. (ed.): Hormonal management in breast cancer. London: Pitman Medical Publ. 1970

Stoll, B. A.: Hypothesis: breast cancer regression under oestrogen therapy. Br. Med. J. *1973 III,* 446

Stoll, B. A.: "False Positive" oestrogen receptor assay in breast cancer. Lancet *1977 II,* 296–297

Tagnon, H. J.: Antioestrogens in treatment of breast cancer. Cancer *39,* 2959–2964 (1977)

Taylor, G. W.: Ovarian sterilisation for breast cancer. Surg. Gynecol. Obstet. *68,* 452 (1939)

Taylor, S. G.: Assessment of response to treatment by retrospective enquiry. In: Clinical evaluation in breast cancer. Hayward, J. L., Bulbrook, R. D. (eds.), pp. 205–214. London, New York: Academic Press 1966

Trams, G., Maass, H.: Specific binding of estradiol and dihydrotestosterone in human mammary cancers. Cancer Res. *37,* 258–261 (1977)

Van Gilder, J. C., Goldenberg, I. S.: Hypophysectomy in metastatic breast cancer. Arch. Surg. *110,* 293–295 (1975)

14. Principles and Indications of Endocrine Treatment of Advanced Breast Cancer

H. T. Mouridsen and T. Palshof

Finsen Institute, RII-RV, Strandboulevarden 49, DK-2100 Copenhagen Ø (Denmark)

Introduction

The systemic treatment available for advanced breast cancer includes chemotherapy and endocrine therapy. With combination chemotherapy remission can be achieved in 50%–70% of cases (CARTER, 1976), while the response rate of endocrine ablative or additive therapy is about 30% (HAYWARD, 1970).

It is now established that response to endocrine therapy is related to the presence of oestrogen or progesterone receptors in the tumour tissue. However, even among the receptor-positive cases, 30%–50% fail to respond to endocrine therapy (McGUIRE et al., 1975, 1977). It has recently been shown by LIPPMAN et al. (1978) that the response rate with chemotherapy is significantly higher in oestrogen receptor-negative (ER^-) tumours than in receptor-positive (ER^+) tumours.

Thus, from a theoretical point of view, it seems rational to combine chemotherapy and endocrine therapy. This is a nonselective approach as regards hormone receptor status. However, the accuracy of the prediction of response to treatments obtained by receptor studies may be further increased and allow better selection of patients for specific therapy.

In this paper we will give a brief summary of the available data on efficacy of endocrine and cytotoxic treatments of premenopausal and postmenopausal patients and present the guidelines for endocrine therapy and cytotoxic chemotherapy used by the Copenhagen Breast Cancer Group.

Advanced Disease in Premenopausal Subjects

The standard initial treatment of advanced disease in premenopausal patients has for many years been ovariectomy, which induces remission in 30% of cases (HAYWARD, 1970). During recent years a number of studies have been initiated and published with the aim of examining

1) whether ovariectomy should be combined with chemotherapy,
2) whether chemotherapy should be added to ovariectomy initially or later, and
3) whether chemotherapy given in addition to ovariectomy should be single-drug or multiple-drug therapy.

BRUNNER et al. (1977) compared a sequential multiple-drug chemotherapeutic regimen (CMFVP) with ovariectomy plus the same chemotherapy. Objective remission (PR + CR) was achieved in 74% of the patients treated with the combination, as against 43% of those treated with the chemotherapy alone, and median survival in the two groups was 19.9 months and 13.2 months, respectively.

VAN DYKE and FALKSON (1971) reported a longer survival in patients treated with ovariectomy plus cyclophosphamide than in patients subjected to ovariectomy alone. These results were later confirmed by AHMANN et al. (1977), who also found ovariectomy plus initial chemotherapy with cyclophosphamide, 5-fluorouracil, and prednisone to be superior to ovariectomy with later chemotherapy in case of progressive disease.

Multiple-drug chemotherapy has proved to be significantly more active than single-drug chemotherapy in postmenopausal women with advanced disease (CANELLOS et al., 1974; LEMKIN and DOLLINGER, 1973; MOURIDSEN, 1977; RUBENS, 1975). In keeping with this, ovariectomy plus single-drug chemotherapy with cyclophosphamide has proved to be significantly less active than ovariectomy plus multiple-drug chemotherapy with CMFCP, as regards both response rate and duration of response (MOURIDSEN et al., in preparation).

These studies suggest that the treatment of premenopausal women, regardless of their hormone receptor status, should take the form of combined endocrine and cytotoxic therapy (Table 1).

However, according to present knowledge, future trials should take into account the hormone receptor status of the tumour. Thus a response rate of about 60% has been reported to endocrine therapy of advanced disease in patients with ER^+ tumours, compared with only about 10% in ER^- tumours.

For ER^+ tumours, ovariectomy should still be the initial standard treatment, and the possible additional effect of combination with tamoxifen and chemotherapy should be examined further (Table 1).

The overall response rate with tamoxifen in premenopausal subjects seems to be comparable to that obtained with ovariectomy (MOURIDSEN et al., 1978). However, few data are available, and knowledge concerning the relationship between response and hormone receptor status is minimal. Future trials should compare rates and duration of responses obtained with (1) ovariectomy alone versus ovariectomy plus tamoxifen, and 2) ovariectomy versus tamoxifen.

As shown by LIPPMAN et al. (1978), chemotherapy induces a response in only some 10% of ER^+ tumours. However, even with these results in mind it is reasonable to evaluate the effect of endocrine therapy combined with chemotherapy in premenopausal patients with hormone receptor-positive tumours.

Table 1. Treatment strategy in premenopausal subjects with advanced breast cancer, based upon ER status

ER status	Treatment
Unknown	Ovariectomy + combination chemotherapy
Positive	Ovariectomy (+ tamoxifen? + chemotherapy?)
Negative	Combination chemotherapy

As regards the receptor-negative tumours, the initial treatment of choice should be combination chemotherapy, whereas endocrine treatment should be reserved for cases that are resistant to this treatment.

Advanced Disease in Postmenopausal Subjects

Endocrine Therapy

Since the 1940s, endocrine treatment of advanced breast cancer in postmenopausal patients has been carried out mainly with oestrogens, gestagens, and androgens. During the last 5 years anti-oestrogens have been substituted for these additive treatments to an increasing extent.

Oestrogens are the hormones that have been administered most widely, and they induce response in up to 30% of the patients treated (Cooperative Breast Cancer Group, 1964; Council on Drugs, 1960; HAYWARD, 1970).

The response rate with different androgens is no higher than 10%–20% (Cooperative Breast Cancer Group, 1964; Council on Drugs, 1960; KENNEDY and YARBRO, 1968). The same response rate has been reported with gestagens (ANSFIELD et al., 1974; GOLDENBERG, 1969; MUGGIA et al., 1968; SEGALOFF et al., 1967; STOLL, 1967), but in studies performed in recent years response rates of up to 40% have been obtained with very high doses (PANUTTI et al., 1976).

Trials with anti-oestrogens were conducted as long ago as the 1960s. In these studies the anti-oestrogens used, clomiphene and nafoxidine, induced response in nearly 30% of patients (LEGHA and CARTER, 1976). During the last few years similar results have been obtained with tamoxifen, and due to its modest toxicity this is the anti-oestrogenic compound most widely used today (MOURIDSEN et al., 1978).

Thus it appears that oestrogen and anti-oestrogen are the most effective of the endocrine treatment alternatives for postmenopausal women. Furthermore, it is now established that the effect of both treatments is related to the presence of oestrogen receptors in the tumour tissue. Thus 50%–70% of ER^+ tumours will respond to treatment with oestrogen or anti-oestrogen, as against less than 10% of ER^- tumours (MCGUIRE, 1975). The response rate with both oestrogen and tamoxifen is highest in patients with soft-tissue disease, and increases with age (Cooperative Breast Cancer Group, 1964; Council on Drugs, 1960; MOURIDSEN et al., 1978). This is to be expected, as the proportion of ER^+ tumours and the level of ER content increases with age (DAEHNFELDT et al., 1978).

Both therapeutic effect and side effects should be considered in the selection of therapy. Due to the apparently lower frequency and milder degree of side effects with tamoxifen (MOURIDSEN et al., 1978) than with oestrogen (CARTER et al., 1977), we prefer tamoxifen.

Cytotoxic Chemotherapy

During the last 5–10 years, single-drug cytotoxic chemotherapy of advanced breast cancer has increasingly been superseded by different multiple-drug combinations. These have proved superior to single-drug treatment (CANELLOS et al., 1974; LEMKIN and DOLLINGER, 1973, MOURIDSEN et al., 1977; RUBENS et al., 1975), inducing response in 40%–70% of cases, (BRODER and TORMEY, 1974; CARTER, 1976). As with endocrine therapy, soft-tissue disease seems to respond better than disease localised to bone and viscera. Few data are available concerning the response-age relationship (BRODER and TORMEY, 1974). The response rate with cyclophosphamide and 5-fluorouracil, seems to decrease with increasing time after the menopause. However, when more than 10 years have passed since the menopause, the rate of response for cyclophosphamide seems to increase again, and the same is the case with adriamycin. The relationship between response to combination chemotherapy and age has not been adequately explained.

Endocrine Therapy or Cytotoxic Chemotherapy

As appears from the two previous sections, we have endocrine and cytotoxic chemotherapy at our disposal for the treatment of postmenopausal subjects with advanced disease. The question arises as to which of these treatments should be preferred. In this respect both the efficacy and the side effects of the specific treatments should be considered.

In general, response rates with endocrine treatment increase with age (Cooperative Breast Cancer Group, 1964; Council on Drugs, 1960; MOURIDSEN et al., 1978), but data concerning the same relationship with combination chemotherapy are not available. However, side effects limit the general application of combination chemotherapy to elderly postmenopausal women. Therefore, in unselected groups of patients, we prefer chemotherapy as the first treatment for patients under 60–70 years of age, and endocrine therapy for elderly patients (Table 2). However, as in the case of premenopausal patients, we believe that future trials should take into account the hormone receptor status of the tumour.

According to the model shown in Table 2, we consider endocrine therapy with tamoxifen to be the therapy of choice in advanced ER^+ tumours. The possible additive effect of combination with other endocrine therapy or with chemotherapy should be further studied in that group of patients. In receptor-negative tumours the first treatment should be chemotherapy.

Table 2. Treatment strategy in postmenopausal subjects with advanced disease, based upon ER status

ER status	Age (years)	First treatment[a]	→PD[b]→	Second treatment[a]
Unknown	< 60–70	C	→	E
	> 60–70	E	Responders →	E
			Nonresponders →	C
Positive		E	Responders →	E
			Nonresponders →	C
Negative		C	→	C

[a] C, chemotherapy (alone or in combination with endocrine therapy); E, endocrine therapy (single-drug or multiple-drug or in combination with chemotherapy).

[b] PD, progressive disease.

Most patients who receive systemic treatment for advanced disease will develop renewed progressive disease. In all age groups, when resistance to chemotherapy is encountered treatment with tamoxifen is indicated. This is supported by the observation that previous chemotherapy does not seem to interfere with the response to subsequent treatment with tamoxifen (Mouridsen et al., 1978).

The choice of treatment for patients resistant to previous treatment with tamoxifen should be guided by the previous response. Thus responders to tamoxifen therapy have a significantly higher chance of responding to other endocrine therapy than do nonresponders (Mouridsen et al., 1978).

Summary

The numerous trials that have been conducted in advanced breast cancer in premenopausal and postmenopausal women have increased the empiric basis for systemic cytotoxic and endocrine treatment. The treatment results have improved but are still very unsatisfactory, and with all the drugs now at our disposal many questions are still unanswered. For instance this applies to the optimal composition and scheduling of endocrine treatment, cytotoxic treatment, and combinations of these two treatments.

During recent years the results of experimental studies have expanded our knowledge of the biology of breast cancer. Future clinical trials should be designed to test and use this information gained from basic research with the aim of improving the rational basis of treatment and obtaining better treatment results in advanced breast cancer.

References

Ahmann, D. L., O'Connell, M. J., Hahn, R. C., Bisel, H. F., Lee, R. A., Edmonson, J. H.: An evaluation of early or delayed adjuvant chemotherapy in premenopausal patients with advanced breast cancer undergoing oophorectomy. N. Engl. J. Med. *297,* 356–360 (1977)

Ansfield, F. J., Davis, H. C., Ellerby, R. A., Ramireg, G.: A clinical trial of megesterol acetate in advanced breast cancer. Cancer *33,* 907–910 (1974)

Broder, L. E., Tormey, D. C.: Combination chemotherapy of carcinoma of the breast. Cancer Treat. Rev. *1,* 183–205 (1974)

Brunner, K. W., Sonntag, R. W., Alberto, P., Senn, H. J., Martz, G., Obrecht, P., Maurice, P.: Combined chemo- and hormonal therapy in advanced breast cancer. Cancer *39,* 2923–2933 (1977)

Canellos, G. P., Taylor, S. G., Band, P., Pocock, S.: Combination chemotherapy for advanced breast cancer: randomized comparison with single drug therapy. In: Proceedings of the 11th International Cancer Congress 1974, p. 596

Carter, A., Sedransk, N., Kelley, R. M., Ansfield, F. J., Raudin, R. G., Talley, R. W., Potter, N. R.: Diethylstilbestrol: Recommended dosages for different categories of breast cancer patients. A Report of the Cooperative Breast Cancer Group. JAMA *237,* 2079–2085 (1977)

Carter, S. K.: Integration of chemotherapy into combined modality treatment of solid tumors. VII. Adenocarcinoma of the breast. Cancer Treat. Rev. *3,* 141–175 (1976)

Cooperative Breast Cancer Group: Results of studies of the cooperative breast cancer group 1961–1963. Cancer Chemother. Rep. *41,* 1–24 (1964)

Council on Drugs. Subcommittee on Breast and Genital Cancer, Committee on Research, American Medical Association: Androgens and estrogens in the treatment of disseminated mammary carcinoma; retrospective study of 944 patients. JAMA *172,* 1271–1284 (1960)

Dæhnfeldt, J. D., Palshof, T., Mouridsen, H. T.: Biochemical characterization of human breast cancer tissue by the determination of steroid receptor protein and cellular proteins under possible hormonal regulation. In: Reviews in endocrine related cancer. Mayer, M., Saez, S., Stoll, B. A. (eds.), p. 76. 1978

Goldenberg, I. S.: Clinical trials of testolactone, medroxyprogesterone-acetate and oxylone acetate in advanced female mammary cancer. A report of the Cooperative Breast Cancer Group. Cancer *23*, 109–111 (1969)

Hayward, J.: Hormones and human breast cancer. Recent Results in Cancer Research, Vol. 24. Berlin, Heidelberg, New York: Springer 1970

Kennedy, B. J., Yarbro, J. W.: Effect of methenolone enenthate in advanced cancer of the breast. Cancer *21*, 197–201 (1968)

Legha, S. S., Carter, S. K.: Antiestrogens in the treatment of breast cancer. Cancer Treat. Rev. *3*, 205–217 (1976)

Lemkin, R., Dollinger, M. R.: Combination versus single drug therapy in advanced breast cancer. Proc. Am. Ass. Cancer Res. *14*, 37 (1973)

Lippman, M. E., Allegra, J. C., Thompson, E. B., Simon, R., Barlock, A., Green, L., Huff, K. K., Hoan, T. D., Aitken, S. C., Warren, R.: The relation between estrogen receptors and response rate to cytotoxic chemotherapy in metastatic breast cancer. N. Engl. J. Med. *298*, 1223–1228 (1978)

McGuire, W. L., Carbone, P. P., Vollmer, E. W. (eds.): Estrogen receptors in human breast cancer. New York: Raven 1975

McGuire, W. L., Raynaud, J.-P., Baullieu, E.-E. (eds.): Progesterone receptors in normal and neoplastic tissues. New York: Raven 1977

Mouridsen, H. T., Palshof, T., Brahm, M., Rahbek, I.: Evaluation of single-drug versus multiple-drug chemotherapy in the treatment of advanced breast cancer. Cancer Treat. Rep. *61*, 47–50 (1977)

Mouridsen, H. T., Palshof, T., Jensen, H. S., Kristensen, D., Rose, C.: Evaluation of oophorectomy plus single drug versus oophorectomy plus multiple drug chemotherapy in the treatment of advanced breast cancer in premenopausal women (in preparation)

Mouridsen, H. T., Palshof, T., Patterson, J., Battersby, L.: Tamoxifen in advanced breast cancer. Cancer Treat. Rev. *5*, 131–141 (1978)

Muggia, F. M., Cassileth, P. A., Ochoa, M., Flatow, F. A., Gellhorn, A., Hyman, G. A.: Treatment of breast cancer with medroxyprogesteroneacetate. Ann. Intern. Med. *68*, 328–337 (1968)

Panutti, F., Martoni, A., Lenaz, G. R., Piana, E., Nanni, P.: Management of advanced breast cancer with medroxyprogesteroneacetate in high doses. Funct. Explor. Sen. 253–256 (1976)

Rubens, R. D., Knight, R. K., Hayward, J. L.: Chemotherapy of advanced breast cancer: a controlled randomized trial of cyclophosphamide versus a four-drug combination. Br. J. Cancer *32*, 730–736 (1975)

Segaloff, A., Cuningham, M., Rice, B. F., Weeth, J. B.: Hormonal therapy in cancer of the breast. XIV. Effect of corticosterone or medroxyprogesterone-acetate on the clinical course and hormonal excretion. Cancer *20*, 1673–1688 (1967)

Stoll, B. A.: Progestin therapy of breast cancer: Comparison of agents. Br. Med. J. *1967 III*, 338–341

Van Dyke, J.-J., Falkson, G.: Extended survival and remission rates in metastatic breast cancer. Cancer *27*, 300–303 (1971)

15. Ablation of the Hypophysis by Radioactive Gold in Metastatic Mammary Carcinoma

W. Piotrowski

Neurochirurgische Klinik, Städtische Krankenanstalten, Theodor-Kutzer-Ufer, D-6900 Mannheim 1 (FRG)

The use of hypophysectomy as a palliative measure in metastatic mammary carcinoma is well-known. This operation has frequently proved to be outstandingly beneficial, especially in the pain due to osseous metastases. Nevertheless the operation is only rarely performed for this indication. This is not due to any reluctance on the part of the neurosurgical clinics, but to the hesitant attitudes of many colleagues, who are insufficiently informed on the benefits of this operation.

The tumour-inhibitory action of hypophysectomy was demonstrated as long ago as the nineteen-thirties in animal experiments (BALL and SAMUELS, 1932, 1938; LACASSAGNE, 1937). LINDER (1948) was able to confirm the favourable effect of oestrogen therapy in carcinoma of the female breast in local patient material. He also found that hormone-independent malignant processes were by no means always therapy-resistant. Thus hypophysectomy was suggested as a central endocrine operation also suitable for application in incurable malignant diseases. Different approaches to the sella turcica are possible:

1) Through a transfrontal or trans-sphenoidal incision,
   or (with considerably lower risk)
2) By percutaneous puncture.

In 1950, K. H. BAUER and E. KLAR (Heidelberg) introduced a devastatingly simple technique, *freehand* percutaneous puncture through the lacrimal bone with an X-ray monitor, using the paranasal, transethmoidal, and trans-sphenoidal route.

Electrocoagulation, initially considered preferable, was replaced in 1955 by the implantation of radioactive gold on the suggestion of the radiologists BECKER and SCHEER (1958). Radioactive gold was preferred to the pure β-emitter yttrium that was formerly used in many centres for this purpose, because:

1) Its predominantly γ-ray irradiation means that it has a greater radiation penetration.
2) Whilst with radioactive gold *unilateral* implantation is sufficient for extensive destruction of the hypophysis in most cases radioactive yttrium had to be deposited *at multiple sites,* which is not easily possible with a single puncture.
3) The bilateral nasal puncture necessary for the use of radioactive yttrium increases the risk of a liquor fistula and meningitis.

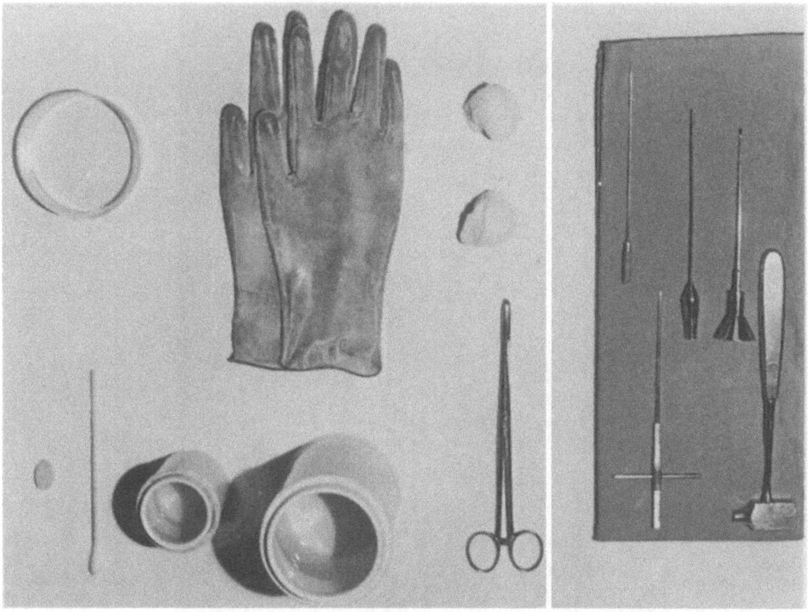

Fig. 1. Instruments needed for extirpation of the hypophysis by means of radioactive gold

The simplicity of the operation is well attested by the simplicity of the instrumentation (Fig. 1). The mean total activity of about 40 mCi per patient is divided amongst 2–4 gold seeds. A review of the fate of 558 patients with metastatic mammary carcinoma who underwent ablation of the hypophysis with radioactive gold (HENNINGSEN and PIOTROWSKI, 1976) showed that objective improvement occurred in 17.4% and subjective improvement in 38% of patients. It can therefore be maintained that about 50% of the women derived some advantage from the operation.

The following beneficial effects are to be expected, either single or combined, from ablation of the hypophysis:

1) Reossification of osteolytic metastases, recalcification of the skeletal system, and resultant healing of spontaneous fractures.
2) Elimination of rheumatoid bone pain, not infrequently soon after awakening from anaesthesia.
3) Improvement of general condition with weight gain.
4) Lifting of the basic attitude to life, with improvement of mood, and a desirable euphoria, which alleviates the distress of the last span of life.
5) Changes in some laboratory findings.

This economical operation can be performed even in the most severe cases of illness, as shown by the case of a 58-year-old woman with skull metastases. The intrasellar gold seeds are recognisable on the X-ray plates (Fig. 2a, b).

There is practically no operative mortality. The incidence of complications is low, liquor fistula and meningitis occurring in less than 5% of cases. Diabetes insipidus is not a real complication, but an indication for associated removal of the posterior lobe of the hypophysis. It soon clears up with no special therapy. There is little question of any late complications, because survival is not prolonged.

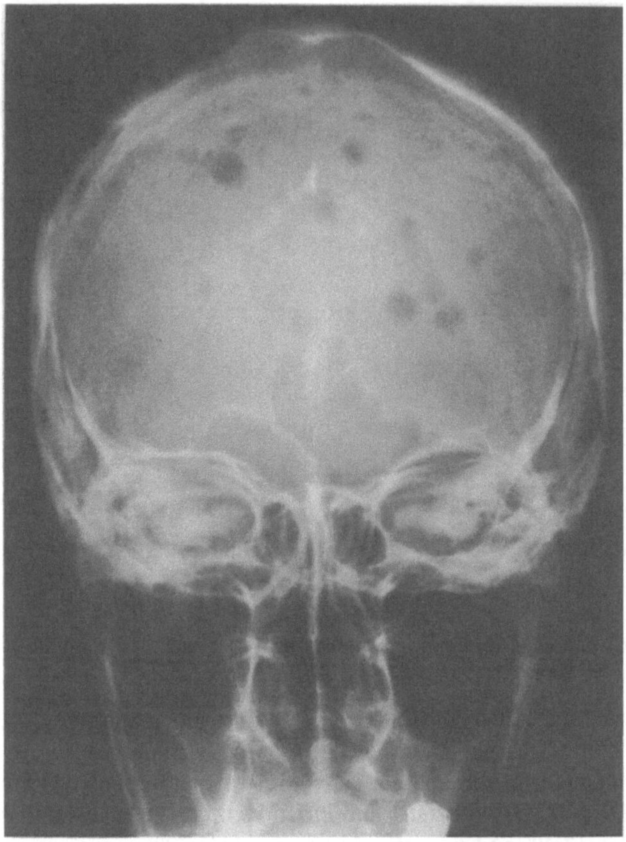

a

Fig. 2 a, b. Skull X-rays in a 58-year-old woman with metastatic mammary carcinoma. Condition after implantation of radioactive gold in the hypophysis. **a** Anteroposterior view

The abrupt relief of pain experienced postoperatively in 5 of the 18 cases who underwent implantation of radioactive gold in Mannheim remains a puzzle. We imagine that it is related to the decrease in oestrogen and to irritation of the neurohypophysis and of the hypothalamus, in particular of the nucleus supraopticus, but this remains hypothetical. TINDALL (1977) thinks that endogenous brain peptides with an action analogous to that of morphine are present in increased amounts after hypophysectomy.

Radioactive extirpation of the hypophysis is indicated in those patients with mammary carcinoma in whom all surgical, radiological, and drug treatments are exhausted, and in whom the disease has become incurable.

The prognosis for successful treatment improves with advancing age of the patients, with increasing duration of the disease-free interval between the primary operation and the detection of metastases, when there are only a few bone –, and no soft-tissue metastases, and when histological examination reveals that the carcinoma is highly differentiated.

Hypophysectomy is therefore not a sensible procedure in all cases. The words of K. H. BAUER (1953) have direct relevance and special significance in this terrible disease:

'Often more knowledge and greater responsibility is needed for the surgeon not to operate than to operate.'

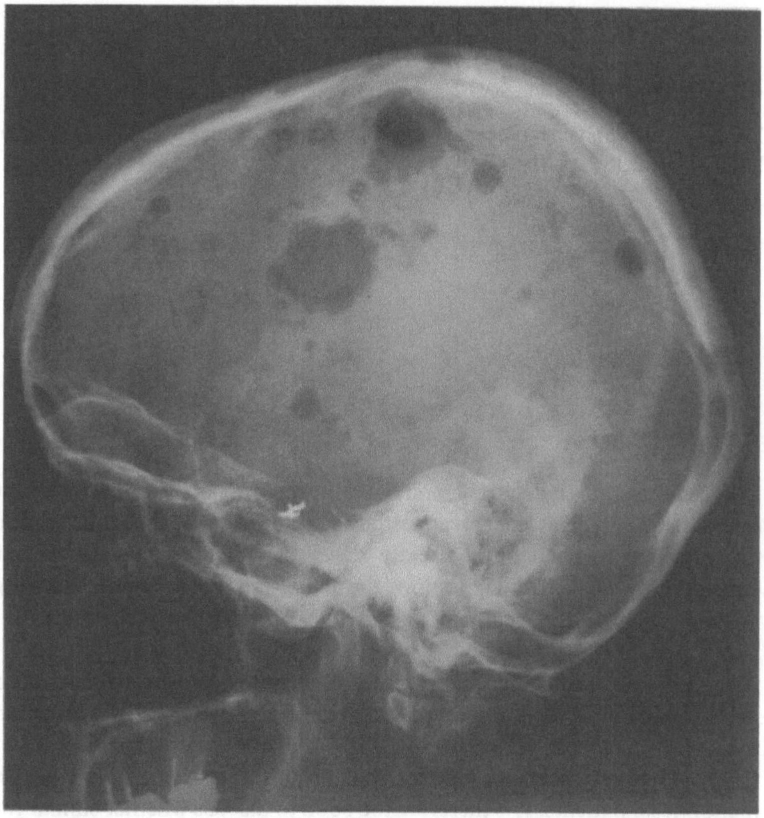

Fig. 2 b.
Lateral view

References

Ball, H. A., Samuels, L. T.: Relation of hypophysis to growth of malignant tumors; effect of hypophysectomy on transplanted mammary carcinoma. Am. J. Cancer *16,* 351–359 (1932)

Ball, H. A., Samuels, L. T.: Relation of hypophysis to growth of malignant tumors; study of influence of nutritional factors on Walker tumor 256 in relation to effect of hypophysectomy. Am. J. Cancer *32,* 50–56 (1938)

Becker, J., Scheer, K. E.: Die radiologische Hypophysenausschaltung bei fortgeschrittenem Krebs. Radiol. Austr. *10,* 119–123 (1958)

Bauer, K. H.: Zur Chirurgie der Hypophyse und der Nebennieren. Langenbecks Arch. Chir. *274,* 606–632 (1953)

Henningsen, B., Piotrowski, W.: Indikationen und Nebenwirkungen der Hypophysenausschaltung zur Therapie des metastasierenden Mammakarzinoms. In: Prophylaxe und Therapie von Behandlungsfolgen bei Karzinomen der Frau. Schmähl, D. (Hrsg.), S. 85–89. Stuttgart: Thieme 1976

Klar, E.: Über neurologische Erfahrungen bei perkutaner Hypophysenausschaltung in über 100 Fällen. Zentralbl. Gesamte Neurol. Psychiatr. *140,* 16–17 (1957)

Lacassagne, A.: Relation between hormones and cancer. Can. Med. Assoc. J. *37,* 112–117 (1937)

Linder, F.: Über die hormonale Behandlung des inoperablen Mammakrebses. Chirurg *19,* 500–506 (1948)

Piotrowski, W.: Historische Entwicklung der Hypophysenchirurgie mit besonderer Berücksichtigung der Heidelberger Technik. Langenbecks Arch. Chir. *331,* 38–47 (1972)

Tindall, G. T.: Totale Hypophysektomie bringt Schmerzfreiheit. (Kongreßbericht) Med. Trib. *12* (36), 33 (1977)

16. *Anti-Oestrogens: An Alternative to Ablative Endocrine Therapy?*

B. Henningsen

Klinikum der Universität Heidelberg, Chirurgische Klinik, Kirschner Straße 1,
D-6900 Heidelberg 1 (FRG)

Ovariectomy, adrenalectomy, and hypophysectomy are surgical interventions, constituting a stress to the patient at least by anaesthesia. This stress must be taken seriously, since normally the patients involved have already developed distant metastases and are consequently considerably weakened. Up to now, the above-mentioned methods have generally been used nonselectively in the treatment of advanced breast cancer, resulting in remission rates of about 30%.

After several years' clinical experience of the anti-oestrogenic agent tamoxifen, it has become necessary to evaluate the therapeutic field of ablative therapy against anti-oestrogen therapy.

Our own experience, like that of most trialists, has been almost exclusively with postmenopausal patients. It is therefore too soon to discuss whether similar remission rates would continue to be achieved if ovariectomy were superseded in its traditional therapeutic function by anti-oestrogen therapy, e.g., tamoxifen.

The situation is rather different when ovariectomy is performed as an adjuvant therapeutic measure. This radical intervention has generally been rejected up to now, since without suitable tests to assess the hormone dependency of the tumour tissue it was a nonselective approach and the number of patients benefiting from it was too small.

The advent of hormone receptor assays and the development of anti-oestrogens led to the resumption of these investigations. Accordingly, the groups of Mouridsen in Copenhagen and Meakin in Toronto are conducting prospective randomised trials to examine adjuvant tamoxifen therapy in premenopausal patients.

Adrenalectomy and hypophysectomy are available as methods of ablative therapy for patients currently undergoing a natural or a chemical menopause. Implantation of radioisotopes (^{198}Au: Bauer, 1956; or ^{90}Y: Forrest, 1956) is probably the least stressful method of pituitary ablation.

Like surgical ablation of the hypophysis, the implantation of radioisotopes must be performed in a neurosurgical centre because of the potential risk of such complications as liquor fistula and meningitis. Visual disturbances are a particularly dreaded complication and cannot be completely avoided after this procedure (the incidence was 1.5% in the Heidelberg study on more than 500 patients).

In the light of the advances achieved in combination chemotherapy, especially since the introduction of anti-oestrogen therapy with tamoxifen, we have restricted the use of hypophysectomy considerably, performing it specifically in patients who have multiple bone metastases causing severe pain. In these circumstances the therapy is not only promising in cases that subsequently show objective tumour remission, but also it often results in subjective improvement due to pain relief even in cases of objective treatment failure.

In our evaluation of the therapeutic field of ablative hormonal therapy of advanced breast cancer we have to ask whether there is still a place for adrenalectomy in the treatment of breast cancer patients.

Since the introduction of bilateral adrenalectomy for the treatment of advanced breast cancer by HUGGINS and DAO (1952), numerous authors have reported remission rates of around 30% with this procedure. However, the quality of the remission is affected by the operative mortality, which cannot be completely eliminated, and also by the continued corticoid substitution required after surgery.

Portalisation of part of the left adrenal gland, an operation method which was perfected by DARGENT and MAYER (1966), did not prove to be a satisfactory solution to the problem of corticoid substitution.

So-called chemical adrenalectomy with aminoglutethimide (SANTEN et al., 1977) is achieved without surgery and thus avoids any operative mortality, but it also requires corticoid substitution.

Many patients have benefited from HUGGINS' splendid idea of eliminating the site of production of the so-called residual oestrogens.

The development of anti-oestrogens, however, has opened up a more elegant approach that is less stressful for the patient. Of course treatment with tamoxifen does not inhibit adrenal oestrogen production, but due to its competitive activity at the oestrogen receptor the effects of the adrenal oestrogens on tumour growth are considerably inhibited.

In patients who might formerly have been selected for adrenalectomy on the basis of their stage of disease, objective tumour remission rates of about 30% were achieved without prior selection by hormonal receptor assays. In our own patients we observed 14 objective tumour remissions in a total of 44 postmenopausal patients.

Tamoxifen and adrenalectomy are similarly effective, but with tamoxifen there is no operative mortality or morbidity and no need for continued corticoid substitution.

Due to the low incidence of side effects following tamoxifen, the quality of remission is superior to that obtained with adrenalectomy. This is why we no longer perform adrenalectomies.

While our statement on the basis of our own experience can only refer to the traditional therapeutic indications, the possibilities of adjuvant adrenalectomy should also be mentioned: these were presented by DAO (1978).

DAO reported a probability of survival for patients having undergone adjuvant adrenalectomy that was strikingly higher than that for historical controls in the same stage of tumour progression but not subjected to adrenalectomy. Admittedly DAO's report concerned only 17 patients. The small number of patients and the use of a historical control group may invite severe criticism. Nevertheless, particularly in view of the disappointing results achieved with adjuvant chemotherapy in postmenopausal patients, more attention should be given to adjuvant hormonal therapy.

It follows logically that positive results might be expected from prospective randomised studies on adjuvant endocrine therapy with tamoxifen in postmenopausal patients.

References

Bauer, K. H.: Über die Hypophysenausschaltung bei inkurablen Krebsfällen mit Hilfe perkutaner, intrasellärer Implantation von radioaktivem Gold. Langenbecks Arch. Chir. *284,* 438–446 (1956)

Dao, T. L.: Endocrine surgery as adjuvant therapy in breast cancer. In: Reviews on endocrine-related cancer. Mayer, M., Saez, S., Stoll, B. A. (eds.) pp. 174–182, 1978

Dargent, M., Mayer, M.: Major endocrine surgery for the treatment of carcinoma of the breast in advanced stages. Lyon: Simep Ed. 1966

Forrest, A. P. M., Peebles Brown, D. A.: Pituitary implant for breast cancer. Lancet *1955 I,* 1054

Huggins, C., Dao, T. L. Y.: Adrenalectomy for mammary cancer; surgical technique for bilateral one stage-adrenalectomy in man. Ann. Surg. *136,* 595 (1952)

Santen, R. J., Samojlik, E., Lipton, A., Harvey, H., Ruby, E. B., Wells, S. A., Kendall, J.: Kinetic, hormonal and clinical studies with aminoglutethimide in breast cancer. Cancer *39,* 2948–2958 (1977)

IV. Anti-Oestrogens in the Treatment of Advanced Breast Cancer

17. Tamoxifen in Advanced Breast Cancer: Experience of the SAKK (Schweizerische Arbeitsgruppe für Klinische Krebsforschung – Swiss Cooperative Oncology Group)[1]

W. P. Jungi, P. Alberto, and F. Cavalli

Kantonspital, Medizinische Klinik C, Abteilung für Onkologie und Hämatologie, CH-9007 St. Gallen (Switzerland)

The Swiss Cooperative Oncology Group has had very wide experience of treating patients with advanced breast cancer, both with endocrine and with cytotoxic therapy. The Swiss Group therefore gratefully accepted the opportunity of testing tamoxifen, as a new and promising, nonsteroid hormone-like substance, in a group of patients with metastatic breast cancer, most of whom had already received some anticancer treatment.

SAKK Protocol 2T/75

This unrandomised, multi-centre phase II-trial was started in 1975 and terminated early in 1977. The characteristics of the patients treated are given in Table 1. Of 91 patients who entered the trial, 82 were evaluable. None of these patients was still menstruating when tamoxifen treatment was started: 36 of the evaluable patients had been premenopausal at the time of first diagnosis of breast cancer, and 46 postmenopausal.
The most frequent sites of metastases were bone and skin. It has to be remembered that many of our patients had more than one metastatic site. All patients had measurable or at least evaluable tumour parameters.

---

1 Participating member institutions of SAKK were:
Onkologische Abteilung, Medizinische Universitätsklinik und -Poliklinik, Kantonsspital, Basel (G. A. Nagel, J. P. Obrecht).
Onkologische Abteilung, Inselspital, Bern (K. W. Brunner, R. W. Sonntag).
Division d'Oncologie-Hématologie, Clinique médicale universitaire, Hôpital cantonal, Genève (P. Alberto, L. Wagenknecht).
Service d'Oncologie, Hôpital des Cadolles, Neuchâtel (P. Siegenthaler).
Abteilung für Onkologie und Hämatologie, Medizinische Klinik C, Kantonsspital, St. Gallen (H. J. Senn, W. F. Jungi).
Servizio d'Oncologia, Ospedale San Giovanni, Bellinzona (F. Cavalli).
Onkologische Abteilung, Medizinische Universitätsklinik, Universitätsspital, Zürich (G. Martz, C. Sauter).
Onkologische Station, Medizinische Poliklinik, Kantonsspital Winterthur (T. Kroner).
Onkologische Station, Medizinische Klinik, Kantonsspital Luzern (H. J. Schmid, F. Riedler).

Table 1. Characteristics of patients included in SAKK study 2T/75 on tamoxifen in advanced breast cancer

Characteristic		No. of patients
Entered		91
Evaluable		82
Menstruating		0
Premenopausal at diagnosis		36
Postmenopausal at diagnosis		46
Tumour sites:	Bone	60
(% of evaluable)	Skin	40
	Lung	27
	Pleura	23
	Lymph nodes	23
	Breast	11
	Liver	10
	CNS	4

Of the 82 evaluable patients, 72 had received some form of previous treatment for their disease, 6 of them only ablative or additive endocrine therapy and 14 only cytostatic drugs. Fifty-two of them had had hormonal and chemotherapy, either in sequence or combined, mostly within the actual study of the Swiss Group at this time, consisting of oophorectomy for the premenopausal or oestrogens for the postmenopausal women, combined with a split variation of the well known Cooper regimen. Tamoxifen[1] was given in a standard dose of 2 × 10 mg/day p.o. The dose was not increased. The drug was discontinued if severe, life-threatening side effects made this necessary. No oestrogen-receptor (ER) determinations were possible at this time in either study.

Response to treatment and any side effects were evaluated according to established criteria by SAKK, specifically by Cancer and Leukemia Group B:

CR, complete remission: complete disappearance of all visible or palpable tumour for a minimum of 3 months.

PR, partial remission: decrease by at least 50% of the original tumour size (measured along two perpendicular diameters if possible) or clear-cut recalcification of osteolytic lesions, both for a minimum of 3 months.

NC, no change: no significant change of the original tumour mass, i.e., less than 50% decrease or increase in size.

PD, progressive disease: more than 50% increase over original tumour size.

Tumour Responses

Table 2 shows the responses achieved in this study. There were 21 complete or partial responses among the 82 evaluable patients, giving a response rate of 25.5%. Another 17 patients, or 20.5%, exhibited stabilisation of their disease, whereas in 44 patients, or 54%, the disease was clearly progressive. When we split these response rates according to menopausal status at the time of diagnosis of breast cancer, there is no difference between premenopausal

1 Tamoxifen was kindly supplied by ICI Switzerland through Mr. Stäuble.

Table 2. Tumour response to tamoxifen in 158 patients with advanced breast cancer in SAKK studies 2T/75 and 2/75

Study	2T/75	2/75
Evaluable patients	82	76
CR + PR	21 (25.5%)	18 (23%)
Mean duration of remission	8 months	10+ months
NC	17 (20.5%)	–
2T/75 + 2/75 combined	CR + PR 39/158 = 25%	

Table 3. Tumour response by site in SAKK study 2T/75 of tamoxifen in advanced breast cancer

Site	%	No.
Breast	22	2/9
Lymph nodes	21	4/19
Skin	21	7/33
Bone	18	9/49
Lung	14	3/22
Liver	12	1/8
Pleura	5	1/19
CNS	0	0/3

and postmenopausal patients. Patients who had received no previous treatment responded somewhat better than patients who had had previous hormonal or chemotherapy. The mean duration of remission was 8 months. The two complete responders are still living and receiving continuous tamoxifen therapy after almost 3 years. The distribution of tumour responses by site is shown in Table 3. The best responses were seen in metastatic lesions in the contralateral breast, lymph nodes, and skin, but there were also quick and valuable remissions in bone and lung metastases, and even one remission in eight patients with liver metastases.

Two of these good remissions are illustrated in Figs. 1 and 2. In the first patient (Fig. 1) there is rapid regression of large metastases in hilar and mediastinal lymph nodes, in the second (Fig. 2), a clear-cut recalcification of osteolytic lesions in the pelvis.

Side Effects

The side effects recorded are shown in Table 4. The drug was generally very well tolerated and had to be discontinued due to unpleasant side effects in very few cases. Nausea and vomiting and exacerbation of preexisting congestive heart failure (resulting in death in one case) were relatively frequent. There were two deaths due to pulmonary embolism, probably attributable to tamoxifen therapy. Four patients exhibited the well-known flaring of bone pain, and there was definite radiological evidence for progressive disease in one of them. Reversible hypercalcaemia was seen in three instances. The other side effects were very rare. In only one case could tumour progression be clearly related to tamoxifen administration.

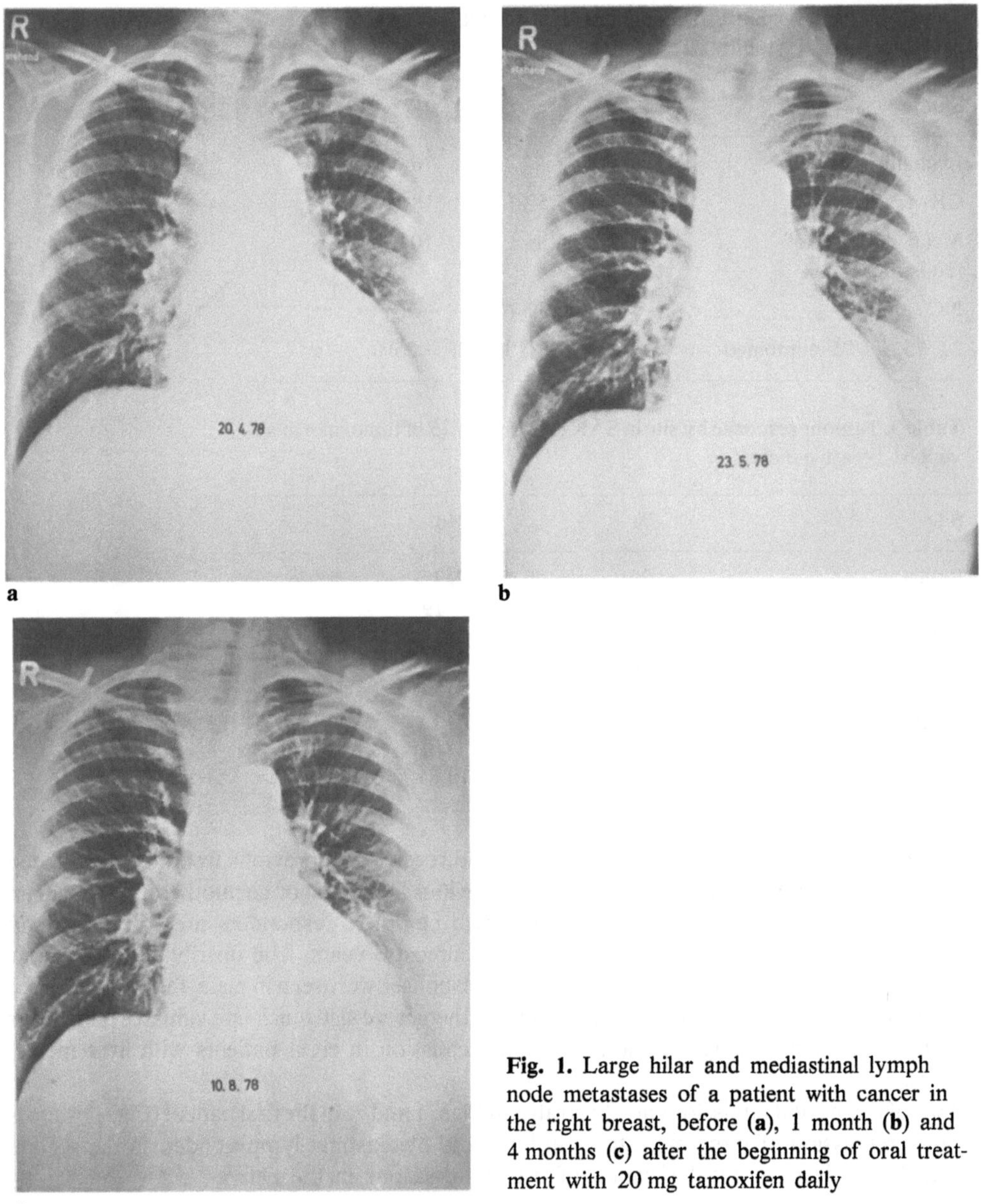

Fig. 1. Large hilar and mediastinal lymph node metastases of a patient with cancer in the right breast, before (**a**), 1 month (**b**) and 4 months (**c**) after the beginning of oral treatment with 20 mg tamoxifen daily

SAKK Protocol 2/75

While the afore-mentioned tamoxifen trial with pretreated patients was in progress, another randomised trial was started in previously untreated pre- and postmenopausal patients by the Swiss Cooperative Group. The design and overall results of this study are presented on page 51 ff. by CAVALLI. Only the results obtained in one half of the postmenopausal patients, who were treated with tamoxifen alone at the same dose of 20 mg per day p.o. until progression, are discussed in this paper. Study 2/75 is a randomized, on-going study involving

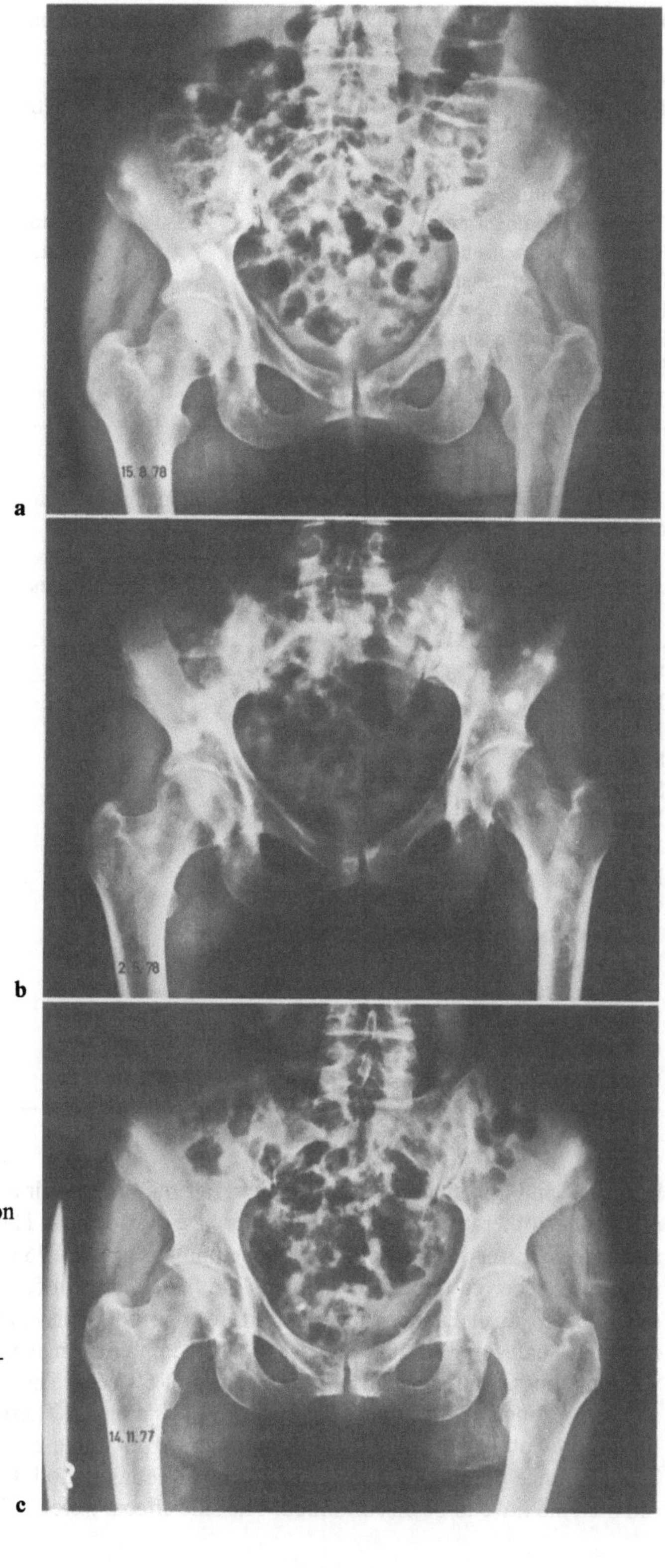

Fig. 2. Massive mixed skeleton metastases, before (a), 6 month (b) and 9 months (c) after the beginning of oral treatment with 20 mg tamoxifen daily. The "pseudo-osteoplastic" progression may be explained as a recalcification of previously undetectable osteolytic metastases. Patient has completely recovered

Table 4. Toxicity in 82 evaluable patients in SAKK study 2T/75 on tamoxifen in advanced breast cancer

Toxic effect	No. of patients affected
Nausea/vomiting	10
Cardiac decompensation	5 (1 fatal)
Pulmonary embolism	4 (2 fatal)
Exacerbation of bone pain ("flaring")	4
Hypercalcaemia (reversible)	3
Elevated serum transaminases	3
Hair loss	2
Thrombocytopenia	1

Table 5. Comparison of published results with tamoxifen in advanced breast cancer

Author	No. of patients	Remissions (%)
VILADIU	31	51
LERNER	25	48
MANNI	31	45
SZEPESI	61	41
SPONZO	12	41
NORDENSKJÖLD	33	39
WARD	68	38
MOSESON	25	36
GOLDER	30	35
HENNINGSEN	35	34
MORGAN	63	33
FERRAZZI	86	32.5
KIANG	69	32
CAVALLI, JUNGI	158	25
COLE	96	18

both pre- and postmenopausal patients. Half the patients first receive endocrine treatment alone, chemotherapy being added when progression occurs. The other half receive endocrine and cytotoxic treatment from the very beginning. There are 76 evaluable postmenopausal patients who received tamoxifen alone as the first treatment for metastatic breast cancer. Of these 76, 18 (23%) responded with complete or partial remissions. There are no patients in the no change category, because in these patients combination chemotherapy was added if there was no remission after an observation period of 6 weeks. The mean duration of remission is somewhat longer in these patients, and is over 10 months. These results combined with those of the previous study, 2T/75, are summarised in Table 2.

The tolerance of tamoxifen in study 2/75 was equally good. Only in 5% of the patients tamoxifen did have to be discontinued. The side effects were similar in nature and extent. The study is still in progress, so that at present no more data are available. For the results obtained with the combination of tamoxifen and chemotherapy, see page 153 of this volume.

Discussion

In published trials tamoxifen has induced tumour responses in as few as 18% (COLE et al., 1971) up to 51% (VILADIU et al., 1977) of treated patients (see Table 5). When our results in the two trials are compared with those published earlier, they are at the bottom of this list. Most of the differences are very probably attributable to widely variable eligibility and evaluation criteria. Whereas in the lower part of the list in Table 5 tumour shrinkage of more than 50% of the original size had been considered a partial remission, in other studies, e.g., that of MANNI et al. (1976), remission criteria were less strict. It has to be stressed also that the three highest remission rates reported (LERNER et al., 1976; MANNI et al., 1976; VILADIU et al., 1977) were seen in small groups consisting of not more than 31 patients treated in single institutions. However, as far as we know, our studies have comprised the first large multi-centre trial so far. Our impression is that the realistic average remission rate achievable with tamoxifen alone in postmenopausal breast cancer patients will be between 25% and 30%. Our treatment results classified by metastatic tumour site are comparable to those of other reports. In agreement with some other authors (LERNER et al., 1976; MANNI et al., 1976; SZEPESI and CZECH 1978; TORMEY et al., 1976) but in contrast to others (FERRAZZI et al., 1977; HENNINGSEN and AMBERGER, 1977; MOSESON et al., 1978), valuable responses have even been achieved in bone metastases. We confirmed the sometimes excellent response of lung metastases to tamoxifen.

The side effects of tamoxifen observed within our two trials are also very similar to those reported previously. There are some differences, however; there are very few cases of hot flushes and undoubted tumour stimulation by the drug in our group. On the other hand, pulmonary embolism and reversible hypercalcaemia seem to be more common in Switzerland. This may reflect climatic differences and special interest in these conditions among our investigators, all of whom are medical oncologists. The standard daily dose of 20 mg tamoxifen was chosen arbitrarily with reference to the results reported and the recommendations of the manufacturer. As there was no possibility of increasing the dose, we cannot tell whether higher doses would have yielded higher remission rates, especially in patients who did not respond to the standard dose or whose response was inadequate. In any case, the daily dose of 20 mg tamoxifen was extremely well tolerated by the great majority of our patients.

At this time it is not possible to postulate the superiority of tamoxifen over traditional additive endocrine treatment with oestrogens in remission induction in postmenopausal breast cancer patients. There is an almost complete paucity of comparative trials, with one notable exception (ROBERTS et al., 1976). The great advantage of tamoxifen over oestrogens lies in the acceptance of the drug by the patients. As oestrogens are sometimes so badly tolerated and tamoxifen is so well accepted, we now give tamoxifen as the first endocrine treatment in postmenopausal patients with metastatic breast cancer. Our studies do not allow any statement on the value of tamoxifen in premenopausal patients or the response to other hormones following tamoxifen failure.

References

Cavalli, F., Alberto, P., Jungi, W. F., Martz, G., Brunner, K. W.: Tamoxifen alone or combined with multiple drug chemotherapy in disseminated breast carcinoma. Proc. 10th Internat. Congress Chemotherapy, Zürich, Vol. II, pp. 1286–1287. Washington: Amer. Soc. Microbiol. 1978

Cole, M. P., Jones, C. T. A., Todd, I. D. H.: A new anti-oestrogenic agent in late breast cancer – an early clinical appraisal of ICI 46474. Br. J. Cancer *25*, 270–274 (1971)

Ferrazzi, E., Cartei, G., De Besi, P., Fornasiero, A., Palù, G., Paccagnella, A., Sperandio, P., Fosser, V., Grigoletto, E., Fiorentino, M.: Tamoxifen in disseminated breast cancer. Tumori *63*, 463–468 (1977)

Golder, M. P., Phillips, M. E. A., Baum, M., Griffiths, K., Fahmy, D. R., Henk, J. M., Jones, V., Preece, P. E.: Hormones in breast cancer patients on tamoxifen. Br. J. Cancer *32*, 246–247 (1975)

Harper, M. J. K., Walpole, A. L.: A new derivative of triphenylethylene: effect on implantation and mode of actions in rats. J. Reprod. Fertil. *13*, 101–119 (1967)

Henningsen, B., Amberger, H.: Antiöstrogene Therapie des metastasierenden Mammakarzinoms. Dtsch. Med. Wochenschr. *102*, 713–716 (1977)

Heuson, J. C.: Current overview of EORTC clinical trials with tamoxifen. Cancer Treat. Rep. *60*, 1463–1466 (1976)

Jordan, V. C.: Antiestrogenic and antitumor properties of tamoxifen in laboratory animals. Cancer Treat. Rep. *60*, 1409–1419 (1976)

Jungi, W. F., Alberto, P., Wagenknecht, L., Cavalli, F., Martz, G., Brunner, K. W.: Antiöstrogene: eine neue endokrine Behandlungsmöglichkeit beim metatasierenden Mammakarzinom. Schweiz. Med. Wochenschr. *108*, 1317–1321 (1978)

Kiang, D. T., Kennedy, B. J.: Tamoxifen (antioestrogen) therapy in advanced breast cancer. Ann. Intern. Med. *87*, 687–690 (1977)

Leclercq, G., Heuson, J. C.: Therapeutic significance of sex-steroid hormone receptors in the treatment of breast cancer. Eur. J. Cancer *13*, 1205–1215 (1977)

Legha, S. S., Carter, S. K.: Antiestrogens in the treatment of cancer. Cancer Treat. Rev. *3*, 205–216 (1976)

Legha, S. S., Davis, H. L., Muggia, F. M.: Hormonal therapy of breast cancer: new approaches and concepts. Ann. Intern. Med. *88*, 69–77 (1978)

Lerner, H. J., Band, P. R., Israel, L., Leung, B. S.: Phase II study of tamoxifen: Report of 74 patients with stage IV breast cancer. Cancer Treat. Rep. *60*, 1431–1435 (1976)

Lippman, M.: Hormone-responsive human cancer in continuous tissue culture. In: Breast cancer. Heuson, J. C., Mattheiem, W. H., Rosencweig, M. (eds.), pp. 111–139. New York: Raven Press 1976

Lippman, M., Bolan, G., Huff, K.: Interactions of antiestrogens with human breast cancer in long-term culture. Cancer Treat. Rep. *60*, 1421–1429 (1976)

Manni, A., Trujillo, J., Marshall, J. S., Pearson, O. H.: Antiestrogen-induced remissions in stage IV breast cancer. Cancer Treat. Rep. *60*, 1445–1450 (1976)

Morgan, L. R., Schein, P. S., Wolley, P. V., Hoth, D., MacDonald, J., Lippmann, M., Posey, L. E., Beazley, R. W.: Therapeutic use of tamoxifen in advanced breast cancer. Cancer Treat. Rep. **60,** 1437–1443 (1976)

Moseson, D. L., Sasaki, G. H., Kraybill, W. G., Leung, B. S., Davenport, C. E., Fletcher, W. S.: The use of antiestrogens tamoxifen and nafoxidine in the treatment of human breast cancer in correlation with estrogen receptor values. Cancer *41*, 797–800 (1978)

Nicholson, R. I., Golder, M. P.: The effects of synthetic antiestrogens on the growth and biochemistry of rat mammary tumors. Eur. J. Cancer *11*, 571 (1975)

Nicholson, R. I., Davies, P., Griffith, K.: Effects of oestradiol-17 and tamoxifen on nuclear oestradiol-17 receptors in DMBA-induced rat mammary tumors. Eur. J. Cancer *13*, 201–208 (1977)

Nordenskjöld, B., Löwhagen, T., Westerberg, H., Zajicke, J.: 3H-Thymidine incorporation into mammary carcinoma cells obtained by needle aspiration before and during endocrine therapy. Acta Cytol. (Baltimore) *20,* 137–143 (1976)

Roberts, M. M., Forrest, A. P. M., Hamilton, T., Langlands, A. O., Lutz, Q., McFayden, J. J., Stewart, H. J.: Preliminary report of a controlled trial in advanced breast cancer comparing tamoxifen with conventional hormone therapy. Cancer Treat. Rep. *60,* 1461–1462 (1976)

Sponzo, R. W., Barkley, J. B., Horton, J., Cunningham, T. J.: Tamoxifen in the management of advanced breast cancer. Proc. Am. Assoc. Cancer Res. *17,* 68 (1976)

Szepesi, T., Czech, W.: Klinische Beurteilung der Anti-Oestrogensubstanz Tamoxifen in der Behandlung des metastasierenden Mammakarzinoms. Wien. Klin. Wschr. *90,* 133–141 (1978)

Tagnon, H. J.: Antiestrogens in treatment of breast cancer. Cancer *39* (Suppl.), 2959–2964 (1977)

Tormey, D. C., Simon, R. M., Lippman, M. J., Bull, J. M., Myers, C. E.: Evaluation of tamoxifen dose in advanced breast cancer: a progress report. Cancer Treat. Rep. *60,* 1451–1459 (1976)

Viladiu, R., Bosch, F. X., Benito, E., Alonso, M. C.: Antiestrogen tamoxifen in the treatment of advanced breast cancer: a series of 31 patients. Cancer Treat. Rep. *61,* 899–900 (1977)

Ward, H. W. C.: Combined anti-prolactin and anti-oestrogen therapy for breast carcinomas. Clin. Oncol. *3,* 1–5 (1977)

Ward, H. W. C.: Anti-oestrogen therapy for breast cancer: a trial of tamoxifen at two dose levels. Br. Med. J. *1978 I,* 13–14

18. *Therapeutic Effect of Tamoxifen Related to Estrogen Receptor Level*

C. Rose, S. M. Thorpe, J. Løber, J. L. Dænfeldt, T. Palshof, and H. T. Mouridsen[1]

The Fibiger Laboratory, Ndr. Frihavnsgade 70, DK-2100 Copenhagen Ø (Denmark)

Introduction

The antioestrogen tamoxifen (TAM) has been shown to be an effective compound in the endocrine therapy of postmenopausal patients with advanced breast cancer. The overall remission rate observed has been found to be 35%–45% in several studies, depending on whether patients have previously received endocrine therapy (KIANG and KENNEDY, 1977; MOURIDSEN, et al., 1978; MOSESON, et al., 1978). This value compares well with that found with other modes of endocrine therapy. A definite advantage of TAM treatment over other forms of endocrine therapy is that side effects are very few and are mild in character (MOURIDSEN et al., 1978).

The predictive value of cytoplasmic oestrogen receptor (ER) determinations for endocrine therapy has been recognised since 1971 (JENSEN et al., 1971). Clinical trials have now revealed that only 10% of patients with an ER-negative (ER–) tumour respond to endocrine therapy, whether in the form of additive or ablative therapy, while about 60% of ER-positive (ER^+) patients respond to endocrine therapy (JENSEN et al., 1975; MCGUIRE et al., 1975). Thus, while ER determinations are valuable in predicting which patients will *not* respond to endocrine therapy, they give, as yet, only equivocal evidence as to which patients will respond to endocrine therapy.

Several previous attempts have been made to investigate whether the predictability of an effect of hormone therapy is increased if the *quantity* of ERs is considered, rather than merely the presence or absence of them. On the basis of results in 123 pre- and postmenopausal patients, JENSEN (1975) concluded that response to endocrine therapy of all kinds is most frequent in the patients with the highest ER values. Although they did not distinguish between pre- and postmenopausal women, both MCGUIRE et al. (1975) and MAASS et al. (1975) found a similar tendency in 45 and 69 patients, respectively, treated with a variety of endocrine treatments. HEUSON et al. (1977) found a positive correlation between the rate of remission and the ER concentration in the tumor biopsies in a study of 34 patients. On the basis of their data they have established a linear logistic model that may be able to predict the probability of response to endocrine treatment in a given patient; this model is based mainly on the ER value of the biopsy.

---

1 Workers at the Fibiger Laboratory were sponsored by the Danish Cancer Society.

In this study of 59 postmenopausal patients with metastatic breast cancer, we investigated whether the therapeutic effect of TAM and/or TAM + medroxyprogesterone acetate (MPA) was related to the patients ER levels.

Materials and Methods

The following studies are discussed in this paper: Study I, in which TAM alone was given; Study II, testing TAM against TAM + MPA; and Study III, testing TAM against TAM + diethylstilboestrol (DES).

Study I involved a consecutive series of patients admitted to Departments R II–R V, Finsen Institute, between 1 February 1976 and 1 August 1976.

Study II involved a consecutive series of patients admitted to Departments R II–R V, Finsen Institute; Department of Oncology, Malmö General Hospital; and Medical Department C, Bispebjerg Hospital, between 1 August 1976 and 1 August 1977.

Study III involved a consecutive series of patients admitted to Departments R II–R V, Finsen Institute; and Medical Department C, Bispebjerg Hospital, between 1 September 1977 and 1 August 1978.

The present material represents a subset of patients from clinical trials designed with the main purpose of comparing the effect of TAM with that of combined treatment with TAM + MPA or TAM + DES (Mouridsen et al., 1979). Data from a small number of patients in a phase II study are included.

Eligibility requirements for the present study were:

1) Prior to therapy, biopsies from histologically verified tumour tissue must had been taken for analysis for cytoplasmic ER protein.
2) The patients were postmenopausal, defined as having had at least 6 months' spontaneous amenorrhoea. Patients who had previously undergone hysterectomy were more than 50 years of age. Patients who had previously undergone oophorectomy could enter the study 3 months after surgical or 6 months after actinic castration.
3) Patients less than 68 years of age were clinically resistant to at least one cytostatic combination regimen. Patients more than 69 years of age could enter the study even when cytostatic treatment had not been attempted.
4) Measurable disease was present.
5) The performance status was ≤ 3.
6) Previous additive endocrine treatment had not been given.
7) The patients had given their verbal informed consent.

Study I was a phase II study and the treatment given was TAM 10 mg three times daily p.o.

In Studies II and III patients were randomly allocated (with the aid of a stochastic array of numbers, closed envelope system) to one of two treatment groups.

Study II patients received treatment with 10 mg tamoxifen three times daily p.o. or treatment with 10 mg tamoxifen three times daily p.o. and 100 mg MPA daily p.o.

Study III patients received treatment with 10 mg tamoxifen three times daily p.o. or treatment with 10 mg tamoxifen three times daily p.o. and 1 mg DES three times daily p.o.

When possible, the treatment was maintained for at least 3 months before the response to treatment was assessed. If at 3 months there was still progressive disease the patient was with-

drawn from the study. If at 3 months there was no change or a remission, the patient continued with the study until progression or relapse.
Pretreatment examinations included physical examination, chest roentgenogram, skeleton survey, laboratory tests (blood cell counts, serum calcium and liver function tests), and estimations of performance status. All visible and palpable lesions were measured to provide a baseline for subsequent examinations, which were performed at intervals of 1–3 months.
Response to treatment was defined according to the UICC criteria (HAYWARD et al., 1977):
Complete remission (CR), complete disappearance of all measurable lesions.
Partial remission (PR), 50%–99% reduction of measurable lesions and/or recalcification of bone lesions.
No change (NC), <50% reduction of measurable lesions and/or no visible changes of bone lesions.
Progressive disease (PD), 50% increase of measurable lesions and/or definite decalcification of bone lesions.
The duration of response was dated from the start of therapy up to PD.

Oestrogen Receptor Determinations

The biopsies taken for ER analyses were obtained less than 1 month prior to therapy in 45 patients, between 1 and 6 months before in ten patients, and more than 6 months before in four patients.
In two patients the tumour material was taken from the primary tumours and in 57 patients from either skin or lymph node metastases.
Biopsies were stored at –80° C until analysis. Cytoplasmic ER concentrations in the tumour specimens were evaluated by measuring [2, 4, 6, 7–^{3}H] oestradiol (AMERSHAM), ^{3}H-oestradiol 17β-binding capacity by a dextran-coated charcoal method (DAEHNFELDT and BRIAND, 1977).

Statistical Analysis

The data were statistically analysed according to the Mann-Whitney rank sum test for unpaired data.

Results

The number of evaluable patients entering Studies I, II, and III were 7, 38, and 29, respectively.
The criteria for eligibility and response were the same in all three clinical trials. When the results were stratified according to age, disease-free interval, dominant disease site, and previous chemotherapy, no significant differences were found. For this reason we found it rational to pool data from all the patients receiving TAM.
The group of patients treated with TAM + DES was too small to evaluate the response and the ER content. As shown in Table 1, the patients treated with TAM + MPA were comparable to those treated with TAM alone in the above-mentioned parameters. Thus a total of 59 patients were evaluated.

Table 1. Patients involved in the study

	TAM	TAM + MPA
Patients (no.)	40	19
Age in years, median (range)	57 (44–74)	60 (53–75)
Disease-free interval in months, median (range)	30 (0–96)	30 (0–96)
Previous chemotherapy	85%	84%
Dominant disease site		
Soft tissue	16	2
Bone	9	7
Viscera	15	10
ER+[a], no./total	21/40	8/19
ER–, no./total	19/40	11/19

[a] ER+, ≥ 20 fmol/mg cytosol protein.

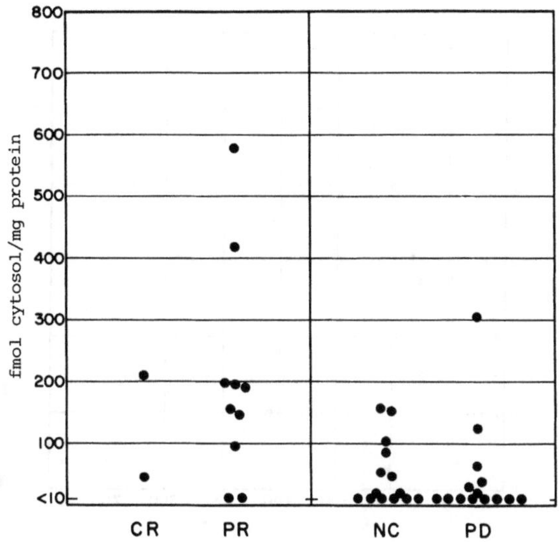

Fig. 1. ER concentration and clinical response to TAM treatment. ER values are plotted in the four response groups CR (complete remission), PR (partial remission), NC (no change), PD (progression of disease). Responders are CR + PR and nonresponders are NC + PD

ER+ and ER– patients are equally represented in this patient material (29/59 ER+ and 30/59 ER–). The individual ER values for all patients are plotted in Figs. 1 and 2 and are grouped according to whether the patients experienced CR, PR, NC, or PD with the TAM or TAM + MPA treatment, respectively. It can be seen from Fig. 1 that 48% (10/21) of the ER+ patients treated with TAM alone responded to treatment (CR + PR). Only 11% (2/19) of the ER– patients responded to therapy. The ER values of the responding patients (mean 171; range < 10–576 fmol cytosol/mg protein) are significantly higher ($P < 0.01$) than the ER values of patients who failed to respond to treatment with TAM (NC + PD); (mean <10; range <10–303 fmol/mg cytosol protein). In contrast, there was no significant difference ($P < 0.1$) between the ER values of responders (mean 86; range <10–757) and nonresponders (mean

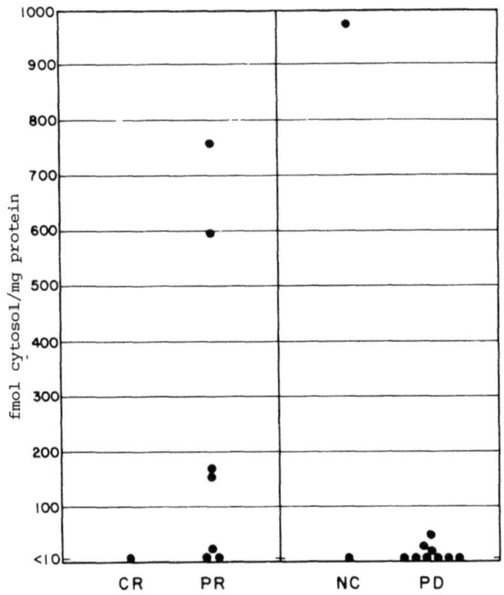

Fig. 2. ER concentration and clinical response to TAM plus MPA treatment. ER values are plotted in the four response groups CR (complete remission), PR (partial remission), NC (no change), PD (progression of disease). Responders are CR + PR and nonresponders are NC + PD

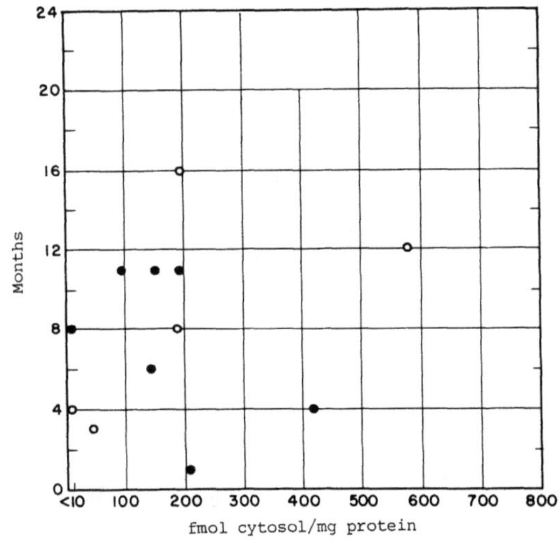

Fig. 3. ER concentration and duration of remission with TAM treatment. ○, patients still in remission; ●, time of onset of progressive disease

<10; range <10–175) when MPA was added to the TAM therapy (Fig. 2). The loss of significant difference is not likely to be due solely to the smaller number of patients in this particular trial. Comparison of the ER values of responders and nonresponders treated with TAM alone in Study II (19 patients) also revealed a significant difference ($P < 0.05$). It appears, therefore, that while there is a correlation between the presence of a high ER concentration in the tumour biopsy and response to treatment with TAM alone, the correlation is lost when TAM is used in combination with MPA.

There is no significant correlation between the ER concentration and the duration of remission ($r = +0.13$) either with TAM therapy (Fig. 3) or in the smaller group treated with TAM + MPA (figure not shown).

No notable differences between responders and nonresponders were found with respect to age, location of dominant site of disease, or previous therapy (no prior treatment, radiation, ablation, chemotherapy).

Discussion

In this unselected population of postmenopausal patients with metastatic breast cancer the overall response rate to TAM treatment is 30% (12/40). This is in keeping with many earlier reports of response rates to all forms of endocrine therapy, and indicates that treatment with TAM equals other forms of endocrine therapy in terms of response rate.

A significant difference in ER concentrations between responders and nonresponders to TAM therapy has been demonstrated in these studies. This difference is still significant even when all ER– patients are excluded from the statistical analysis.

Although the response rate to TAM + MPA was as good as that to TAM alone, there was no significant difference in ER concentrations between the responders and nonresponders in the group receiving TAM + MPA. Perhaps this is due to pharmacodynamic interactions between the two drugs at the receptor level.

No significant correlation was found between the ER concentration and the duration of remission in the present data. This finding is in contrast to that reported by MOSESON et al. (1978), who demonstrated a positive correlation between ER concentration and duration of remission in nine patients treated with anti-oestrogen therapy.

Attempts have been made to improve the predictive value of ER determination by setting rational rather than arbitrary limits for ER+ and ER– values. Thus JENSEN et al. (1975) found that when the critical level below which a patient is considered to be ER– was raised, the response rate of ER+ patients increased from 57% to 74%, with only a slight increase in the number of negatives. Two other approaches have been based on examination of the character of the ER in the target tissues. Both the 4–5 S and the 8–9 S forms of ERs are found in some biopsies. SAVLOV et al. (1977) have presented data suggesting an association between presence of 8–9 S ER and response to endocrine therapy. LAING et al. (1977) investigated whether the ER was found in the nucleus as well as in the cytoplasm, and found that when receptors were found in both cell fractions the response rate was higher than when only cytoplasmic receptors were found. Finally, evidence has been presented that estimation of a parameter indicative of a functioning ER, namely the progesterone receptor, would allow more accurate prediction of response to endocrine therapy (HORWITZ and MCGUIRE, 1977). The accuracy of prediction of response to endocrine therapy could also conceivably be increased by correlating the ER determination to endocrine therapy that is strictly related to the oestrogen hormone itself, e.g., ovariectomy, high-dose oestrogen, or anti-oestrogen therapy. In the present study we have investigated whether ER values are correlated to response to treatment with TAM. The response rate of ER+ patients is 48% (10/21). This value is reached with the arbitrary value of 20 fmol/mg cytosol protein; this is currently being used in our laboratory as the cut-off value between an ER+ and an ER– sample. Examination of the data reveals that if the cut-off level is raised to 75 fmol/mg cytosol protein, the predictive value of the ER determination is increased to 60% (9/15), at the cost of one additional false-negative patient. None of these response rates differs significantly from those previously reported for ER+ patients to TAM (MORGAN et al., 1976; MOSESON et al., 1978) or to various other modes of endocrine therapy (MCGUIRE et al., 1975; JENSEN et al., 1975).

One possible explanation for the lack of response to endocrine therapy in a large proportion of ER+ patients may be that the tumours contain hormone-independent as well as hormone-dependent cells. This appears to be the case in at least some experimental animal tumours (SLUYSER and VAN NIE, 1974). Immunofluorescent studies of ER content in human mammary cancer biopsies also indicate that this is the case in human mammary carcinomas (PERTSCHUK, 1976; NENCI et al., 1976).
Evidence has been presented by LIPPMAN et al. (1978) that there is a very close correlation between absence of ER receptors and response to chemotherapy. With both this and the possible heterogeneous nature of the tumour in mind, it may be prudent to combine chemotherapy with endocrine therapy.
Attempts have previously been made to combine various types of additive endocrine therapy. In two studies in which TAM was used in combination with antiprolactin or androgens, these combined therapies were shown to give slightly better results than treatment with TAM alone (WARD, 1977; TORMEY et al., 1976).
In our own studies (MOURIDSEN et al., 1979) in which TAM was used in combination with MPA or DES, no additive effect of treatment was observed. It therefore seems that to achieve an increased effect with combined endocrine therapies, endocrine treatments with different modes of action must be selected.

Summary

Cytoplasmic oestrogen receptor (ER) determinations were performed in 59 postmenopausal patients with metastatic breast cancer. Fifty percent of the patients were found to be ER+. Forty patients were treated with tamoxifen (TAM) and 19 patients were treated with tamoxifen plus medroxyprogesterone acetate (MPA).
The response rate of TAM-treated patients was 30% (12/40). Of the 21 ER+ patients, ten (48%) responded to therapy. The ER values of these patients were significantly higher than the ER values of nonresponders ($P < 0.01$). No correlation could be found between the ER value and the duration of remission in TAM-treated patients.

References

Dæhnfeldt, J. L., Briand, P.: Determinations of high-affinity gestagen receptors in hormone-responsive and hormone-independent GR mouse mammary tumors by an exchange assay. In: Progesterone receptors in normal and neoplastic tissues. McGuire, W. L., Raynaud, J. P., Baulien, E.-E. (eds.), p. 59. New York: Raven Press 1977

Hayward, J. L., Carbone, P. P., Heuson, J.-C., Kumaoka, S., Segaloff, A., Reubens, R. D.: Assessment of response to therapy in advanced breast cancer. Eur. J. Cancer *13,* 89–94 (1977)

Heuson, J. C., Longeval, E., Mattheiem, W. H., Deboel, M. C., Sylvester, R. J., Leclercq, G.: Significance of quantitative assessment of estrogen receptors for endocrine therapy in advanced breast cancer. Cancer *39,* 1971–1977 (1977)

Horwitz, K. V., McGuire, W. L.: Estrogen and progesterone: their relationship in hormone-dependent breast cancer. In: Progesterone receptors in normal and neoplastic tissues. McGuire, W. L. et al. (eds.), p. 103. New York: Raven Press 1977

Jensen, E. V.: Estrogen receptors in hormone-dependent breast cancers. Cancer Res. *35,* 3362–3364 (1975)

Jensen, E. V., Block, G. E., Smith, S., Kyser, K., Desombre, E. R.: Estrogen receptors and breast cancer response to adrenalectomy. Natl. Cancer Inst. Monogr. *34,* 55–70 (1971)

Jensen, E. V., Polley, T. Z., Smith, S., Block, G. E., Ferguson, D. J., Desombre, E. R.: Prediction of hormone dependency in human breast cancer. In: Estrogen receptors in human breast cancer. McGuire, W. L., Carbone, P. P., Vollmer, E. P. (eds.), p. 37. New York: Raven Press 1975

Kiang, D. T., Kennedy, B. J.: Tamoxifen (antiestrogen) therapy in advanced breast cancer. Ann. Intern. Med. *87,* 687–690 (1977)

Laing, L., Smith, M. G., Calman, K. C., Smith, D. C., Leake, R. E.: Nuclear oestrogen receptors and treatment of breast cancer. Lancet *1977* II, 168–169

Lippman, M. E., Allegra, J. C., Thompson, E. B., Simon, R., Barlock, A., Green, L., Huff, K. K., Do, H. M. T., Aitken, S. C., Warren, R.: The relation between estrogen receptors and respone rate to cytotoxic chemotherapy in metastatic breast cancer. N. Engl. J. Med. *298,* 1223–1228 (1978)

Maass, H., Engel, B., Trams, G.: Steroid hormone receptors in human breast cancer and the clinical significance. J. Steroid Biochem. *6,* 743–749 (1975)

McGuire, W. L., Pearson, O. H., Segaloff, A.: Predicting hormone responsiveness in human breast cancer. In: Estrogen receptors in human breast cancer. McGuire, W. L., Carbone, P. P., Vollmer, E. P. (eds.), p. 17. New York: Raven Press 1975

Morgan, L. R., Jr., Schein, P. S., Woolley, P. V., Hoth, D., Macdonald, J., Lippmann, M., Posey, L. E., Beazley, R. W.: Therapeutic use of tamoxifen in advanced breast cancer: Correlation with biochemical parameters. Cancer Treat. Rep. *60,* 1437–1443 (1976)

Moseson, D. L., Sasaki, G. H., Kraybill, W. G., Leung, B. S., Davenport, C. E., Fletcher, W. S.: The use of antiestrogens, tamoxifen and nafoxidine in the treatment of human breast cancer in correlation with estrogen receptor values. Cancer *41,* 797–800 (1978)

Mouridsen, H. T., Palshof, T., Patterson, J., Battersby, L.: Tamoxifen – a review of its efficacy in advanced breast cancer. Cancer Treat. Rev. *5,* 131–141 (1978)

Mouridsen, H. T., Palshof, T., Rose, C.: Therapeutic effect of tamoxifen alone versus tamoxifen in combination with gestagen or estrogen in advanced breast cancer. In: Endocrine treatment of breast cancer – A new approach. Henningsen, B., Linder, F., Steichele, C. (eds.), p. 169–177. Berlin, Heidelberg, New York: Springer 1980

Nenci, I., Beccati, M. D., Piffanelli, A., Lanza, G.: Detection and dynamic localisation of estradiol-receptor complexes in intact target cells by immunofluorescence technique. J. Steroid Biochem. *7,* 505–510 (1976)

Pertschuk, L. P.: Detection of estrogen binding in human mammary carcinoma by immunofluorescence: a new technique utilizing the binding hormone in a polymerized state. Res. Commun. Chem. Pathol. Pharmacol. *14,* 771–774 (1976)

Savlov, E. D., Wittliff, J. L., Hilf, R.: Further studies of biochemical predictive tests in breast cancer. Cancer *39,* 539–541 (1977)

Sluyser, M., Van Nie, R.: Estrogen receptor content and hormone-responsive growth of mouse mammary tumors. Cancer Res. *34,* 3253–3257 (1974)

Tormey, D. C., Simon, R. M., Lippman, M. E., Bull, J. M., Myers, C. E.: Evaluation of tamoxifen dose in advanced breast cancer: A progress report. Cancer Treat. Rep. *60,* 1451–1459 (1976)

Ward, W. W. C.: Combined antiprolactin and antiestrogen therapy for breast carcinoma. Clin. Oncol. *3,* 91–95 (1977)

19. Results of Tamoxifen Therapy in Patients with Breast Cancer

N. Firusian, S. Öhl, and R. Becher

Universitätsklinikum der Gesamthochschule Essen, Westdeutsches Tumorzentrum, Hufelandstraße 55, D-4300 Essen (FRG)

Oestrogens have been shown to accelerate the growth of some human breast cancers. This effect may be due to a direct hormonal action on the tumour cell, since oestrogen receptors have been found in a high percentage of these cancers (McGuire et al., 1975). An ablative hormone therapy, as demonstrated by the beneficial effect of oophorectomy (Kennedy, 1974), might lower the circulating oestrogen levels in the patient, but does not totally abolish oestrogen secretion. Nonsteroidal anti-oestrogens such als tamoxifen have been introduced, and may act by competitive binding to the oestrogen receptors on the target tissue (Cole et al., 1971). Recent clinical trials of anti-oestrogens have shown that objective remissions can be induced in women with advanced metastatic breast cancer (Ward, 1973; Kiang and Kennedy, 1977).

In this paper we summarize our experience with tamoxifen in a series of women with stage IV breast cancer at the West German Tumour Centre, Essen, correlating its effectiveness with previous hormonal procedures.

Materials and Methods

In all, 104 patients were treated with tamoxifen from July 1975 to August 1978. Twenty had an inadequate trial period of less than 2 months, five suffered from severe nausea and vomiting, and fifteen patients died within the first month of tamoxifen therapy, leaving only 84 evaluable cases. The majority of our patients had received hormone therapy previously and all were postmenopausal, 44 of them because of previous castration. The daily tamoxifen dosage was 30 mg in 67, and 20 mg in 17 patients. To determine oestrone, oestradiol, and prolactin levels, sera were assayed by radioimmuno-assay methods up to 12 weeks after the start of tamoxifen therapy.

Results

Thirty-six patients responded (complete remission 16/84 = 19,0%, partial remission 20/84 = 23.8%), with a mean duration of remission of 9.2 months (Table 1). Skin and nodal lesions improved with tamoxifen in 30% of cases, pleural and liver metastases in 39%, and bone lesions in 15.4% (Table 2). One notable group of patients showed long-lasting stable conditions with

Table 1. Response to tamoxifen in 84 patients with advanced breast cancer

Response	Patients	Duration of response
Complete regression	16/84 = 19.0%	9.2 months
Partial regression	20/84 = 23.8%	
Stable disease	17/84 = 20.0%	
Progressive disease	31/84 = 36.9%	

Table 2. Response to tamoxifen according to site of metastases

Site		No.	Responds (%)
Locoregional		45	18/45 = 40.0
Visceral	pleuropulmonary 38 hepatic 3	41	16/41 = 39.0
Bone		39	1/39 = 15.4

Table 3. Patients with no objective change, accompanied by subjective improvement of symptoms during tamoxifen therapy

Patient no.	Type of metastases	Duration of "no change" condition (months)
5	Bone	5
14	Bone	13
32	Bone	7
44	Bone + locoregional	11
45	Bone + locoregional	17
48	Bone	19
49	Bone	14
53	Bone	4+
56	Bone	3+
64	Pleuropulmonary	13+
66	Bone + locoregional	25+
68	Bone	4+
71	Bone	5+
73	Bone	9+
74	Pulmonary	5+
76	Bone	4+
78	Bone	3+

subjective improvement of their symptoms. The majority of these patients had generalized bone metastases (Tables 1 and 3).

Correlation with History of Hormonal Response

Sixteen of 36 patients who showed improvement had responded to previous ablative or additive hormonal treatment. In eight patients the anti-oestrogen therapy was the first hormonal therapy to lead to a remission. Five patients with objective remissions had failed to respond to previous castration.

Side Effects

In 9.5% of the patients there were no remarkable complications during therapy. We observed initial nausea and vomiting in 8.3%, genital pruritus in 6.0%, and ichthyosis in 4.8% of our patients. Transient thrombocytopenia (1.2%) and cardiovascular side effects (1.2%) were observed occasionally (Table 4).

Discussion

Tamoxifen is an amino-ether derivative of polycyclic phenols, with a basic structure close to that of diethylstilboestrol. The anti-oestrogenic effect of this compound might be due to its competition with oestradiol at the cytoplasmic receptor sites (JORDAN, 1974). The fate of the oestrogen receptor complex after translocation into the nuclei is still not known. However, other anti-oestrogens, such as nafoxidine, have been shown to remain in the nucleus for a long time and to interfere with the regeneration of oestrogen receptors.

Table 4. Side effects and complications in 84 patients with advanced breast cancer during tamoxifen therapy

Side effect/complication	Affected	
	No.	%
Ichthyosis	4/84 =	4.8
Pruritus of genital tract	5/84 =	6.0
Initial nausea, vomiting	7/84 =	8.3
Persistent vomiting	1/84 =	1.2
Hot flushes	8/84 =	9.5
Hypercalcaemia syndrome (bone met.)	1/84 =	1.2
Transient thrombocytopenia	1/84 =	1.2
Persistent thrombocytopenia	1/84 =	1.2
Leucopenia	1/84 =	1.2
Cardiovascular complications	1/84 =	1.2
Totals	29/84 =	34.5

The results summerised in this paper are comparable with results from other centres (Kiang and Kennedy, 1977; Ward, 1973; Cole et al., 1971).
The side effects of tamoxifen are less severe than those of other additive hormonal therapies. Most side effects were related to "oestrogen depletion" due to the basic pharmacological action; for instance, when tamoxifen occupied the oestrogen receptor sites and blocked the peripheral function of oestrogens, postmenopausal symptoms occurred in some patients. The most worrying side effect was the development of an acute cardiovascular complication in one patient who had previously received polyvalent chemotherapy.

References

Cole, M. P., Jones, C. T. A., Todd, I. D. H.: A new anti-oestrogenic agent in late breast cancer. An early clinical appraisal of ICI 46,474. Br. J. Cancer *25,* 270–275 (1971)

Heuson, J. C., Engelsman, E., Blonk van der Wijst, J. Maass, H., Drochmans, A., Michel, J., Nowakowski, H., Gorins, A.: Comparative trial of nafoxidine and ethinyloestradiol in advanced breast cancer; an EORTC study. Br. Med. J. *1975 II,* 711–713

Jordan, V. C.: Antitumor activity of antiestrogen (tamoxifen) in the dimethylbenzanthracene (DMBA) induced rat mammary carcinoma model. J. Steroid Biochem. *4,* 354 (1974)

Kennedy, B. J.: Hormonal therapies in breast cancer. Semin. Oncol. *1,* 119–130 (1974)

Kiang, D. T., Kennedy, B. J.: Tamoxifen (antiestrogen) therapy in advanced breast cancer. Ann. Intern. Med. *87,* 687–690 (1977)

McGuire, W. L., Carbone, P. P., Sears, M. E., Escher, G. C.: Estrogen receptors in human breast cancer: On overview. In: Estrogen receptors in human breast cancer. McGuire, W. L., Carbone, P. P., Vollmer, E. P. (eds.), pp. 1–7. New York: Raven Press 1975

Sinha, D., Cooper, D., Dao, T. L.: The nature of estrogen and prolactin effect on mammary tumorigenesis. Cancer Res. *33,* 411–414 (1973)

Ward, H. W. C.: Anti-oestrogen therapy for breast cancer: A trial of tamoxifen at two dose levels. Br. med. J. *1973 I,* 13–14

20. Results with Tamoxifen in Advanced Mammary Carcinoma

R. Kolb, R. Jakesz, and H. Reiner

Chirurgische Universitätsklinik, Alser Straße 4, A-1087 Wien (Austria)

Introduction

In recent years, important results have been obtained with tamoxifen (TAM) in the treatment of relapsing mammary carcinoma (Henningsen and Amberger, 1977; Hanni et al., 1976). This compound appears to be particularly effective when hormone-sensitive tumours can be selected by hormone receptor determination (Terenius, 1974) and when the therapy is reserved for postmenopausal patients, although isolated positive results have also been reported in menstruating women (Manni et al., 1976).

This paper presents the results of a controlled study of the use of anti-oestrogens in advanced mammary carcinoma.

Patients and Methods

So far 62 patients have been treated with the anti-oestrogen TAM and in 44 it is possible to evaluate the treatment results to date.

Patients were admitted to the study if their lesions were verified histologically or could be clearly defined radiologically as metastases. The course of the disease was documented photographically, by means of X-rays, and by measurements. In 17 of 44 evaluable cases oestrogen receptors (ER) content was determined by the method of Wagner (1972), in addition to histological examination of the tumour tissue. A result was taken to be positive when more than 15 fmol receptor protein/mg cytosol protein was present.

Of the 44 patients, more than 5 years had passed since the last menstrual period in 37, whilst in the remaining seven the last menstrual period was less than 5 years before.

The daily dose of TAM was 3 × 10 mg. The patients were examined every 2—3 weeks during the first 3 months of therapy, and thereafter every 2 months. In addition to a thorough clinical examination, appropriate other examinations (X-ray, conventional laboratory diagnostic tests) were carried out.

The results were evaluated according to the rules of the British Breast Group (Hayward et al., 1977).

Results

Of the 44 patients evaluated, 24 showed remission, whilst in 20 progression of the lesions was recorded. The remission group included 11 patients with a local recurrence and 13 with

Table 1. Results of treatment with TAM in breast cancer patients with local recurrences or metastases (n = 44)

	Local recurrence	Metastases
Remission (partial)	11	13
Progression	3	17
	14	30

Table 2. Effects of TAM treatment on metastases (n = 30)

Site of metastases	Remission	Progression
Soft tissue	3	4
Bone	7	10
Generalised	3	3
	13	17

Table 3. Results of TAM treatment classified by ER status (n = 17)

	ER+	ER−
Remission (partial)	9	1
Progression	3	4
	12	5

metastases, whilst three patients with local recurrences and 17 with metastases were found among those with progression (Table 1). The duration of remission in 11 patients varied between 2 and 14 months.

In the presence of distant metastases (Table 2), there was no clear difference in the results of treatment with TAM. However, the objective response rate of bone metastases seems to be considerably lower than that of soft tissue metastases, although during the treatment with TAM women with bone metastases showed clear signs of alleviation of pain, combined with improvement in the psychological condition.

Oestrogen receptor determinations were performed in the tumour tissue of 17 patients (Table 3). Twelve women were classified as receptor-positive (ER^+) and five as receptor-negative (ER^-). Of the ER^+ cases, nine showed remission and three progression, whilst in the ER^- cases there was a remission in one case and progression in four cases.

Discussion

With a total remission rate of 54%, our results are among the most favourable in the data so far published (HENNINGSEN and AMBERGER, 1977).

If, however, the results of the ER determinations are taken into account in the therapeutic regimen, this remission rate can be increased further for the selected cases. In our small sample of cases, nine of 12 ER^+ cases showed remissions, corresponding to a percentage of 75%.

Thus hormonal therapy with anti-oestrogens provides a real alternative to polychemotherapy for ER^+ postmenopausal patients. In addition, it should be mentioned here that in our case material none of the known side effects, which in the literature are slight compared with those seen with chemotherapy, were experienced with TAM.

Furthermore, it should be noted that in premenopausal patients ovariectomy should be the first therapeutic step in metastatic ER^+ carcinoma, although even menstruating patients showed a favourable response to TAM.

Summary

The results of a study with tamoxifen (TAM) (10 mg three times daily) in advanced breast cancer are reported. Of 44 patients, 24 showed a remission and 20 a progression. Of the 17 patients in whom an oestrogen receptor (ER) determination in tumour tissue had been carried out, 12 were receptor-positive (ER^+) and five receptor-negative (ER^-).

Nine of the 12 ER^+ cases (75%) responded to the treatment with TAM. Of the five ER^- patients, one showed remission and four progression.

References

Hayward, J. L., Carbone, P. P., Heuson, J. C., Kumaoka, S., Segaloff, A., Rubens, R. D.: Assessment for response to therapy in advanced breast cancer. Eur. J. Cancer *13,* 89 (1977)

Henningsen, B., Amberger, H.: Antiöstrogene Therapie des metastasierenden Mammakarcinoms. Dtsch. Med. Wochenschr. *102,* 713 (1977)

Manni, A., Trujillo, J., Pearson, O. H.: Antiestrogen-induced remissions in stage 4 breast cancer. Proc. Amer. Assoc. Cancer Res. *17,* 279 (1976)

Terenius, L.: Anti-estrogens and their role in mammary cancer. In: Mammary cancer and neuroendocrine therapy. Stoll, B. A. (ed.). London: Butterworth 1974

Wagner, R. K.: Characterization and assay of steroid hormone receptors and steroid-binding serum proteins by agargel electrophoresis at low temperature. Hoppe-Seylers Z. Physiol. Chem. *353,* 1235 (1972)

21. *The Significance of Tumour "Stimulation" by Tamoxifen*

B. A. Stoll

St. Thomas' Hospital, Department Oncology, London SE1 7EH (U.K.)

Several publications on tamoxifen therapy in advanced breast cancer have reported a "flare" in the tumour soon after the onset of therapy. Although it is said to occur in about 10% of cases, it leads to withdrawal of patients from tamoxifen therapy in less than 0.5% of treated patients (PATTERSON and BAUM, 1978). In this brief presentation, I would like to consider three questions: What is this flare? What does it indicate? Is it safe to continue tamoxifen therapy when it occurs?

The term "flare" has been applied to three different manifestations occurring soon after the onset of tamoxifen therapy in breast cancer. The first is an increase in pain, swelling, or erythema in soft tissue deposits of breast cancer; the second is an increase in pain associated with bone metastases; the third is the onset of hypercalcaemia soon after the start of therapy. A flare usually appears between 1 and 3 weeks after the start of treatment, but in one report of a patient who had three separate flares following attempts at tamoxifen therapy, they seemed to appear after increasingly short intervals (MCINTOSH and THYNNE, 1977).

Does a flare indicate acceleration of growth? JORDAN (1976) has reported that when tamoxifen is administered to rats with DMBA-induced mammary cancer, it may show no effect on tumour growth, it may cause immediate regression of the tumour, or there may be a period of continuing growth before regression appears. Similarly, in the case of the human tumour regressing after tamoxifen therapy, NORDENSKJÖLD (1975) has shown that the tumour diameter may start to decrease immediately or it may continue to increase at its normal rate before starting to decrease.

Even more significant, TORMEY has recorded serial measurements of tumour area in lesions that showed a so-called flare after tamoxifen therapy. He showed that although some of the tumours continued to grow at the same rate after tamoxifen therapy was started none showed a faster clinical growth rate than before therapy (TORMEY et al., 1976)

It therefore appears that a soft tissue flare has nothing to do with stimulation of tumour growth.

Does a flare predict the likelihood of tumour regression later? According to MORGAN, lesions with a positive oestrogen receptor assay (ER^+ lesions) tend to show a delayed increase in erythema and oedema before showing tumour regression (MORGAN et al., 1976). TORMEY has reported that of patients showing flares in soft tissue lesions or bone pain, the continuation of treatment led to subsequent tumour regression in about half (TORMEY et al., 1976).

The onset of hypercalcaemia during the course of breast cancer is thought to reflect excessive calcium mobilisation associated with lytic bone metastases. Many would regard hypercalcaemia as evidence of tumour stimulation when it occurs within 1 or 2 weeks of the onset of tamoxifen therapy. Yet there is evidence that the tumour may regress subsequently on tamoxifen therapy. The majority of hypercalcaemia cases occur when the tumour is ER^+ (VELDHUJS, 1978), and the hypercalcaemia often disappears despite continuation of the treatment (HENNINGSEN and AMBERGER, 1977). It may be followed by recalcification of bone metastases (ENGELSMAN, 1978). POWLES (1977) has suggested that the appearance of bone pain in association with hypercalcaemia may possibly be related to prostaglandin release. This may apply to the soft tissue flare also.

MINTON has reported a patient in whom hypercalcaemia followed tamoxifen therapy but later subsided on prednisolone therapy (MINTON et al., 1978). I myself have reported a patient who developed a soft tissue flare within 2 weeks of starting tamoxifen therapy, yet nevertheless persisted with treatment. Within only 4 weeks, she was rewarded by almost complete regression of her skin metastases (STOLL, 1975).

To sum up, therefore, a flare in soft tissue lesions or in bone pain following tamoxifen therapy is thought to indicate a local reaction to the tumour. There is no evidence that it reflects can acceleration of tumour growth, although the pre-existing growth may continue for several weeks before regression becomes manifest. The onset of hypercalcaemia is often a hormone-precipitated condition. It appears safe to continue tamoxifen therapy in the presence of a flare or of hypercalcaemia, although corticosteroids may be added for a few weeks to control the symptoms. Finally, it appears that the flare phenomenon tends to be followed by tumour regression in the majority of cases.

References

Engelsman, E. (1978) Personal communication

Henningsen, B., Amberger, H.: Antioestrogene Therapie des metastasierenden Mammakarzinoms. Dtsch. Med. Wochenschr. *102,* 713–716 (1977)

Jordan, V. C.: Antiestrogenic and antitumor properties of tamoxifen in laboratory animals. Cancer Treat. Rep. *60,* 1409–1419 (1976)

McIntosh, J. H., Thynne, G. S.: Tumour stimulation by anti-oestrogens. Br. J. Surg. *64,* 900–901 (1977)

Minton, M. J., Cantwell, B. M. J., Knight, R. K., Rubens, R. D., Hayward, J. L.: Safety of tamoxifen. Lancet *1978 I,* 396–397

Morgan, L. R., Schein, P. S., Woolley, P., Vhoth, D., MacDonald, J., Lippmann, M., Posey, L. E., Beazley, R. W.: Therapeutic use of tamoxifen in advanced breast cancer. Cancer Treat. Rep. *60,* 1437–1443 (1976)

Nordenskjöld, B.: [^{3}H] thymidine incorporation into DNA of mammary carcinoma before and after endocrine therapy. Proc. Symp. 'The Hormonal Control of Breast Cancer', pp. 43–52. Alderly Park: I.C.I., Pharmaceuticals Division 1975

Patterson, J., Baum, M.: Safety of tamoxifen. Lancet *1978 I,* 8055

Powles, T. J.: Factor influencing metastasis in bone. In: Secondary spread in breast cancer. Stoll, B. A. (ed.), p. 81. London: Heinemann Medical 1977

Stoll, B. A.: Discussion, Proc. Symp. 'The Hormonal Control of Breast Cancer', pp. 57–58. Alderley Park: I.C.I., Pharmaceuticals Division 1975

Tormey, D. C., Simon, R. M., Lippmann, M. E., Myers, C. E.: Evaluation of tamoxifen dose in advanced breast cancer. Cancer Treat. Rep. *60,* 1451–1459 (1976)

Veldhuis, J. D.: Tamoxifen and hypercalcemia. Ann. Intern. Med. *88,* 574–575 (1978)

V. Combination Therapy of Advanced Breast Cancer

22. *Simultaneous Hormone- and Chemotherapy, Compared with Hormone Therapy Followed by Chemotherapy in the Treatment of Metastasising Mammary Carcinoma – Preliminary Results of a Current Study*

F. Cavalli, P. Alberto, W. F. Jungi, G. Martz, L. Barrelet, J. P. Obrecht, and K. W. Brunner[1]

Servizio Oncologico, Ospedale San Giovanni, CH-6500 Bellinzona (Switzerland)

Introduction

It is undisputed that in the majority of patients the course of the disease of mammary carcinoma in the metastasising stage has been decisively influenced through the results of modern cytostatic combination therapy (Brunner u. Martz, 1976; Fey, 1978).
Our current protocol (SAKK 2/75) is designed to determine whether it is better to combine primary polychemotherapy with a hormonal treatment, or whether cytostatic therapy should be introduced alone when the failure of hormonal therapy is certain. At the same time, three different polychemotherapeutic regimes (a "mild", a "standard", and a "maximal" cytostatic treatment) are compared with one another.
This paper gives the preliminary results of these as yet incomplete studies.

Patients and Methods

Between 1 September 1975 and 15 February 1978 (time of the last clinical assessment), 258 patients were admitted to the study (Protocol SAKK 2/75).
Sixty patients were considered to be premenopausal and 192 postmenopausal. On the basis of the localisation of metastases and the interval between mastectomy and the establishment of metastases, the patients were classified into a "low-risk" group of 66 patients and a "high-risk" group of 192 cases. None of the patients had received cytostatic or hormone treatment. The therapeutic plan is summarised in Fig. 1; after stratification, the patients were randomised into two groups, A and B.
In Group A the patients received polychemotherapy combined with hormone treatment from the outset. The hormone treatment given consisted of ovariectomy for premenopausal patients, and 20 mg tamoxifen (TAM) daily p.o. for postmenopausal patients (Cavalli et al., 1978). In Group B, on the other hand, only the appropriate hormone therapy was carried out at first. The polychemotherapy was not begun until 6 weeks later, and then only when the measurable tumour mass had not decreased up to this time. If this was the case (i.e., if remission occurred in response to hormonal therapy), the cytostatic therapy was first

1 Schweizerische Arbeitsgruppe für Klinische Krebsforschung (SAKK) (Swiss working-group for Clinical Cancer Research).

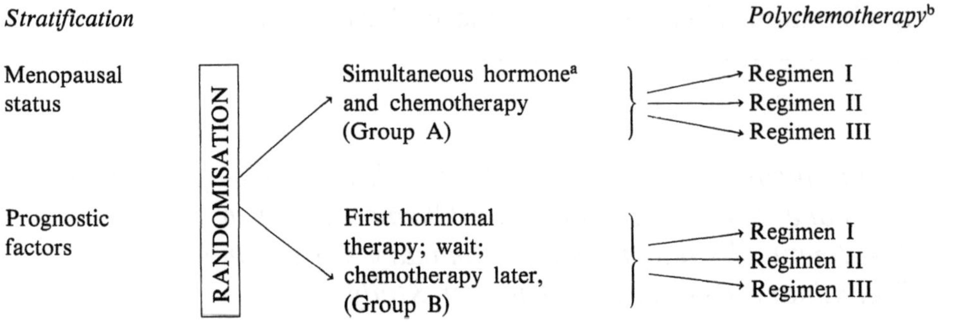

[a] *Hormonal therapy* was ovariectomy (premenopausal patients) or (mild): tamoxifen p.o. (postmenopausal patients).

[b] *Polychemotherapy:* Regimen I chlorambucil, methotrexate, 5-fluorouracil, prednisone. Regimen II (standard): chlorambucil (L) p.o., methotrexate p.o., prednisone, alternating with 5-fluorouracil i.v., vincristine i.v., prednisone. Regimen III (maximal): doxorubicin i.v., alternating with high-dose LFMP, chlorambucil p.o., methotrexate, 5-fluorouracil i.v., and prednisone p.o.

Fig. 1. Therapy plan for untreated metastasising mammary carcinoma study protocol SAKK

introduced from the time of renewed progression of the measurable tumour. All patients were randomised to one of the three polychemotherapy regimens.

Regimen I. Patient randomised to Regimen I received intermittent mild polychemotherapy with 5 mg chlorambucil/m^2 p.o. daily, 10 mg methotrexate/m^2 p.o. once weekly, 500 mg 5-fluorouracil/m^2 p.o. once weekly, and prednisolone in decreasing doses. This treatment was given for 2 weeks, and after each treatment cycle there was a 2-week pause before the next.

Regimen II. The standard therapy of SAKK (Brunner et al., 1977) was given as Regimen II. For the first 14 days of the month the patients received chlorambucil as in Regimen I, 15 mg methotrexate/m^2 weekly p.o. distributed over 3 days, and prednisolone. In the second half of the month the treatment was changed for vincristine i.v. once weekly (maximal dose 2.0 mg) and 5-fluorouracil (500 mg/m^2) i.v. once weekly.

Regimen III. As maximal cytostatic treatment, the patients received in monthly rotation either 60 mg doxorubicin/m^2 i.v. once every 4 weeks or high-dose LMF, consisting of chlorambucil as in Regimen I, 40 mg methotrexate/m^2 i.v. once weekly and 600 mg 5-fluorouracil/m^2 i.v. once weekly. The high-dose LMF was administered only during 2 weeks per month.

The course of the therapy was assessed according to the following objective criteria:

Progression (P): increase of measurable tumour mass and/or occurrence of a more recent tumour lesion.

No change (NC): stationary maintenance of tumour parameters or decrease of the same to less than 25%.

Improvement (PR < 50%): decrease of the measurable tumour size (product of the two longest diameters) by less than 50%.

Partial remission (PR > 50%): decrease of the measurable tumour size (product of the two longest diameters) by more than 50%.

The survival time was calculated by the use of the principle of cumulative survival curves after the method of Kaplan and Meier (1958).

Table 1. Remission rate after chemotherapy regimen (n = 194)

Regimen	n	PR > 50%	PR < 50%	Total
I	68	19 (= 28%)	13	32 = 47%
II	62	32 (= 52%)	7	39 = 62%
III	64	41 (= 64%)	3	44 = 69%

Results

Of the 258 patients admitted to this study by 15 February 1978, 210 were evaluable with reference to response to treatment.

Twenty-five cases were not evaluable on account of serious flaws in the protocol. In 23 cases the minimum time for evaluation (1 month of treatment) had not yet exspired. Of 210 evaluable cases, 63 were premenopausal, and 147 postmenopausal women. In the premenopausal group, 24 out of 36 cases in Group A (remission rate 66%) showed PR > 50%. In Group B ovariectomy induced tumour regression in six of 27 cases (remission rate 22%); in nine further patients PR > 50% was not induced until polychemotherapy was instituted. The remission rate for Regimen B thus amounted to a total of 55% (15/27).

Of the postmenopausal patients, 33 of 71 cases in Group A (remission rate = 45%) attained PR > 50%. In this age group, 76 patients were randomised to Group B. In 18 of these patients TAM alone produced tumour regression (remission 23%), and 11 of these TAM-induced remissions still persist, giving a projected median duration of remission of more than 10 months (10 +). The remission rates obtained with the three different chemotherapeutic regimens (I, II, III) are summarised in Table 1. The present evaluation relating to chemotherapy is based on 194 patients (210 evaluable, less 16 lasting remissions with hormone therapy in Group B). In the 68 patients treated according to Regimen I, 19 (28%) attained PR > 50%, whilst in 13 women the remission was objectively less good. Regimen II has so far been administered to 62 patients, 32 of whom attained PR > 50% (52%). In seven further cases the measurable tumour size decreased by less than 50%.

Of the 64 patients receiving Regimen III, 41 (64%) attained PR > 50%. With this regimen only three further cases showed PR < 50%. Comparison of the rate of PR > 50% obtained with Regimen I and that with Regimen III reveals that the difference is statistically highly significant ($P < 0.01$). All other differences so far have been statistically nonsignificant. In these preliminary evaluations of the study the toxicity of the chemotherapy has not yet been finally analysed, but it seems to be more marked than in the other therapeutic procedures used. In this group two patients died of heart failure, possibly caused by doxorubicin.

Consideration of the cumulative survival curve reveals that so far neither the pre – nor the postmenopausal cases show any significant difference between Group A and Group B. At the time of the present evaluation, the course of the survival curve is also similar for all three chemotherapeutic regimens.

Discussion

With the treatment options currently available, about one-third of patients with untreated metastasising mammary carcinoma can experience a complete or good partial (> 50%) remis-

sion that persists for a mean of 9–12 months (BRUNNER and MARTZ, 1976). In the last SAKK study, BRUNNER and MARTZ (1976) were able to show that a simultaneous hormone and chemotherapeutic treatment yields better results than polychemotherapy alone. The present SAKK protocol was designed to investigate two questions in particular:
1) The point when hormonal and cytotoxic chemotherapy should be combined.
2) The necessary intensity of polychemotherapy. Both problems are currenty considered to be unsolved (TATTERSALL and TOBIAS, 1977). The evaluations so far available from our study, which is still in progress, do not allow a definite answer to either question.
Hitherto we have been unable to establish a difference in the course of the two groups in which chemotherapy is instituted simultaneously with hormone therapy or later, after failure of hormonal therapy has been established.
A clear answer to this question is obviously impossible without a longer observation time. But it will be especially necessary in the definitive analysis of this study to divide the whole patient sample into different subgroups with homogeneous prognostic factors (FEY, 1978) to facilitate the observation of possible differences, which will probably balance each other over the whole collective.
With regard to chemotherapy, we already have an indication that intensive cytostatic treatment induces a higher remission rate, so far without a significant prolongation of survival. Should this trend persist we might have to deal with a surprising and portentous finding. However, before we can form a definite opinion we require a longer observation time.
A conclusive analysis must also investigate the significance of "secondary therapy" (i.e., treatment after actual progression within the study) to explain a possible absence of difference in the survival curve.

Summary

The preliminary results of an on-going SAKK study on metastasising mammary carcinoma are reported. At the time of writing 210 cases are already evaluable. This study seeks to investigate the question of the necessary intensity of polychemotherapy and also the problem of whether cytostatic therapy should be begun at the same time as hormonal therapy or just after failure of this measure. At present no definite answer is available. The results point to a new, possibly important aspect of the treatment of metastasising mammary carcinoma.

References

Brunner, K. W., Martz, G. A.: Das Mammakarzinom. In: Internistische Krebstherapie. Brunner, K. W., Nagel, G. A. (Hrsg.), S. 250. Berlin, Heidelberg, New York: Springer 1976

Brunner, K. W., Sonntag, R. W., Alberto, P., Senn, H. J., Martz, G., Obrecht, P., Maurice, P.: Combined chemo- and hormonal therapy in advanced breast cancer. Cancer *39,* 2923 (1977)

Cavalli, F., Alberto, P., Jungi, F., Martz, G., Brunner, K. W.: Tamoxifen alone or combined with multiple drug chemotherapy in disseminated breast cancer. Proc. 10th Internat. Congr. Chemother. 1978, Vol. II, p. 1286

Fey, M.: Prognostische Faktoren beim metastasierenden Mammakarzinom. Dissertation, Bern, 1978

Kaplan, E. L., Meier, P.: Nonparametric estimation from incomplete observations. J. Am. Stat. Assoc. *53,* 457 (1958)

Tattersall, M. H. N., Tobias, J. S.: Are dose-response relationships relevant in clinical cancer chemotherapy? In: Recent advances in cancer treatment, Vol. 3. Tagnon, H. J., Staquet, M. J. (eds.), p. 227. New York: Raven Press 1977

23. *Lack of Estrogen Receptor Associated with an Increased Response Rate to Cytotoxic Chemotherapy in Metastatic Breast Cancer?*

M. E. Lippman and J. C. Allegra

Medicine Branch, National Cancer Institute, National Institutes of Health, Building 10, Room 6B02, Bethesda, MD 20014 (USA)

Recent advances in the management of metastatic breast cancer have led to a significant improvement in patient care. A variety of new kinds of endocrine therapy, such as antiestrogen administration or medical adrenalectomy with aminoglutethimide, have reduced the toxicity of endocrine therapy. The use of steroid receptor determinations has improved the selection of patients for endocrine therapy enormously, such that about 75% accuracy in patient assignment for or against endocrine therapy can be anticipated.

With the advent of combination chemotherapy, a large number of women, perhaps as many as two-thirds, will benefit from drug therapy. Unfortunately, these cytotoxic therapies involve significant hazards and virtually unavoidable toxicity. Clearly, the higher response rate to chemotherapy than to endocrine therapy is no justification for the indiscriminate application of the former to women as primary therapy. In view of the less than perfect response rate to chemotherapy combined with the obvious toxicity, we wondered whether there might not be some means of selecting patients for chemotherapy on a more scientific basis than clinical impression.

Several lines of reasoning suggested that estrogen receptor (ER) determination might be of significant help. First, it is known that tumors that are ER-negative (ER^-) tend to have higher thymidine labeling indices and higher mitotic indices (MEYER et al., 1977). More rapidly growing tumors might be expected to respond more favorably to chemotherapy that is cell cycle phase-specific. Second, premenopausal women, who tend to have more rapidily growing tumors, shorter disease-free intervals, and better responses to chemotherapy, at least in the adjuvant setting, are more frequently ER^- (ALLEGRA et al.; KNIGHT et al., 1977; FISHER et al., 1975; BONNADONNA et al., 1977). Thirdly, the response rates to secondary endocrine or chemotherapy tend generally to be lower than are obtained when these procedures are used as primary therapy, implying that tumors tend to respond to one form of therapy and not the other. Finally, in leukemia, glucocorticoid receptor levels tend to correlate with slower-growing tumors with more prolonged responses to chemotherapy (KONIOR et al., 1977).

Thus, we studied the relationship of ER to response rate to cytotoxic chemotherapy in a cohort of 70 women.

The study methods employed have been described in detail elsewhere (LIPPMAN et al., 1978). The most important features of the design are as follows. First, all patients had ER assays performed on metastatic foci immediately before the institution of cytotoxic chemotherapy. Second, an arbitrary cut-off of 10 fmol per mg cytoplasmic protein was chosen in advance. Third, uniform and widely accepted response criteria were employed, requiring a minimum of

Table 1. Characteristics of the patients treated with cytotoxic chemotherapy as a function of ER status

	RE+	ER−	*P* value ER+ vs ER−
Number of patients	25	45	
Mean estrogen receptor content (fmol/mg cytoplasmic protein)	56	2	
Age (mean ± SD)	50 ± 10	52 ± 11	> 0.1
Menopausal status			
Pre	6/25 (24%)	13/45 (28%)	> 0.1
Post	19/25 (76%)	32/45 (72%)	
Karnofsky index (mean ± SD)	89 ± 10	88 ± 10	> 0.1
Disease-free interval (months) (mean ± SD)	17 ± 11	22 ± 12	> 0.1
Number of sites involved			
1	7	15	
2	5	13	> 0.1
3	13	17	
Prior therapy	7/25 (28%)	9/45 (20%)	> 0.1
Endocrine	7/25 (28%)	9/45 (20%)	> 0.1
Chemotherapy	1/25 (4%)	1/45 (2%)	> 0.1
Median time from first recurrence to chemotherapy trial (months)	1.5	3.0	> 0.1

50% regression of all measurable disease for 2 months and the appearance of no new lesions. Fourth, response rate was assessed by investigators unaware of the ER results. Fifth, as an additional control, response to endocrine therapy as a function of ER status was assessed in an entirely unrelated group of 85 patients (ALLEGRA et al.). In this group, ER positivity predicted response for 34 of 52 patients (65%) whereas ER negativity was associated with absence of response in 30 of 33 patients (91%). Thus, we are confident that the ER assay as performed in our laboratory (LIPPMAN et al., 1978) gives expected predictive accuracy and is therefore valid.

Obviously many prognostic variables may influence response rates to chemotherapy. Thus, it is critical to evaluate whether or not ER^+ and ER^- patients are similar with respect to important clinical features known to influence clinical outcome. Patient characteristics are shown in Table 1. As shown, patient age, menopausal status, Karnofsky performance index, number of sites involved with metastatic disease, proportion receiving prior therapy, and disease-free interval are similar.

Sites involved with metastatic disease are shown in Table 2. While basically similar numbers of each site are shown, there is a significantly higher number of patients with visceral involvement. This potential bias quite probably arose because of a tendency on the part of clinicians managing these patients to advance them directly to chemotherapy trials if they had

Table 2. Sites of involvement of patients treated with cytotoxic chemotherapy

Tumor site	ER+	ER–	*P* value ER+ vs ER–
Skin	15/25	28/45	> 0.1
Soft tissue	12/25	16/45	> 0.1
Node	6/25	11/45	> 0.1
Lung	12/25	13/45	> 0.1
Pleura	4/25	3/45	> 0.1
Ascites	–	1/45	> 0.1
Brain	1/25	2/45	> 0.1
Liver	12/25	10/45	< 0.05
Bone	14/25	19/45	> 0.1
Bone marrow	2/25	4/45	> 0.1

Table 3. Chemotherapy regimens[a] employed in evaluating response as a function of ER status

Therapy	ER+ (n = 25)	ER– (n = 45)
Adriamycin-containing therapies		
A	1	0
A-V	1	2
A-M-F	0	1
A-D-V	2	1
C-A-V	2	0
C-A	1	0
C-A-F	9	9
C-A-M-F	0	15
C-M-F-A-D-V	0	2
P-A-V	0	2
	16 (64%)	32 (71%) $P > 0.1$
Therapies without adriamycin		
C-F	1	0
C-M-F	7	9
C-M-F-V	0	3
Platinum	0	1
Cytembena	1	0
	9 (36%)	13 (29%) $P > 0.1$

[a] A, adriamycin; C, cytoxan; D, dibromodulcitol; F, 5-fluorouracil; M, methotrexate; P, L-phenylalanine mustard; V, vincristine.

Table 4. Response rate to cytotoxic chemotherapy as a function of ER status

	Response rate
ER+	3/25 (12%)
ER–	34/45 (76%)

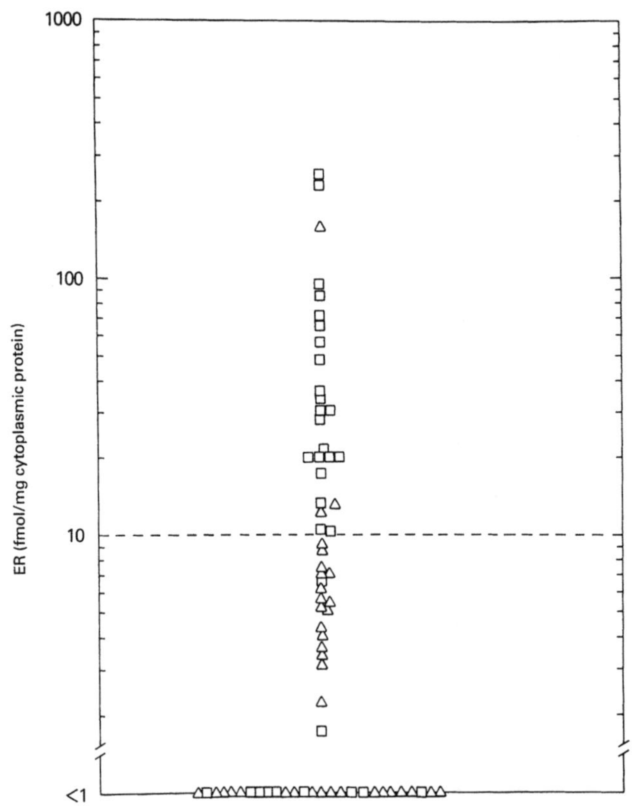

Fig. 1. The influence of ER status on objective response rate to cytotoxic chemotherapy in metastatic breast cancer. Responders include those with complete and those with partial responses. The 37 responders are shown by *triangles* (△) and the 33 nonresponders by squares (□). The *dashed line* at 10 fmol/mg cytoplasmic protein is the cutoff employed in this study for separating ER^+ from ER^- patients

extensive visceral disease, irrespective of ER status. Later it will be shown that the higher proportion of ER^+ patients with visceral disease does not influence the results.

The therapies administered are shown in Table 3. As can be seen, a large number of combinations and single agents were employed. Basically, the proportion of patients receiving a combination with or without adriamycin is identical. In addition, median white blood cell nadirs were identical in the ER^+ and ER^- groups receiving therapy. Only one patient in each group received a minimally active single agent (cytembena or *cis*-platinum). No patient received less than two cycles of chemotherapy before being termed a nonresponder. All patients in the ER^+ and the ER^- groups who were receiving the same therapy, e.g., CMF, were treated according to an identical protocol with identical dosage modifications. Finally, although 15 patients in the ER^- group received a CAMF combination not used in the ER^+ group (because of a hierarchy of other protocols employed at the NCI); the response rate in

Table 5. Response rates to cytotoxic chemotherapy of different sites as a function of ER status

Tumor site	ER+	ER−	*P* value ER+ vs ER−
Skin	1/15	20/28	< 0.0001
Soft tissue	0/12	9/16	< 0.001
Node	0/6	8/11	< 0.0001
Lung	2/12	6/13	> 0.1
Pleura	0/4	3/3	< 0.01
Ascites		0/1	
Brain	0/1	0/2	
Liver	0/12	2/10	> 0.1
Bone	1/14	13/19	< 0.005
Bone marrow	0/2	2/4	

Table 6. Response rates to cytotoxic chemotherapy as a function of type of chemotherapy and status

	Drug combinations containing adriamycin	Drug combinations without adriamycin	Single agents	Total
ER+	3/16	0/8	0/1	3/25
ER−	26/32	8/12	0/1	34/45
	$P < 0.005$	$P < 0.025$		$P < 0.0001$

this subset of patients will be shown to be no different from that in the ER^- group as a whole.

The overall response rate to cytotoxic chemotherapy is shown in Table 4. Thirty-four of 45 ER^- and 3 of 25 ER^+ patients had an objective response to chemotherapy ($P < 0.001$). The overall response rate is 37 of 70 patients (53%), and is typical of what one might expect for such a varied group of chemotherapy.

The distribution of responders and nonresponders as a function of ER concentration is shown in Fig. 1. When the distribution of responders and nonresponders is examined with respect to ER status by Wilcoxan rank sum analysis there is a significant difference ($P < 0.005$). No retrospectively chosen cut-off value for ER concentration positivity yields better discrimination than the one chosen prospectively.

The response rate as a function of site involved is shown in Table 5. There are more sites than patients since most patients had more than one site involved with metastatic disease. In addition, not every site actually regressed in a patient termed a responder, since criteria of response allow that some sites remain stable while others regress. Nonetheless, it is apparent that patients with visceral involvement respond no differently from patients with soft tissue or bone involvement, provided that they are members of the same ER subset.

Response as a function of type of therapy is summarised in Table 6. Regardless of therapy, ER^- patients respond more frequently to cytotoxic chemotherapy than ER^+ patients. Furthermore, if the 15 patients in the ER^--group receiving CAMF are subtracted from the 34 of 45 ER^- responders, the resultant 30-patient group contains 25 responders, and this response rate is not different from that of the initial group.

It is interesting to note that all responders in the ER^+ group received a combination containing adriamycin. We firmly believe that receptor status is not directly related to chemotherapy response. That is, ER is a necessary, albeit insufficient, requirement for a hormone response. The receptor is a direct mediator of hormone action. On the other hand, we believe that the association between lack of receptor and response to chemotherapy is indirect and possibly due to a correlation between receptor status and tumor kinetics. Thus we could expect that a variety of factors, such as certain types of chemotherapy, chemotherapy schedules, prior therapy with its selective pressure on tumor cell populations and tumor bulk (adjuvant versus advanced disease setting) might all significantly alter the usefulness of the ER test in predicting response to cytotoxic chemotherapy. This may explain some of the controversy in the literature that has sprung up subsequent to the publication of our initial results (LIPPMAN et al., 1978). FRENNING et al. (1978) have shown opposite results. That is, they claim that ER^+ patients respond to chemotherapy more often. This study is not yet available for detailed analysis. In contrast, other authors have published their results, which show that ER^- patients respond twice as frequently to chemotherapy as ER^+ patients (JONAT and MAASS, to be published). Obviously, further analyses with careful attention to details of therapy and other prognostic variables will be required for the true nature of the association between ER and chemotherapy response rate to be understood.

We believe our data do have certain implications, however. Our data suggest that ER status is an important variable and as such should be considered as a stratification criterion prospectively in randomized trials, or the distribution of ER^+ and ER^- patients in each arm should be determined retrospectively as a source of potential bias. Second, our data suggest a testable hypothesis as to why some patients (ER^+) show resistence to chemotherapy. Conceivably, less cell cycle-specific therapy or efforts to recruit ER^+ cells with endocrine therapy may significantly aid in the chemotherapy of ER^+ patients. Third, on the assumption that many tumors are heterogeneous mixes of ER^+ and ER^- cells (MERCER et al., 1978), our data predict that at least some patients may convert from ER^- to ER^+ status following cytotoxic chemotherapy, presumably on the basis of selection of relatively resistant ER^+ cells. Finally, our data may help to explain why results with cytotoxic chemotherapy are relatively unrewarding in postmenopausal females in the adjuvant setting. These women are more frequently ER^+ (well over 80% in some series) and thus possibly less responsive to drug therapy. Clearly adjuvant data need to be analysed in the light of receptor status.

References

Allegra, J. C., Lippman, M. E., Thompson, E. B.: Estrogen receptor status is the most important prognostic variable in predicting response to endocrine therapy in metastatic breast cancer. Eur. J. Cancer (submitted)

Allegra, J. C., Lippman, M. E., Thompson, E. B.: The frequency, distribution, and quantitative analysis of steroid hormone receptors in patients with breast cancer. Cancer Res. (submitted)

Bonadonna, G., Rossi, A., Valagussa, P., Banti, A., Veronesi, U.: The CMF program for operable breast cancer with positive axillary nodes: Updated analysis on the disease free interval, site of relapse, and drug tolerance. Cancer *39,* 2904–2915 (1977)

Fisher, B., Carbone, P., Economou, S. G., Frelick, R., Glass, A., Lerner, H., Redmond, C., Zelen, M., Band, P., Katrych, D. L., Wolmark, N., Fisher, E. R.: L-phenylalanine mustard (L-PAM) in the management of primary breast cancer. A report of early findings. N. Engl. J. Med. *292,* 117–122 (1975)

Frenning, D. H., Kennedy, B. J., Vosika, J.: Correlation of estrogen receptors and response to chemotherapy in advanced breast cancer. Proc. Am. Soc. Clin. Oncol., Abstract C-162 (1978)

Jonat, W., Maass, H.: Some comments on the necessity of receptor determination in human breast cancer. Cancer Res. (to be published)

Knight, W. A., Livingston, R. B., Gregory, E. J., McGuire, W. L.: Estrogen receptor as an independent prognostic factor for early recurrence in breast cancer. Cancer Res. *37,* 4669–4671 (1977)

Konior, G. S., Lippman, M. E., Johnson, G. E.: Correlation of glucorticoid receptor levels and complete remission duration in "poor prognosis" acute lymphoblastic leukemia. Proc. Am. Soc. Clin. Oncol., Abstract C-346 (1977)

Lippman, M. E., Huff, K. K.: A demonstration of androgen and estrogen receptors in human breast cancer using a new protamine sulfate assay. Cancer *38,* 868–874 (1976)

Lippman, M. E., Allegra, J. C., Thompson, E. B., Simon, R., Barlock, A., Green, L., Huff, K. K., Do, H. M. T., Aitken, S. C., Warren, R.: The relation between estrogen receptors and response rate to cytotoxic chemotherapy in metastatic breast cancer. N. Engl. J. Med. *298,* 1223–1228 (1978)

Mercer, W. D., Wahl, T. M., Carlson, C. A.: Identification of estrogen receptors in human breast cancer cells by immunofluorescence. Proc. Am. Soc. Clin. Pathol., Abstract No. 28 (1978)

Meyer, J. S., Rao, B. R., Stevens, S. C., White, W. L.: Low incidence of estrogen receptor in breast carcinomas with rapid rates of cellular replication. Cancer *40,* 2290–2298 (1977)

24. *The Influence of a Polychemotherapeutic Regimen on the Female Endocrine Control Mechanisms in Mammary Carcinoma Patients*

K.-D. Schulz, P. Schmidt-Rhode, P. Weymar, H. J. Künzig, and W. Geiger

Universitäts-Frauenklinik, Kerpener Straße 34, D-5000 Köln 41 (FRG)

Since chemotherapy was introduced into the treatment of malignant tumours, cytostatically induced amenorrhoea has been repeatedly described as an undesirable endocrine side effect in sexually mature women.

Since various malignancies, such as mammary carcinoma, endometrial carcinoma, and in some cases also ovarian carcinoma, react sensitively to a change of endocrine milieu due to their endocrine dependency, a detailed investigation of the hypothalo-hypophyseo-ovarian axis under the influence of carcinostatic polychemotherapy seemed necessary.

Only exact knowledge of endocrine changes will permit a rational combination of hormonal and chemotherapeutic treatment measures in respect of patients suffering from the above-mentioned tumours.

Three groups of patients with metastasising mammary carcinomas were studied within the scope of the present examination:

1) Sexually mature women with intact, undisturbed, ovarian function.
2) Menopausal patients with disorders of ovarian function characteristic of this time of life.
3) Postmenopausal patients, who had had their last menstrual periods at least 5 and not more than 15 years before.

All patients received a polychemotherapeutic regimen, either the combination of adriamycin and cyclophosphamide described by SALMON-JONES (1974) or the slightly modified regimen described by BONADONNA et al. (1976), involving a combination of cyclophosphamide, methotrexate, and 5-fluorouracil. In both cases the interval therapeutic scheme was used.

According to the development of haematotoxicity, the actual treatment cycle lasting 1—2 weeks was followed by a therapy-free interval of 2—3 weeks.

The analysis of plasma samples obtained from all the patients for their content of FSH, LH, prolactin, 17β-oestradiol, testosterone, and progesterone was carried out with the aid of radioimmunological determination methods. Since it was at first unknown when and in what form disorders of the ovarian cycle control would occur during polychemotherapy, we initially limited ourselves to the analysis of clinical data, such as menstrual history and basal temperature curves, in the sexually mature and menopausal patients.

Table 1 shows that after an average treatment duration of 4—5 months, disorders of ovarian function invariably occurred in all 15 mature patients investigated. These disorders were ap-

Table 1. Beginning and type of ovarian functional disorder during cytostatic treatment in women with intact ovarian function before treatment

No.	Pat.	Age	Type of ovarian functional disorders	Duration of therapy before onset of ovarian disorders (months)	Total dose of cytostatic drugs befor onset of ovarian disorders
1	IF	37	Luteal insufficiency	6	455 mg adriamycin/ 5.6 g cyclophosphamide
2	IU	37	Luteal insufficiency	9	600 mg adriamycin/ 7.6 g cyclophosphamide
3	WH	32	Luteal insufficiency anovulatory cycles	1	60 mg adriamycin/ 0.8 g cyclophosphamide
4	MB	40	Luteal insufficiency	4	180 mg adriamycin/ 1.8 g cyclophosphamide
5	PJ	38	Luteal insufficiency; oligomenorrhoea	4	260 mg adriamycin 2.6 g cyclophosphamide
6	GV	39	Oligomenorrhoea; anovulatory cycles	3	195 mg adriamycin/ 1.8 g cyclophosphamide
7	CF	40	a) Anovulatory oligomenorrhoea	2.5	160 mg adriamycin/ 1.8 g cyclophosphamide
			b) Amenorrhoea	5	260 mg adriamycin/ 3.0 g cyclophosphamide
8	MH	39	a) Luteal insufficiency	2	160 mg adriamycin/ 1.8 g cyclophosphamide
			b) Amenorrhoea	4	280 mg adriamycin/ 3.0 g cyclophosphamide
9	HF	32	Luteal insufficiency	5.5	10.5 g cyclophosphamide 10 g 5-fluorouracil 300 mg methotrexate
10	IK	42	Anovulatory cycles	5	10.5 g cyclophosphamide 10 g 5-fluorouracil 300 mg methotrexate
11	IB	28	a) Anovulatory oligomenorrhoea	8	14.7 g cyclophosphamide 14 g 5-fluorouracil 420 mg methotrexate
			b) Amenorrhoea	11	23.1 g cyclophosphamide 22 g 5-fluorouracil 660 mg methotrexate

Table 1 (continued)

No.	Pat.	Age	Type of ovarian functional disorders	Duration of therapy before onset of ovarian disorders (months)	Total dose of cytostatic drugs befor onset of ovarian disorders
12	IR	37	a) Oligomenorrhoea and luteal insufficiency b) Amenorrhoea	3	6.3 g cyclophosphamide 6 g 5-fluorouracil 180 mg methotrexate 8.4 g cyclophosphamide 8 g 5-fluorouracil 240 mg methotrexate
14	DS	33	Luteal insufficiency	6	10.5 g cyclophosphamide 10 g f-fluorouracil 300 mg methotrexate
15	AK	30	Oligomenorrhoea	2.5	4.2 g cyclophosphamide 4 g 5-fluorouracil 120 mg methotrexate

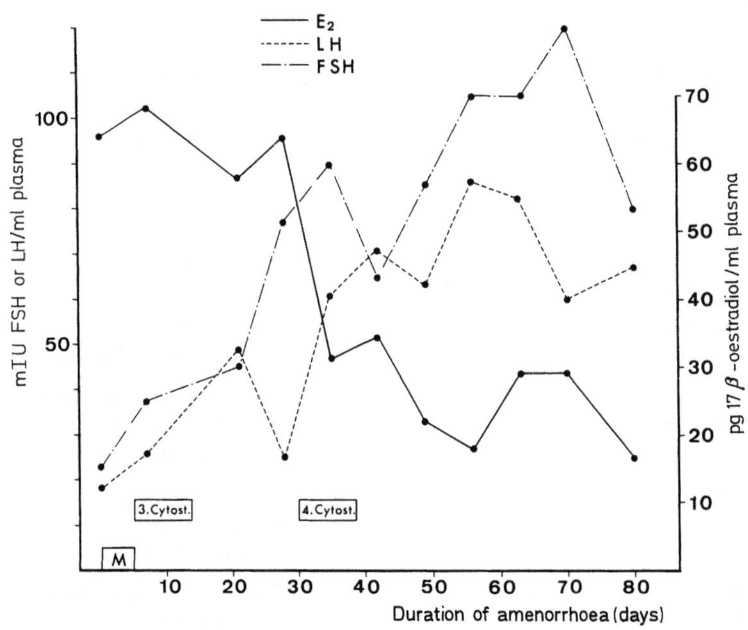

Fig. 1. Endocrine characterisation of chemotherapeutically induced amenorrhoea. ——, E_2; – – –, LH; – - –, FSH

parent chiefly in the form of oligomenorrhoea, polymenorrhoea, anovulatory cycles, or corpus luteum insufficiency.

Consecutive amenorrhoea was only observed in four cases. The endocrine characterisation of this amenorrhoea can be deduced from a typical example presented in Fig. 1. After the end of

Table 2. Onset and type of ovarian functional disorder apparent in amenorrhoea during cytostatic treatment in premenopausal patients

No.	Pat.	Age	Characteristics of the menstrual cycle before therapy	Duration of therapy before onset of amenorrhoea (months)	Dose of cytostatic drugs given before onset of amenorrhoea
1	GG	50	21/35 days, anovulatory	3	180 mg ADM; 1.8 g cyclophosphamide (3 cycles ADM/ cyclophosphamide)
2	US	50	28/30 days, anovulatory	1	130 mg ADM; 1.6 g cyclophosphamide (2 cycles ADM/ cyclophosphamide)
3	KH	50	24/30 days, anovulatory	2	140 mg ADM; 1.2 g cyclophosphamide (2 cycles ADM/ cyclophosphamide)
4	DK	48	22/30 days, corpus luteum insufficiency	1	130 mg ADM; 1.2 g cyclophosphamide (2 cycles ADM/ cyclophosphamide)
5	SM	45	28/36 days, corpus luteum insufficiency	2.5	195 mg ADM; 2.4 g cyclophosphamide (3 cycles ADM/ cyclophosphamide)
6	RS	48	22/37 days, irregular, sometimes anovulatory cycles	3	4.2 g cyclophosphamide 4 g 5-FU; 120 mg MTX (3 cycles CMF)
7	JB	45	28/40 days, luteal insufficiency	2	4.2 g cyclophosphamide, 4 g 5-FU; 120 mg MTX (3 cycles CMF)

the last menstruation, there is a very rapid reduction in ovarian oestradiol synthesis. The values obtained from plasma analysis are similar to those obtained in ovariectomised or postmenopausal patients. In contrast to this there is a considerable increase of hypophyseal gononadotropin secretion. This hypergonadotropic situation continues despite continuation of the chemotherapy.

The investigation permits the conclusion that disorders in the ovarian regulatory cycle evoked by cytostatic treatment take place primarily in the ovary itself. Only then does the decline in plasma oestradiol concentration lead to a secondary increase of FSH and LH liberation from the hypophysis through a negative feedback control of the hypothalamus.

Table 3. Hormonal parameters in premenopausal women after 2–3 months' cytostatic treatment

No.	Patient	Age	pg E_2/ml plasma	mIU FSH/ml plasma	mIU LH/ml plasma
1	KD	48	42	60	31
			33	58	54
			39	65	49
2	GG	50	42		52
			18		51
			11		38
3	US	50	23	82	65
			26	95	54
			18	59	76
4	SM	45	18		54
			31		84
			11		75
5	RS	48	35		107
			20		88
			52		96

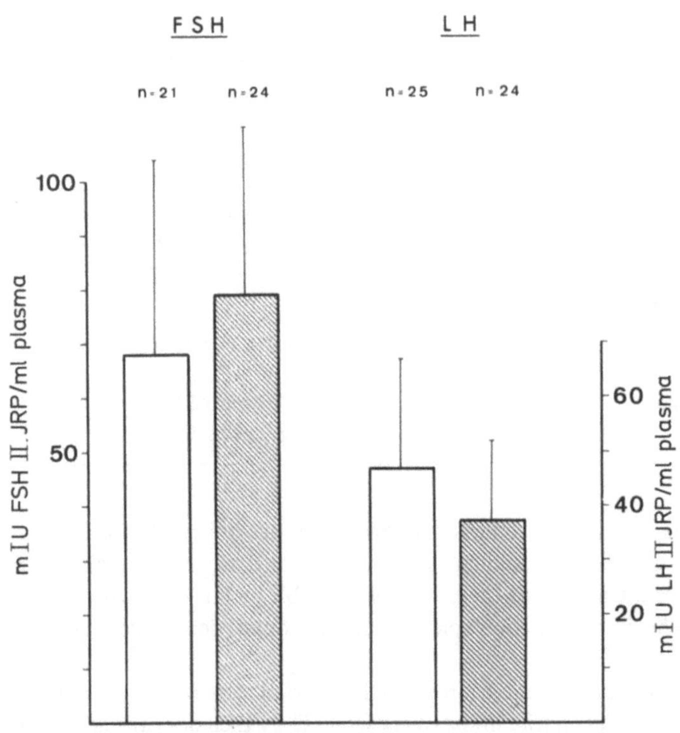

Fig. 2. Comparative studies of the FSH and LH plasma concentrations in healthy postmenopausal women (□) and in postmenopausal patients with metastasising mammary carcinoma (▨)

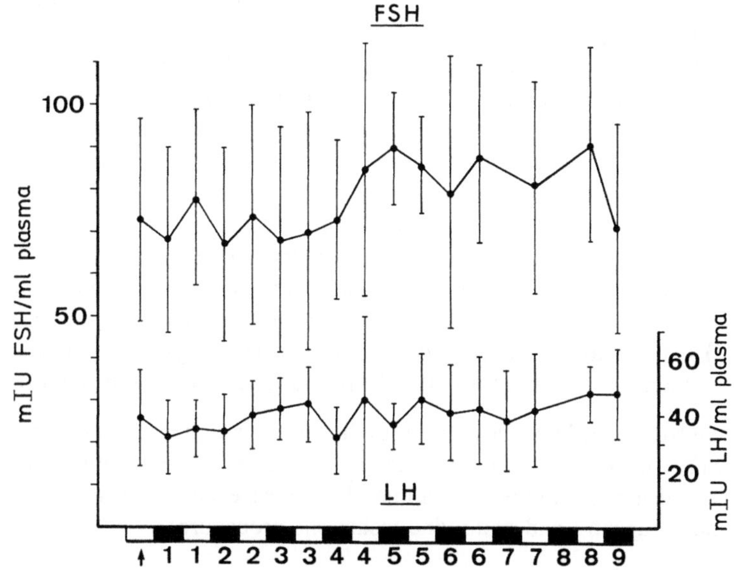

Fig. 3. The behaviour of hypophyseal FSH and LH secretion in postmenopausal patients during polychemotherapy. ●—●, number of treatment cycles; ● — ●, number of therapy-free intervals. *Arrow* indicates untreated control

Table 2 shows observations made in the seven menopausal patients. In these cases there were already disorders of ovarian function before therapy, such as luteal insufficiency, oligomenorrhoea, polymenorrhoea, or anovulatory cycles. The hormonal characteristics of the ovarian functional disorders typical of this phase of life have recently been presented by different groups of workers (SHERMAN et al., 1976; KAISER et al., 1977). In these patients amenorrhoea occurred very early in the polychemotherapeutic regimen. In all cases an effect of this kind occurred after 1–3 months' treatment. Table 3 shows that hypergonodotropic amenorrhoea develops as a sign of primary damage to the female gonads. The ovary seems to be far more sensitive in this age group than in younger women. In the course of our further investigations the influence of cancerostatic polychemotherapy on the endocrine system of postmenopausal women was investigated. First a comparison of the different hormonal parameters in healthy women and in patients of the same postmenopausal age with metastasising mammary carcinoma was carried out. As Fig. 2 shows, there is no significant difference between the two groups in hypophyseal FSH and LH secretion. Identical values were obtained for the plasma concentrations of prolactin, 17β-oestradiol, progesterone, and testosterone in both groups.

After high-dose chemotherapy for over 9 months, no change of the hypophyseal gonadotropin liberation could be demonstrated in postmenopausal patients with disseminated mammary carcinoma (Fig. 3). Nor did the prolactin, 17β-oestradiol, progesterone, and testosterone values in the plasma show any statistically significant reaction to the cytostatic regime. In summary, it has been shown that:

1) An *intermittent carcinostatic polychemotherapeutic regimen* is capable of producing sustained functional derangement of the hypothalamo-hypophyseo-ovarian axis. However, effects of this kind occur only in sexually mature patients. During the menopause there is no change of the above-mentioned hormonal parameters.

2) The *type of disorder* ranges from corpus luteum insufficiency through anovulatory cycles to amenorrhoea.
3) The *primary* and *most essential point of attack* of the cytostatic drugs investigated appears to be the ovary alone. The controlling regulatory centres, such as the hypothalamus and the hypophysis, show marked resistance. No cytostatically induced suppression of the gonadotropin secretion can be recognised. The negative feedback control of the hypothalamic region is preserved.
4) The *ovary of any patients with stable, intact cycles* is apparently relatively insensitive to chemotherapy. Although cycle disorders of different kinds do arise in all patients, only in a few cases are these functional changes finally transformed into amenorrhoea. This only takes place after long-lasting administration of cytostatics in high doses.
5) If there are *pretherapeutic disorders of ovarian function,* in these sense of menopausal changes, amenorrhoea usually results after short-term low-dose therapy.

It is to be hoped that the present results, together with receptor determination in tumour tissue, will prove to be of decisive assistance in the realm of therapeutic planning for patients with metastasising mammary carcinoma. This is especially relevant for the combination of chemotherapeutic and endocrine treatment procedures.

References

Bonadonna, G., Bursamolino, E., Valagussa, P., Rossi, A., Brugnatelli, L., Brambilla, C., De Lena, M., Tanani, G., Bajetta, E., Musumeci, R., Veronesi, U.: Combination chemotherapy as an adjuvant treatment in operable breast cancer. N. Engl. J. Med. *294,* 405 (1976)

Kaiser, R., Geiger, W., Künzig, H. J., Weymar, P.: Hormonanalytische Untersuchungen bei Zyklen in der Prämenopause. Arch. Gynaekol. *223,* 213 (1977)

Salmon, S. E., Jones, S. E.: Chemotherapy of advanced breast cancer with a combination of adriamycin and cyclophosphamide. Proc. Am. Assoc. Cancer Res. *15,* 359 (1974)

Sherman, B. M., West, J. H., Korenman, S. G.: The menopausal transition: analysis of LH, FSH, oestradiol and progesterone concentrations during menstrual cycles of older women. J. Clin. Endocrinol. *42,* 629 (1976)

25. *Therapeutic Effect of Tamoxifen Alone Versus Tamoxifen in Combination with Gestagen and Oestrogen in Advanced Breast Cancer*

H. T. Mouridsen, T. Palshof, and C. Rose

Finsen Institute, RII-RV, Strandboulevarden 49, DK-2100 Copenhagen Ø (Denmark)

Introduction

The treatments used in postmenopausal women with advanced breast cancer include additive endocrine therapy. Due to the same or better efficacy as with other preparations and to the mild side effects, most authors now believe that the anti-oestrogen compound tamoxifen (TAM) is the drug of choice when additive endocrine treatment is indicated (MOURIDSEN et al., 1978; TAGNON, 1977).

In unselected patient populations the response rate with TAM is about 35%, but in patients not previously treated with hormones the response rate is even higher, about 45%. The median duration of remission is about 12 months (MOURIDSEN et al., 1978).

It is now well established that the response rate with TAM is related to the presence of cytoplasmatic oestradiol receptor (ER) protein in the tumour (BARNES et al., 1977; KING, 1975; LECLERCQ and HEUSON, 1977; MOSESON et al., 1978; MOURIDSEN et al., 1978). Thus the response rate in ER-positive (ER^+) patients is about 60%, as against less than 10% in patients with ER-negative (ER^-) tumours. However, about 40% of patients with ER^+ tumours still fail to respond to treatment with TAM. The explanation for this is not known. Determination of nuclear receptor concentrations may increase the accuracy of response prediction, and the presence or absense of other steroid hormone receptors, such as gestagen and androgen receptor proteins, may also be considered.

With the aim of increasing the therapeutic effect of TAM we conducted two prospective clinical trials in which TAM was compared with TAM and medroxyprogesterone acetate (MPA) or TAM and diethylstilboestrol (DES). Only two similar studies have been published (TORMEY et al., 1976; WARD, 1977); in these combined treatment with TAM and androgen (TORMEY et al., 1976) or TAM and antiprolactin (WARD, 1977) was found to be only slightly superior to treatment with TAM alone.

Gestagen has been reported to induce remissions in 15%–45% of cases (ANSFIELD et al., 1974; GOLDENBERG, 1969; MUGGIA et al., 1968; PANNUTI et al., 1976; SEAGALOFF et al., 1967; STOLL, 1967). Although progesterone is generally considered to be an oestrogen antagonist (HSUEH et al., 1975), the mechanism of action in human breast cancer is not clear.

Administration of pharmacological doses of oestrogens to postmenopausal patients with advanced breast cancer can induce remission in about 30% of cases (HAYWARD, 1970). The mechanism of this action is also unknown.

It has been reported that about 70% of patients who had previously responded to endocrine therapy were able to achieve a second response to TAM (Kiang and Kennedy, 1977; Manni et al., 1976).

The aim of the present study was to compare the therapeutic effect of TAM alone with the effect of combined treatment with TAM + MPA and TAM + DES in postmenopausal patients with advanced breast cancer.

Material and Methods

From this point onward, Study I indicates the study comparing TAM and TAM + MPA, and Study II, the one comparing TAM and TAM + DES.

The patients in Study I were a consecutive series admitted to Departments R II–R V, Finsen Institute, the Department of Oncology, Malmö General Hospital, and Medical Department C, Bispebjerg Hospital, between 1 August 1976 and 1 August 1977.

The patients in Study II were a consecutive series admitted to Departments R II–R V, Finsen Institute, and Medical Department C, Bispebjerg Hospital between 1 September 1977 and 1 August 1978.

Eligibility requirements for the two studies were:

1) The patients must be postmenopausal, i.e., must have experienced at least 6 months' spontaneous amenorrhoea. Patients who had previously undergone hysterectomy must be more than 50 years of age. Patients who had previously undergone ovariectomy could enter the study 3 months after surgical or 6 months after actinic castration.
2) Patients less than 68 years of age must be clinically resistant to at least one cytostatic combination regimen. Patients more than 68 years of age could enter the study despite clinical resistance to cytostatic treatment.
3) There must be measurable disease.
4) The performance status must be ≥ 3.
5) Previous additive endocrine treatment must not have been given.
6) The patients should have given their verbal informed consent.

The patients were randomly allocated (using a stochastic array of numbers, closed envelope system) to one of two treatment groups.

Study I

Patients in Study I received treatment with 10 mg TAM three times daily or treatment with 10 mg TAM three times daily and 100 mg MPA daily p.o. as a single dose.

Study II

Patients in Study II received treatment with 10 mg TAM three times daily or treatment with 10 mg TAM three times daily and 1 mg DES three times daily.

Wherever possible, the treatments were maintained for at least 3 months before the response to treatment was assessed. If at 3 months there was still progressive disease the patient was withdrawn from the study. If at 3 months there was no change or a remission the patient continued in the study until progression or relapse.

Pretreatment examinations included physical examination, chest roentgenogram, bone survey, laboratory tests (blood cell counts, serum calcium and liver function tests), and estimations of performance status. All visible and palpable lesions were measured to provide a baseline for subsequent examinations. These were repeated at 1- to 3-months intervals.

Furthermore, whenever possible, biopsies from tumour tissue were taken for analyses of ER protein by the dextran-charcoal method (Daehnfeldt and Briand, 1977) prior to therapy.

Response to treatment was defined according to the UICC criteria (Hayward et al., 1977), as follows:

Complete remission (CR): complete disappearance of all measurable lesions.

Partial remission (PR): 50%–99% reduction of measurable lesions and/or recalcification of bone lesions.

No change (NC): <50% reduction of measurable lesions and/or no visible changes in bone lesions.

Progressive disease (PD): 50% increase of measurable lesions and/or definite decalcification of bone lesions.

Duration of response was dated from the start of therapy up to PD.

Results

Study I

Study I involved 101 patients, and their characteristics are shown in Table 1: 46 patients were randomised to treatment with TAM and 55 patients to the combined treatment with TAM + MPA. One patient treated with TAM was lost to follow-up before she had been treated for 3 months and is therefore considered nonevaluable.

The patients randomised to the two regimens were comparable as regards age, length of disease-free interval, previous treatment with cytotoxic agents, and dominant metastatic site.

Table 1. TAM versus TAM + MPA in advanced breast cancer. Patients

		TAM	TAM + MPA
Patients entered	(n)	46	55
Patients not evaluable	(n)	1	0
Patients evaluable	(n)	45	55
Age, median	(years, range)	60 (44–81)	61 (49–81)
Disease-free interval, median	(months, range)	18 (0–144)	18 (0–120)
Previous chemotherapy	(%)	71	65
Patient with dominant disease site	(n)		
Soft tissue		16	18
Bones		13	16
Viscera		17	21
ER+[a]	(n/total)	11/20	9/21
ER–	(n/total)	9/20	12/21

[a] ER+ indicates an ER protein concentration of ≥ 20 fmol/mg protein.

Table 2. TAM versus TAM + MPA in advanced breast cancer

	TAM	TAM + MPA
PD[a]	18/45 = 40%	25/55 = 46%
NC	7/45 = 16%	16/55 = 29%
PR	16/45 = 35%	10/55 = 18%
CR	4/45 = 9%	4/55 = 7%
PR + CR	20/45 = 44%	14/55 = 26%

[a] PD includes patients with progressive disease at the time of assessment of results after 3 months' treatment and patients with rapidly progressive disease and death before this time.

Table 3. TAM versus TAM + MPA in advanced breast cancer. Duration of remission in months in patients with PR + CR

	TAM			TAM + MPA		
	n	Median	Range	n	Median	Range
PR	16	10	6 – 14+	10	9	4 – 16+
CR	4	9	6 – 15+	4	12+	8+ – 17+

Oestrogen receptor determinations were performed in 20 of the patients receiving TAM only and 21 of the patients receiving the combined therapy. ER^+ and ER^- tumours are equally distributed in the two patient groups (Table 1).

At the time of analysis 10 months had passed since entry of the last patient.

The results of therapy are shown in Table 2. Statistical analysis revealed no significant difference ($P > 0.2$) (Mann–Whitney rank sum test, unpaired data) between the two treatment regimens. However, remission (PR + CR) was obtained in 20 patients (45%) with TAM, compared with 14 patients (26%) with TAM + MPA. The 95% confidence limits of the difference between the remission rates ($d \pm 0.2$ SED) is 0%–38% (WULF, 1973), indicating that treatment with TAM will at best, induce PR + CR in 38% more of the patients than TAM + MPA. At worst, treatment with TAM will induce the same number of remissions as treatment with the combination.

The median duration of remission did not differ significantly between the two treatments, and so far there is no difference between duration of remission in patients achieving PR and in those achieving CR (Table 3).

Response rates correlated with ER, as shown in Table 4. The response rates in the ER^+ patients are the same with TAM alone as with combined TAM and MPA ($P > 0.1$).

Side effects occurred in 12 patients, evenly distributed in the two treatment groups. Three patients had hot flushes, three oedema, one hypercalcaemia, one loss of hair, and one headache. Three patients had vaginal bleeding and treatment with TAM and MPA had to be discontinued in one of these patients. Otherwise the treatments were extremely well tolerated.

Table 4. TAM versus TAM + MPA in advanced breast cancer. Relationship between response (PR + CR) and ER content

	TAM	TAM + MPA
ER+	7/11 (~63%)	4/9 (~44%)
ER−	2/9 (~22%)	2/12 (~17%)

Table 5. TAM versus TAM + DES in advanced breast cancer

		TAM	TAM + DES
Patients entered	(n)	49	40
Too early to evaluate	(n)	8	6
Patients not evaluable	(n)	3	2
Patients evaluable	(n)	38	32
Age, median	(years, range)	69 (42–83)	69 (46–82)
Disease-free interval, median	(months, range)	30 (6–204)	30 (0–108)
Previous chemotherapy	(%)	50	50
Patient with dominant disease site	(n)		
Soft tissue		16	13
Bones		6	8
Viscera		16	11
ER+[a]	(n/total)	4/11	4/11
ER−	(n/total)	7/11	7/11

[a] ER+ indicates an ER protein concentration of ≥ 20 fmol/mg protein.

Study II

Study II involved 89 patients (Table 5). It was too early to evaluate the results in 14 of these patients, and five of them were not evaluable. In four of these cases (two in each group) the patients themselves discontinued treatment due to side effects before 3 months had passed, and one patient was lost to follow-up. Of the other 70 patients, 38 were randomised to treatment with TAM and 32 to treatment with TAM + DES. As Table 5 shows the two groups of patients were comparable with respect to age, disease-free interval, previous chemotherapy, and localisation of the dominant disease. Analysis for ER was performed in 11 of the evaluable patients in each group and ER^+ and ER^- tumours were equally distributed.

The response to treatment is shown in Table 6. No difference between the two groups in the numbers of responders and nonresponders was observed ($P > 0.8$). The observation period was too short to allow calculation of the median duration of remission, as more than 50% of the responders were still in remission when the results were analysed.

Only very few data are available concerning the relationship between frequency of response and ER content (Table 7), but in agreement with other studies most of the responders are found among the ER^+ patients.

Side effects occurred most frequently and were most pronounced with the combined treatment (Table 8). Two patients in each group discontinued treatment due to nausea after

Table 6. TAM versus TAM + DES in advanced breast cancer

	TAM	TAM + DES
PD	11/38 = 29%	11/32 = 34%
NC	11/38 = 29%	9/32 = 28%
PR	12/38 = 32%	6/32 = 19%
CR	4/38 = 11%	6/32 = 19%
PR + CR	16/38 = 42%	12/32 = 38%
Duration of remission (months), median (range)	6+(3+–12+)	5+(3–11.5+)

Table 7. TAM versus TAM + DES in advanced breast cancer. Relationship between response (PR + CR) and ER content

	TAM	TAM + DES	Total
ER+	3/4	1/4	4/8
ER–	0/7	1/7	1/14

Table 8. TAM versus TAM + DES in advanced breast cancer. Side effects

	TAM	TAM + DES
Nausea	4	8
Vaginal bleeding	0	2
Thrombophlebitis	0	1
Breast pain	0	3
Leg cramps	0	1
Total	4/41	15/34

1–2 months of treatment. Vaginal bleeding occurred in two patients after 7 and 8 months of treatment with TAM + DES. Both patients were in remission at that time and continued treatment with TAM alone. No cases of biochemical or haematological side effects were observed.

Discussion

The results of this study give no evidence for an improvement in response rate when TAM is combined with MPA or DES at the particular dose levels examined. On the contrary, it seems that treatment with TAM alone can give a higher remission than treatment with TAM +

MPA. The rate of remission in response to treatment with TAM + DES is equal to that with TAM alone.

The lack of an additive effect with either combination might be explained by interference with the pharmacokinetics of TAM by MPA or DES, resulting in decreased absorption in the gastrointestinal tract, altered metabolism, or decreased uptake in the tumour cell. Because a valid assay for TAM is not at our disposal we have not been able to elucidate these questions.

In the case of the combination TAM + MPA, another possible explanation is pharmacodynamic interaction. It seems reasonable to believe that such interactions would take place at the receptor level.

Experimental (Milgrom et al., 1973) and clinical data (McGuire and Horwitz, 1977; Stoll, 1967b) support the hypothesis that synthesis of the progesterone receptor in mammary tumour tissue needs an actively functioning ER. Anti-oestrogen given at the same time as progesterone will therefore have indirect antiprogesterone effects.

In general, progesterone acts as an oestrogen antagonist, reducing the amount of ER in the target tissues (Hsueh et al., 1975) and decreasing the time the ER complex is in the nucleus (Hsueh et al., 1976).

Experimental results with DMBA-induced rat mammary tumours suggest that TAM possibly exerts its effect in the same manner, namely by opposing the replenishment of the cytoplasmic ER (Nicholson et al., 1976).

However, with the mature rat uterus as a target tissue it has recently been shown (Koseki et al., 1977) that TAM does allow replenishment of the ER in the cytoplasm. Furthermore, TAM causes elevated nuclear ER levels. This may indicate that the TAM–receptor complex acts by way of a more profound alteration at the transcriptional level. If, therefore, progesterone can reduce the time the TAM–receptor complex remains in the nucleus, progesterone may oppose the action of TAM.

As mentioned earlier, the mode of action of DES remains unknown. Theoretically, TAM and DES should not antagonise each other at the receptor level, and the present data support this idea.

Evidence obtained with the human cell line MCF-7 indicates that the effect of high doses of oestrogens is nonspecific and not mediated through the ER (Lippman, 1976). Preliminary data from an on-going clinical adjuvant study (Palshof et al., 1978) support this observation. Thus it seems that the effect of adjuvant treatment with DES is independent of the ER status of the primary tumour.

However, in the present study any difference as regards mode of action of TAM and DES, has not resulted in any additive effect of treatment with the two drugs in combination.

In conclusion, the two studies indicate that neither combined treatment with TAM and MPA nor combined treatment with TAM and DES is better than treatment with TAM alone.

Summary

Postmenopausal patients, of whom all those under 68 years of age were resistant to chemotherapy, entered two clinical studies.

In Study I 46 patients were randomised to treatment with 10 mg tamoxifen (TAM) three times daily and 55 to treatment with 10 mg TAM three times daily and 100 mg medroxyprogesterone acetate (MPA) once daily. Remission (PR + CR) was obtained in 20 patients (45%)

with TAM, as against 14 patients (26%) with TAM + MPA; however, this difference is not significant ($P > 0.2$). Nor was the median duration of remission significantly different with the two treatments: 6–15 months with the single drug compared with 4–17 + months with the combined treatment. Response rates correlated with the presence of oestrogen receptor (ER), with no differences in the two treatment groups. Side effects occurred in 12 patients.

In Study II the results have so far been evaluated in 38 patients randomised to treatment with 10 mg TAM three times daily and in 32 randomised to treatment with 10 mg TAM three times daily plus 1 mg DES three times daily. Remission (PR + CR) was achieved in 16 patients (42%) with TAM, as against 12 patients (38%) with the combined treatment ($P > 0.8$). The median duration of remission with the two treatments was 6+ and 5+ months, respectively. Response rates were related to the presence of ER. Side effects occurred in four patients treated with TAM and in 15 patients treated with TAM + DES.

References

Ansfield, F. J., Davis, H. C., Jr., Ellerby, R. A., Ramireg, G.: A clinical trial of megesterol acetate in advanced breast cancer. Cancer *33*, 907–910 (1974)

Barnes, D. M., Ribeiro, G. G., Skinner, L. G.: Two methods of measurements of oestradiol-17β and progesterone receptors in human breast cancer and correlation with response to treatment Eur. J. Cancer *13*, 1133–1145 (1977)

Dæhnfeldt, J. L., Briand, P.: Determination of high affinity gestagen receptors in hormone responsive and hormone-independent GR mouse mammary tumors by an exchange assay. In: Progesterone receptors in normal and neoplastic tissues. McGuire, W. L., Raynaud, J.-P., Baulieu, E.-E. (eds.), p. 59. New York: Raven Press 1977

Goldenberg, I. S.: Clinical trials of testolactone, medroxy-progesterone-acetate and oxylone acetate in advanced female mammary cancer. A report of The Cooperative Breast Cancer Group. Cancer *23*, 109–111 (1969)

Hayward, J.: Hormones and human breast cancer. Recent results in cancer research. Berlin, Heidelberg, New York: Springer 1970

Hayward, J. L., Carbone, P. P., Heuson, J.-C., Kumaoka, S., Segaloff, A., Rubens, R. D.: Assessment of response to therapy in advanced breast cancer. Eur. J. Cancer *13*, 89–94 (1977)

Hsueh, A. J. W., Peck, E. J., Clark, J. H.: Progesterone antagonism of the estrogen receptor and estrogen-induced uterine growth. Nature *254*, 337–339 (1975)

Hsueh, A. J. W., Peck, E. J., Clark, J. H.: Control of uterine estrogen receptor levels by progesterone. Endocrinologia *98*, 438–444 (1976)

Kiang, D. T., Kennedy, B. J.: Tamoxifen (antiestrogen) therapy in advanced breast cancer. Ann. Intern. Med. *87*, 687–690 (1977)

King, J. B.: Clinical relevance of steroid-receptor measurements in tumors. Cancer Treat. Rev. *2*, 273–295 (1975)

Koseki, Y., Zava, D. T., Chamness, G. G., McGuire, W. L.: Estrogen receptor translocation and replenishment by the antiestrogen tamoxifen. Endocrinologia *101*, 1104–1110 (1977)

Leclercq, G., Heuson, J.-C.: Therapeutic significance of sexsteroid hormone receptors in the treatment of breast cancer. Eur. J. Cancer *13*, 1205–1217 (1977)

Lippman, M.: Hormone-responsive human breast cancer in continuous tissue culture. In: Breast cancer: trends in research and treatment. Heuson, J.-C., Mattheiem, W. H., Rozencweig, M. (eds.), p. 111. New York: Raven Press 1976

Manni, A., Trujillo, J., Marshall, J. S., Pearson, O. H.: Antiestrogen-induced remissions in stage IV breast cancer. Cancer Treat. Rep. *60*, 1445–1450 (1976)

McGuire, W. L., Horwitz, K. B.: A role for progesterone in breast cancer. Ann. N.Y. Acad. Sci. *286,* 90–100 (1977)

Milgrom, E., Luu This, M., Atger, M., Baulieu, E. E.: Mechanisms regulating the concentration and the conformation of progesterone receptors in the uterus. J. Biol. Chem. *248,* 6366–6374 (1973)

Moseson, D. L., Sasaki, G. H., Kraybill, W. G., Leung, B. S., Davenport, C. E., Fletcher, W. S.: The use of antiestrogens tamoxifen and nafoxidine in the treatment of human breast cancer in correlation with estrogen receptor values. A phase II study. Cancer *41,* 797–800 (1978)

Mouridsen, H. T., Palshof, T., Patterson, J., Battersby, L.: Tamoxifen in advanced breast cancer. Cancer Treat. Rev. *5,* 131–141 (1978)

Muggia, F. M., Cassileth, P. A., Ochoa, Jr., M., Flatow, F. A., Gellhorn, A., Hyman, G. A.: Treatment of breast cancer with medroxyprogesterone-acetate. Ann. Intern. Med. *68,* 328–337 (1968)

Nicholson, R. I., Golder, M. P., Davies, P., Griffiths, K.: Effects of estradiol-17β and tamoxifen on total and accessible cytoplasmic estradiol-17β receptors in DMBA-induced rat mammary tumors. Eur. J. Cancer *12,* 711–717 (1976)

Palshof, T., Mouridsen, H. T., Dæhnfeldt, J.: Adjuvant endocrine therapy of breast cancer in premenopausal (placebo versus tamoxifen) and postmenopausal (placebo versus tamoxifen versus diethylstilboestrol) subjects In: Endocrine treatment of breast cancer. A new approach. Henningsen, B., Linder, F., Steichele, C. (eds.). Berlin, Heidelberg, New York: Springer 1980

Pannuti, F., Martoni, A., Lenaz, G. R., Piana, E., Nanni, P.: Management of advanced breast cancer with medroxyprogesteroneacetate (NSC 26386) in high doses. Functional exploration of serology, pp. 253–256 (1976)

Segaloff, A., Cuningham, M., Rice, B. F., Weeth, J. B.: Hormonal therapy in cancer of the breast. XIV – effect of corticosterone or medroxyprogesterone-acetate on the clinical course and hormonal excretion. Cancer *20,* 1673–1688 (1967)

Stoll, B.: Progestin therapy of breast cancer: Comparison of agents. Br. Med. J. *1967a III,* 338–341

Stoll, B.: Vaginal cytology as an aid to hormone therapy in postmenopausal cancer of the breast. Cancer *20,* 1807–1813 (1967b)

Tagnon, H. J.: Antiestrogens in the treatment of breast cancer. Cancer *39,* 2959–2964 (1977)

Tormey, D. C., Simon, R. M., Lippman, M. E., Bull, J. M., Myers, C. E.: Evaluation of tamoxifen dose in advanced breast cancer: A progress report. Cancer Treat. Rep. *60,* 1451–1459 (1976)

Ward, H. W. C.: Combined antiprolactin and antiestrogen therapy for breast carcinoma. Clin. Oncol. *3,* 91–95 (1977)

Wulf, H. R.: Confidence limits in evaluating controlled therapeutic trials. Lancet *1973 II,* 969

VI. Adjuvant Endocrine Therapy of Breast Cancer

26. *Is There a Place for Adjuvant Endocrine Therapy of Breast Cancer?*[1]

J. W. Meakin

The Princess Margaret Hospital and the University of Toronto, 500 Sherbourne Street, Toronto, M4X 1K9 (Canada)

Introduction

Is there a place for adjuvant endocrine therapy of breast cancer? The answer is not clear, but is probably "yes". More investigation needs to be done to define the role of adjuvant endocrine therapy. This paper is a summary of the present position and a consideration of future work.

Ovarian Ablation

As early as 1889, SCHINZINGER suggested that ovariectomy might be useful in the primary treatment of patients with breast cancer, but it was not until 1948 that the first prospective, randomized trial of the value of prophylactic ovarian irradiation was started in Manchester (COLE, 1968). This trial, in premenopausal patients with positive and negative axillary nodes, demonstrated delay in recurrence but no prolongation of survival at 10 years.
A subsequent trial of prophylactic ovarian irradiation in Oslo by NISSEN-MEYER (1964), and his colleagues showed some value in delaying recurrence and prolonging survival in premenopausal patients with positive axillary nodes, and in postmenopausal patients with positive or negative axillary nodes.
The NSABP trial in the United States demonstrated no value in surgical ovariectomy at 3–5 years of follow-up (RAVDIN et al., 1970).

Prednisone

NISSEN-MEYER also demonstrated in a group of patients that prednisone, added to castration, prolonged survival beyond that in historical castrated and non-castrated controls (NISSEN-MEYER, 1964).

Toronto-London Trial

A trial based on these data was carried out from 1965 to 1972 in patients with operable breast cancer. After surgery and postoperative radiotherapy, patients were randomized to no further

1 This work was supported by the Ontario Cancer Treatment and Research Foundation, and by the Imperial Cancer Research Fund.

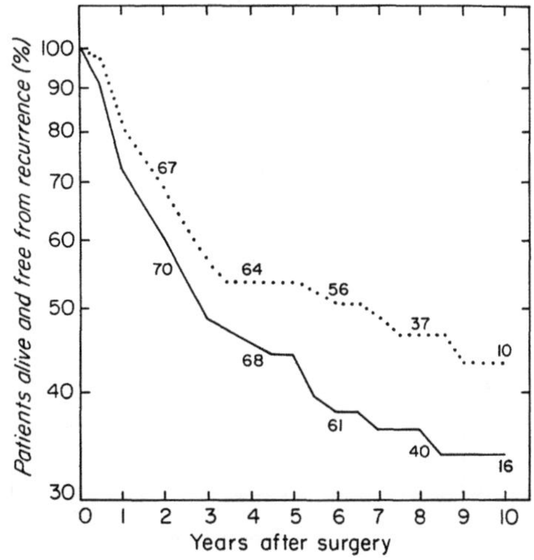

Fig. 1. Premenopausal patients less than 45 years old. ———, NT (70 patients); · · · · · · · ·, R (67 patients) (NT vs R, $P = 0.13$). Numbers of patients followed to specific times are recorded on the graphs

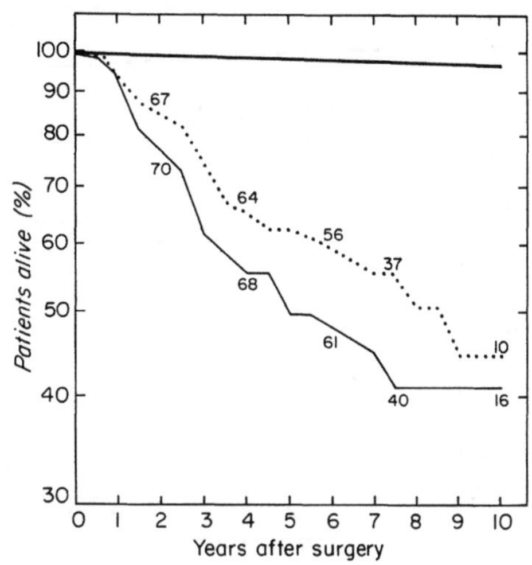

Fig. 2. Premenopausal patients less than 45 years old. ———, NT (70 patients); · · · · · · · ·, R (67 patients) (NT vs R, $P = 0.19$). The natural survival for age range is shown by the *heavy line* at the top. Numbers of patients followed to specific times are recorded on the graphs

treatment (NT), ovarian irradiation (R: 2000 rads in 5 days), or, in the case of patients aged 45 years or over, ovarian irradiation plus prednisone (R + P: prednisone 2.5 mg three times daily). The 1976 results have been published elsewhere (MEAKIN et al., 1977). The results of the 1977 update of 705 evaluable patients are as follows, and has been reported elsewhere (MEAKIN et al., in press).

Premenopausal Patients under 45 Years of Age

This group (35–44 years) embraced clinical stages (TNM) I, II, and III, and the patients were randomized only between NT and R. The two groups were comparable for age and stage. Histologically positive axillary lymph nodes were identified in 83% of the NT group and in 91% of the R group.

Figures 1 and 2 present the curves for recurrence-free interval and survival (actuarial). The numbers of patients followed to specific times are recorded on the graphs. While there is a per-

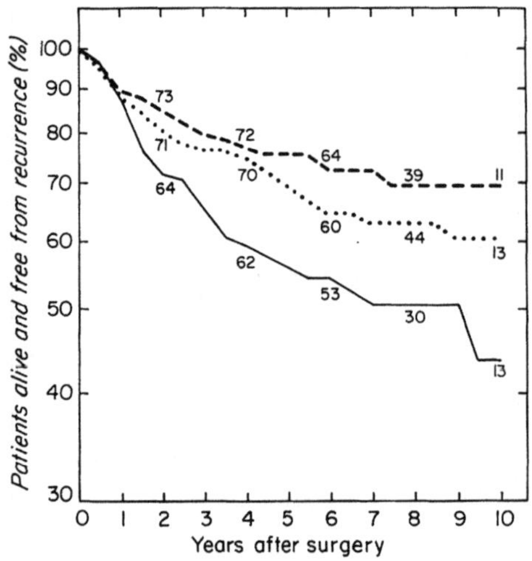

Fig. 3. Premenopausal patients 45 years old or over. ——, NT (64 patients); ········, R (71 patients); -------, R + P, (73 patients) (NT vs R, $P = 0.18$; NT vs R + P, $P = 0.02$; R vs R + P, $P = 0.31$). Numbers of patients followed to specific times are recorded on the graphs

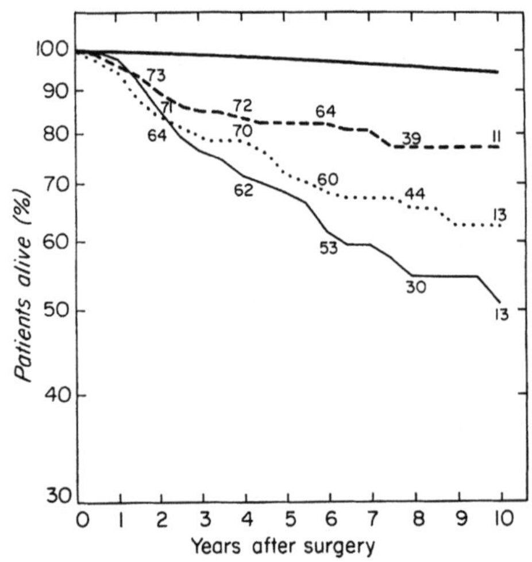

Fig. 4. Premenopausal patients 45 years old or over. ——, NT (64 patients); ········, R (71 patients); ------, R + P (73 patients) (NT vs R, $P = 0.44$; NT vs R + P, $P = 0.02$; R vs R + P, $P = 0.11$). The natural survival for age range is shown by the *heavy line* at the top. Number of patients followed to specific times are recorded on the graphs

sistent delay in recurrence and a prolongation of survival, the differences are not statistically significant ($P = 0.13$ for Fig. 1 and $P = 0.19$ for Fig. 2).

Separate analysis of the histologically node-positive patients only from Fig. 1 and 2 reveals a similar degree of delay in recurrence and improvement in survival between the NT and R groups, as follows:

(a) Fig. 1, $P = 0.12$; (b) Fig. 2, $P = 0.17$.

Premenopausal Patients 45 Years of Age or Over

In this group, clinical stages (TNM) I, II, and III were randomized to NT, R, or R + P. The three groups were comparable for age and stage. Histologically positive axillary nodes were identified as follows: NT, 69%; R, 66%; R + P, 71%.

The actuarial curves for recurrence-free interval and survival are shown in Figs. 3 and 4. The numbers of patients followed to specific times are recorded on the graphs.

Figure 3 shows that while R and R + P delay recurrence, only R + P does so to a statistically significant degree (NT vs R + P, $P = 0.02$).
In Fig. 4, R and R + P are seen to prolong survival, but only R + P to do so significantly compared with the NT group ($P = 0.02$).
If only the patients in Figs. 3 and 4 who had histologically positive axillary nodes are analyzed, the significance of the difference between the NT and R + P groups decreases to $P = 0.04$ (Fig. 3) of $P = 0.06$ (Fig. 4).

Postmenopausal Patients

No differences in time to recurrence or in survival could be demonstrated among the NT, R, and R + P groups.

Discussion

These data are in agreement with the results of the Manchester (COLE, 1968) and Oslo trials (NISSEN-MEYER, 1968) in demonstrating an apparent delay in recurrence and prolongation of survival after adjuvant ovarian irradiation alone, but the changes were not statistically significant in this study.
The lack of agreement with the results of the NSABP trial (RAVDIN et al., 1970) of prophylactic ovariectomy is possibly due to chance, or perhaps an irradiated ovary may result in a different physiologic state from that after a surgical ovariectomy. Alternatively, further follow-up data from the NSABP trial (RAVDIN et al., 1970) may demonstrate some value in surgical ovariectomy, for it may be noted that the effect of ovarian ablation in our study did not become firm until after 3—5 years of follow-up.
However, the data drawn from this study indicate that the addition of small doses of prednisone to ovarian irradiation produces a significant delay in recurrence and prolongs survival in premenopausal patients. Whether the prednisone produced its effect by suppressing estrogen of adrenal origin or by some other mechanism is not known. Other possible mechanisms include a reduction in prolactin secretion (perhaps mediated by reduced estrogen production), immunologic factors, or direct antitumor effects. Again it is emphasized that the effect of ovarian irradiation plus prednisone did not become definite until after 3 years of follow-up.
One of the important features of these data is that ovarian ablation and prednisone were effective in premenopausal patients with histologically positive axillary nodes to a degree comparable to the published data for adjuvant melphalan (FISHER et al., 1977) and CMF (cyclophosphamide, methotrexate, 5-fluorouracil) in premenopausal patients (BONADONNA, 1977). Thus it would seem rational in future studies to examine the role of adjuvant hormonal therapy, both as a complement and as an alternative to adjuvant chemotherapy.

A View of the Current Position of Adjuvant Endocrine Therapy

Because of the established value of endocrine therapy in advanced breast cancer it seems reasonable to use such an approach in an adjuvant setting, providing one can establish by experiment benefit, safety, and means of selection of patients with residual, hormone-responsive disease.
The current evidence for benefit consists of: (1) the marginal value of ovarian ablation; (2) the enhancement of the value of ovarian ablation by the addition of prednisone; and (3) the con-

tinuing observations that adjuvant, cytotoxic chemotherapy is more effective in premenopausal women, suggesting that at least part of the effect is hormone-mediated by means of ovarian suppression.

With some exceptions, the morbidity of hormone therapy is less than that for cytotoxic chemotherapy with respect to both quality of life and mortality. Furthermore, the economic cost of delivering endocrine therapy is generally lower. Therefore the potential benefit: cost ratio for endocrine therapy is high, a desirable feature for any therapeutic procedure.

Reasonable methods of patient selection for endocrine therapy have now been established for advanced disease (steroid receptors, rate of growth, tissue distribution, etc.). It remains to be shown whether or not similar criteria can be applied in the adjuvant setting (1) to select patients with residual disease, especially those with negative axillary nodes; and (2) to determine whether or not the residual disease is hormone-responsive.

Because endocrine therapy in advanced disease has generally been viewed as controlling, but not eliminating disease, there has been a tendency in the past to prefer cytotoxic, cell-kill methods in adjuvant therapy. There is now some evidence that endocrine approaches can have a cell-kill effect for neoplastic cells; briefly, this evidence includes (1) wellknown lympholytic effects of glucocorticoids, which may have immunotherapeutic implications in breast cancer; (2) survival of patients treated with ovarian ablation and prednisone approaching the survival expectancy of the normal population (see above, Fig. 4); and (3) the death in tissue culture of hormone-responsive cells deprived of hormones and/or treated with antihormones (LIPPMAN, 1976 and personal communication). The mechanisms of cell kill involved may include cell lysis, interference with the synthesis of essential cellular components, and diversion of tumor cells into a state of differentiation, with exhaustion of the proliferating, stem cell compartment.

Endocrine therapy may have to be combined with cytotoxic chemotherapy for two reasons: (1) because of the outgrowth of hormone-insensitive cells; and (2) to stimulate hormone-responsive cells into a cycling state, making them more susceptible to cytotoxic chemotherapy.

In summary, the place of adjuvant endocrine therapy in the management of breast cancer is partially established, but a number of investigations, laboratory and clinical, are required for further definition. To this end a number of proposals for investigations are outlined below.

Proposed Clinical Research into the Use of Adjuvant Endocrine Therapy in Breast Cancer

As a high priority, the value of adjuvant ovarian irradiation and prednisone, as observed in the Toronto-London Trial, needs to be tested by another group.

A number of trials are under way, but some additional proposals are as follows:

Patients with Operable Disease, Positive Axillary Nodes and EBP (Estrogen-Binding Protein)-positive Tumors

Do Hormone (H) Therapy and Cytotoxic (C) Chemotherapy Complement Each Other? Three types of experimental designs are:

a) In *premenopausal patients* with the intention of determining whether or not endocrine and chemotherapeutic tumor-inhibiting approaches are complementary, randomize to H (e.g., ovarian ablation + prednisone or tamoxifen), C (e.g., CMF), or H + C.

b) In *postmenopausal patients,* with the intention of determining whether or not endocrine and chemotherapeutic tumor-inhibiting approaches are complementary, randomize to tamoxifen (T) or T + C (e.g., CMF).
c) In *postmenopausal patients,* with the intention of determining whether or not hormone stimulation of tumor growth can enhance cytotoxic chemotherapy, randomize to H (e.g., estrogen in low doses) + C (e.g., CMF) or C alone. This proposal is based on the possibility that the failure of C in postmenopausal patients may be due to a noncycling state of tumor cells because of low estrogen levels.

How Complete or Intensive Must Hormone Therapy be to be Effective?

a) *Premenopausal Patients.* In view of the enhancement of the results of ovarian ablation (O) by prednisone (P), a study should be performed to find whether the effect obtained can be further enhanced by tamoxifen (T), patients being randomized to O + P, O + P + T, or T. This proposal is in part dependent on the outcome of current trials of the value of T as an adjuvant agent in premenopausal patients.
b) *Postmenopausal Patients.* If current trials of the adjuvant use of T fail to show value, this may be due to a failure of T to block all estrogen of adrenal and ovarian (residual) origin, and under such circumstances it would be reasonable to randomize between T and T + P.

Patients with Operable Disease, Positive Axillary Nodes, and EBP-negative or EBP-unknown Tumors

Primary tumors may be erroneously labeled EBP-negative because of innate heterogeneity of distribution of EB proteins in the neoplastic tissue or because of errors of sampling, storage, and technique. An assay for EBP may not have been done at all.
If there is reason to believe the primary tumor is genuinely EBP-negative, some investigators may be reluctant to enter premenopausal patients on trials from which cytotoxic chemotherapy is omitted. However, until the data are firmer it seems reasonable to enter all patients, but especially those with tumors whose EBP status is uncertain or unknown, on the same trials as EBP-positive patients, as suggested above. Patients should be stratified by EBP status.

Does Adjuvant Endocrine Therapy Affect the Phenotype of the Residual Tumor in an Unfavorable Manner?

To date there is minimal evidence for an unfavorable effect of adjuvant endocrine therapy, but it is theoretically possible that hormone therapy might allow the outgrowth of disease, which is more or less difficult to control with chemotherapy. Therefore it would be of value to incorporate an assessment of steroid-binding proteins in recurrent disease tissue and of survival from first recurrence into clinical trials.

Patients with Operable Disease and Negative Axillary Nodes

As it is recognized that this class of patient has a good prognosis, very little clinical research into the value of adjuvant therapy has been carried out. The problem has been to identify those patients with residual disease whom one might expect to benefit from adjuvant therapy. Two types of trials are suggested:
Can a High-Risk Group be Identified? In trials directed at the identification of a high-risk group, prospectively and retrospectively postulated indicators of prognosis should be col-

lected, including: auxometric parameters preoperatively, tumor size, tumor steroid-binding proteins, internal mammary node scan, and tumor markers such as CEA (carcinoembryonic antigen).

Does Adjuvant Therapy Affect Prognosis? In studies designed to test whether the prognosis is affected by adjuvant therapy, the patients should be stratified for the parameters given in the last section and randomized as follows:

EBP +: Control (i.e., no postoperative therapy); hormone therapy (e.g., tamoxifen); or hormone therapy + chemotherapy (e.g., CMF);

EBP −: Control, chemotherapy, or hormone therapy + chemotherapy.

References

Bonadonna, G., Rossi, A., Valagussa, P., Banfi, A., Veronesi, U.: Adjuvant chemotherapy with CMF in breast cancer with positive axillary nodes. In: Adjuvant therapy and cancer. Salmon, S. S., Jones, S. E. (eds.), pp. 83–94. Amsterdam: North-Holland 1977

Cole, M. P.: Suppression of ovarian function in primary breast cancer. In: Prognostic factors in breast cancer. Forrest, A. P. M., Kunkler, P. B. (eds.), pp. 146–156. Edinburgh: Livingston 1968

Fisher, B., Redmond, C.: Studies of the National Surgical Adjuvant Breast Project (NSABP). In: Adjuvant therapy and cancer. Salmon, S. S., Jones, S. E. (eds.), pp. 67–81. Amsterdam: North-Holland 1977

Lippman, M. E.: Hormone-dependent human breast cancer in long-term tissue culture. In: Hormones and cancer. Komanduri, K. N., Charyulu, A. (eds.), pp. 219–231. Miami: Symposia Spezialist 1979

Lippman, M. E.: Personal communication

Meakin, J. W., Allt, W. E. C., Beale, F. A., Brown, T. C., Bush, R. S., Clark, R. M., Fitzpatrick, P. J., Hawkins, N. V., Jenkin, R. D. T., Pringel, J. F., Rider, W.: Ovarian irradiation and prednisone following surgery for carcinoma of the breast. In: Adjuvant therapy of cancer. Salmon, S. S., Jones, S. E. (eds.), pp. 95–99. Amsterdam: North-Holland 1977

Meakin, J. W. et al.: Ovarian irradiation and prednisone following surgery and radiotherapy for carcinoma of the breast. Can. Med. Assoc. J. (in press)

Nissen-Meyer, R.: Prophylactic endocrine treatment of carcinoma of the breast. Clin. Radiol. *15,* 152–160 (1964)

Nissen-Meyer, R.: Suppression of ovarian function in primary breast cancer. In: Prognostic factors in breast cancer. Forrest, A. P. M., Kunkler, P. B. (eds.), pp. 139–145. Edingburgh: Livingston 1968

Ravdin, R. G., Lewison, E. F., Slack, N. H.: Results of a clinical trial concerning the worth of prophylactic oophorectomy for breast cancer. Surg. Gynecol. Obstet. *131,* 1055–1064 (1970)

Schinzinger, A.: Über Carcinoma mammae. Verh. Dtsch. Ges. Chir. *18,* 28–29 (1889)

27. *Adjuvant Endocrine Therapy of Breast Cancer – A Controlled Clinical Trial of Oestrogen and Anti-Oestrogen: Preliminary Results of the Copenhagen Breast Cancer Trials*

T. Palshof, H. T. Mouridsen, and J. L. Dæhnfeldt

The Fibiger Laboratory, Ndr. Frihavnsgade 70, DK-2100 Copenhagen (Denmark)

Introduction

Advanced breast cancer is known to respond to endocrine therapy (Co-operative Breast Cancer Group, 1964; Hadow et al., 1944; Huggins and Dao, 1953; Luft and Olivecrona, 1953), and determinations of steroid hormone receptor proteins in tumour tissue have proved to be of value in predicting the therapeutic response to endocrine manipulations (King, 1975; Singhakowinta et al., 1975).

The aim of the present studies is to evaluate the effect of adjuvant endocrine therapy. Any prolongation of the disease-free interval will be correlated retrospectively with the type of endocrine therapy and the content of oestrogen and progesterone receptors in tumour biopsies. In the case of recurrent disease, steroid hormone receptor content in accessible metastatic lesions will be compared with that in the primary tumour.

Materials and Methods

Since 1 March, 1975, 343 consecutive patients admitted to three University Hospitals in Copenhagen (Dept. R, Gentofte, Dept. D, Glostrup and Dept. L. Bispebjerg Hospital) have entered the study. The primary treatment given is simple mastectomy and postoperative irradiation. Patients admitted to the study are those in stages I–III, i.e., patients with no evidence of distant metastases revealed by physical examination, X-ray of chest and skeleton, bone scintigraphy, and bone marrow biopsy.

Inclusion Criteria

1) Patients should be under 70 years of age.
2) Primary treatment should be simple mastectomy and postoperative irradiation.
3) Staging procedures, including X-ray of the chest, bone survey, bone scintigraphy, and bone marrow biopsy should all give normal results, i.e., tumours should be of categories T1–T4, N0–N3, and M0.
4) There should be no concomitant malignancy, excluding carcinoma in situ outside the breast.
5) Postmenopausal patients should have had no previous thromboembolic or chronic hepatic diseases.

6) Patients should not be pregnant.
7) In case of hypertension or congestive heart failure, entry may take place only after proper correction of these disorders.

Definitions

1) Patients with at least 5 years spontaneous amenorrhea are postmenopausal.
2) Patients who have previously undergone hysterectomy or ovariectomy or in whom cyclic hormone administration still causes menstrual bleeding are defined as postmenopausal after the age of 55 years.
3) All other patients are regarded as premenopausal or menopausal.

Treatment

In both trials the treatment is double blind and starts 2 weeks after surgery. Patients classified as postmenopausal are randomised to treatment with 10 mg tamoxifen three times daily, 1 mg diethylstilboestrol (DES) three times daily, or one placebo tablet three times daily. In both groups treatment is continued for 2 years. Patients classified as premenopausal are randomised to 10 mg tamoxifen three times daily, or one placebo tablet three times daily. Treatment is discontinued in the case of severe or life-threatening side effects or in the case of recurrent disease. Patients are considered nonevaluable until the duration of treatment exceeds 3 months.
Clinical and biochemical examinations are performed in each patients in the outpatient department every 3 months, and bone scintigraphy once a year. After 2 years of follow-up patients will be monitored every 6 months for the next 3 years.

Results

Entry to the studies was closed in March 1978. 211 premenopausal patients and 132 postmenopausal patients have entered the trial. Tumour biopsies for oestradiol receptor protein determination were obtained in 78% of the cases. In the premenopausal group the ratio between positive (i.e., > 20 fmol/mg protein) and negative receptor protein content was found to be 0.7. In the postmenopausal patients the corresponding figure was 1.0 and for all patients it was 0.8. The lower values in the premenopausal group may be due to blocking by endogenous hormones (Table 1).

Table 1. Cytoplasmic oestradiol receptor protein determinations in the Copenhagen Breast Cancer Trials

	ER+	ER–	ER?	Ratio ER+/ER–	Total
Premenopausal and menopausal	62	95	54	0.7	211
Postmenopausal	56	54	22	1.0	132
All patients	118	149	76	0.8	343

Table 2. Distribution of 343 patients according to treatment and oestrogen receptor status in the Copenhagen Breast Cancer Trials

	Treatment group	ER+	ER–	ER?	Total
Premenopausal and menopausal	Tamoxifen	32	53	28	113
	Placebo	30	42	26	98
Postmenopausal	Tamoxifen	23	16	8	47
	DES	13	18	6	37
	Placebo	20	20	8	48
All patients		118	149	76	343

Table 3. Distribution of relapses recorded among 343 patients in the Copenhagen Breast Cancer Trials

	Treatment group	ER+	ER–	ER?	Total	Frequency (%)
Premenopausal and menopausal	Tamoxifen	7	9	3	19	17
	Placebo	6	7	6	19	19
Postmenopausal	Tamoxifen	0	4	3	7	15
	DES	2	2	1	5	14
	Placebo	2	8	1	11	23
	Total	17	30	14	61	
	Frequency (%)	14	20	18	18	

Table 4. Statistical estimation of median disease-free intervals (years) based on disease-free intervals in 343 patients in the Copenhagen Breast Cancer Trials

	Treatment group	ER+	ER–	ER?	All
Premenopausal and menopausal	Tamoxifen	6.1	7.7	15.6	8.3
	Placebo	7.7	7.7	7.5	7.6
Postmenopausal	Tamoxifen	8	4.7	3.9	9.7
	DES	7.9	13.9	10.2	10.8
	Placebo	13.3	3.5	17.0	6.5

Table 2 shows the distribution of patients according to type of endocrine therapy and receptor status.

Table 3 gives the distribution of recurrent disease recorded up to May 1978 according to treatment groups and receptor status; this shows that the overall frequency of recurrence is about 14% in the ER+ patients, 20% in the ER– patients and 18% in the ER– unknown group. This

covers a total number of 61 cases of recurrence, with an average observation time of nearly 2 years.
Table 4 shows the statistical estimation of median disease-free intervals. It is not yet possible to draw any conclusion on correlations between the rate of recurrences and type of treatment.
Before entry to the studies all patients are informed about possible side effects and nearly all patients have told the investigators immediately when these have occurred. Side effects have been mild or moderate and treatment has been discontiued in less than 10% of cases. It should be emphasised that the treatment is double blind and thus the analysis of side effects in relation to treatment cannot be finally evaluated.

Discussion

The Copenhagen Breast Cancer Trials were designed to improve the accuracy with which the response to endocrine adjuvant treatment can be predicted and to evaluate the efficiency and quality of such treatments.
At present the preliminary results do not permit final conclusions.
Results in the premenopausal group indicate that adjuvant treatment with tamoxifen is no better than placebo, regardless of the receptor status.
In the postmenopausal grop, adjuvant treatment with tamoxifen seems to be effective in the ER+ group. Furthermore, the ER– group seems to benefit from treatment with DES, which might support the observation by Lippman (1978) that the effect of DES is not receptor-mediated.
The median disease-free interval in the placebo-treated ER– group is short and is currently being tested for statistical significance.
In the postmenopausal group, ER+ tumours seem to be less aggressive than ER– tumours, irrespective of treatment.
The present results of the Copenhagen Breast Cancer Trials thus confirm our early preliminary results (Palshof et al., 1977; 1978).

Summary

In an attempt to clarify the value of adjuvant endocrine therapy as an alternative to other treatment modalities, we have started two controlled, prospective, double-blind trials, the Copenhagen Breast Cancer Trials.
In these studies postmenopausal women are randomised after primary local treatment to treatment with DES, tamoxifen, or placebo. Premenopausal women are similarly randomised to receive treatment with tamoxifen or placebo.
Entry to the trials was closed in March 1978, when 343 patients had entered the studies. The preliminary results indicate that postmenopausal patients with ER+ tumours benefit from adjuvant treatment with tamoxifen.
Adjuvant treatment with DES seems to be effective in ER– postmenopausal patients. In postmenopausal patients the ER+ tumors have a lower rate of recurrence. At present these preliminary results do not permit definite conclusions.

Acknowledgements

This investigation was supported by grants from the Danish Cancer Society (scholarship no. 38/76 for T. Palshof), the Danish Medical Research Council.

Grants were also received from Mrs. AGATHE NEYE. Imperial Chemical Industries generously supplied the drugs for these studies. Workers at the Fibiger Laboratory were sponsored by the Danish Cancer Society.

References

Co-operative Breast Cancer Group: Results of studies of the co-operative breast cancer group 1961–1963. Cancer Chemother. Rep. *41* (Suppl.) (1964) 1

Haddow, A. L., Watkinson, J. M., Paterson, E.: Influence of synthetic oestrogens upon advanced malignant disease. Br. Med. J. *1944 II,* 393–398

Huggins, C., Dao, T. L. Y.: Adrenalectomy and oophorectomy in treatment of advanced carcinoma of the breast. JAMA *151,* 1388 (1953)

King, R. J. B.: Clinical relevance of steroid-receptor measurement in tumors. Cancer Treat. Rev. *2,* 273–293 (1975)

Lippman, M. E., Allegra, J. C., Thompson, E. B., Simon, R., Barlock, A., Green, L., Huff, K. K., Hoan, T. D., Aitken, S. C., Warren, R.: The relation between estrogen receptors and response rate to cytotoxic chemotherapy in metastatic breast cancer. N. Engl. J. Med. *298,* 1223–1228 (1978)

Luft, R., Olivecrona, H.: Experiences with hypophysectomy in man. J. Neurosurg. *10,* 301 (1953)

Palshof, T., Dæhnfeldt, J. L., Mouridsen, H. T.: Adjuvant endocrine therapy of breast cancer. A controlled clinical trial of estrogen and anti-estrogen. Preliminary report on the Copenhagen Breast Cancer Trials. Reviews on endocrine-related cancer (Suppl.), pp. 168–173. April 1978

Palshof, T., Mouridsen, H. T., Dæhnfeldt, J. L.: Preliminary results of The Copenhagen Breast Cancer Trials: Adjuvant additive endocrine treatment of pre- and postmenopausal women. Symposium on Breast Cancer. Reviews on endocrine-related cancer (Suppl.) pp. 57–59. Oct. 1978

Singhakowinta, A., Mohindra, R., Brooks, S. C., Vaitkevicius, Brennan, M. J.: Clinical correlation of endocrine therapy and estrogen receptor. In: Estrogen receptors in human breast cancer. McGuire, W. L., Carbone, P. P., Vollmer, E. P. (eds.), pp. 131–156. New York: Raven Press 1975

VII. Principles of Clinical Trials

28. Principles of Clinical Trials

Ludwig Breast Cancer Study Group[1]

Ludwig Institut für Krebsforschung, Inselspital, CH-3010 Bern (Switzerland)

Summary

Proper design and conduct of a clinical trial requires the consideration of a set of principles. These principles include the collaborative effort, consideration of both a medical and a statistical plan, and development of a data network. The Ludwig Breast Cancer Study Group with international participants has been formed according to these principles. This represents an approach to clinical trials which is designed to maximize the scientific pay-off. The goal is

---

1 The Study Group comprises: Drs. J. Stjernswärd, C. Jordan (Ludwig Institute for Cancer Research, Berne, Switzerland); M. Zelen, K. Stanley, R. Gelber, M. Isley (Frontier Science and Technology Research Foundation, Inc., Boston, USA); P. Helman, A. Hacking, A. L. Brown, A. White, A. C. Harrison, E. Dowdle (Cape Town Breast Cancer Group, Cape Town, South Africa); C. G. Schmidt, R. Zschaber, H. Ludwig, R. Callies, L. D. Leder (West Germany Cancer Research Center, Essen, Germany); C.-M. Rudenstam, E. Cahlin, B. Risberg, L. Ivarsson, O. Ruusvik, L. Mattsson, C.-G. Bäckström, S. Dahlin, Y. Hessman, O. Thoren, M. Suurküla, C. Johnsén (Swedish Western Breast Cancer Group, Göteborg, Sweden); J. Lindtner, J. Novak, M. Naglas, J. Cevek, A. Vodnik, E. Majdic, P. Mavec, R. Golough, J. Lamovec, S. Sebek (The Institute of Oncology, Ljubljana, Yugoslavia); S. Parbhoo, K. Hobbs, E. Boesen, D. Skeggs, B. Stoll, F. Sennanayake, B. Scott (The Royal Free Hospital, London, England); K. Griffith (Tenevus Cancer Institute, Cardiff, Wales, United Kingdom); N. Diederich, M. Di Cato, F. Schoetter (Groupe Luxembourgeois de Chimiotherapie, Luxembourg); H. Cortés-Funes, F. Martinez Tello, F. Cruz Caro, R. Perez Carrion, A. Die Goyanes, A. Marazuela, B. L. Madrigal, I. Requena, F. Calero, J. Lizon, S. Mallagray, P. Espana, R. Inchausty, M. A. Figueras (Madrid Breast Cancer Group, Madrid, Spain); I. Russell, M. A. Schwarz, J. F. Forbes, P. R. B. Kitchen, R. C. Bennett, E. Guli, R. Reed, J. Funder (Anti-Cancer Council of Victoria, Melbourne, Australia), K. Brunner, H. Cottier, A. Zimmermann (Inselspital, Berne, Switzerland); F. Cavalli (Ospedale San Giovanni, Bellinzona, Switzerland); W.-F. Jungi (Kantonsspital, St. Gallen, Switzerland); G. Martz (Kantonsspital, Zurich, Switzerland); P. Siegenthaler (Hôpital des Cadolles, Neuchâtel, Switzerland); M. H. N. Tattersall, R. Fox, R. Wood, D. Glenn, F. Niesche, R. West, S. Renwick, D. Green, J. Donovan, P. Duval, T. Jelihovsky, Z. Kronowski (Ludwig Institute for Cancer Research, Sydney, Australia); J. S. Simpson, E. C. Watson, C. T. Collins, A. J. Gray, J. W. Logan, J. J. Landreth, L. Holloway, P. Cairney (Wellington Hospital, Wellington, New Zealand).

to determine the optimal treatment for every identifiable prognostic subgroup of patients.

Introduction

A well-conducted clinical trial provides great potential for the advancement of medical science. Far too often, however, small or poorly designed trials are started, which not only dissipate the resources of society and the scientific community, but may also be misleading.

The Ludwig Breast Cancer Study Group was created in January 1977 to search for optimal adjuvant therapies in operable breast cancers. The group includes members from Melbourne and Sydney, Australia; London and Cardiff, United Kingdom; Essen, Germany; the Grand Duchy of Luxembourg; Wellington, New Zealand; Capetown, Port Elizabeth, and East London, South Africa; Göteborg, Sweden; Berne, Tessin, Neuchâtel, St. Gallen, and Zurich, Switzerland; and Ljubljana, Yugoslavia; recently centres in Madrid, Spain joined the group. Patients are entered centrally via the Coordinating Centre in Switzerland by means of telephone or telex facilities. The Statistical Centre is located in Boston. This organisational structure emphasises the flexibility of communications available to current clinical research.

Localisation of a clinical trial is no longer necessary. It is possible to devise a system that makes it almost as easy to conduct a multinational trial as a single-institution study.

This group has activated a series of four related studies based upon the principles given in Table 1. The application of these principles in the development of the studies is discussed in the later sections of this paper.

Collaborative Effort

It must be ensured that sufficient accrual can be raised to answer the medical question within a realistic time. We know from our observations that many individuals enhance their research funding opportunities by conducting small trials. Unfortunately, such trials are potential sources of false-positive or false-negative results. In a recent analysis (FREIMAN et al., 1978),

Table 1. Principles of Clinical Trials

Collaborative effort
Medical plan
Review of recent results
Control arm selection
Key study questions
Sub-group considerations
Statistical plan
Decisive study end point results – positive or negative
Accrual in 2–3 years
Data network

in 94% of a set of "negative" trials (67 of 71 studies) the risk of missing a true 25% therapeutic improvement was over 10%. Clinical research should be based upon reproducibility of results.

The value of a collaborative effort in clinical trials is evident. Advantages include standardisation of the criteria of disease, end point evaluation, and application of therapy; the existence of a forum for discussion and evaluation of the latest progress in therapy; and the opportunity to make a substantial scientific contribution. There are a great many instances where definitive progress towards an objective can only be made by a cooperative group. The Ludwig Breast Cancer Study Group is a true cooperative group, working in line with the principle "one for all and all for one".

When resources are pooled, a trial will give new information on the biology of the disease. The outcome of the therapeutic effect of the different treatment arms may perhaps be of lesser importance than the new information about the disease that can be gained by additional studies, whether in the laboratory, by pathology, or in vivo. Against the background of a large, well-controlled, clinical study where work-up, therapy and follow-up have been standardised, it may be useful to do extra studies where the effort is rewarded by the possibility of adding to the knowledge of the disease.

Medical Plan

A clearly written scientific planning document is the cornerstone of any scientific investigation. This document and the associated data forms ensure standardisation as to the entry of patients, application of therapy, evaluation, and monitoring: it also provides the basis for reproducibility, an essential element of a clinical trial. It is important that biostatisticians and clinicians work together *before* a clinical trial is activated, so that the biological background and hypothetical therapeutic differences can be interfaced with the statistical plan and analysis objectives.

Determination of the treatment arms is a fundamental step. The evaluation of treatments requires a control or standard arm to serve as a basis for comparisons. Thorough research and evaluation of previous results is required before a study design is conceived, inclusion of the best-known-therapy arm being a moral requirement. Next, the question of importance must be determined. The initiation of a study without a "burning question" is also a dissipation of resources. The medical question should dictate the therapy arm to be compared with the standard or control arm, not vice versa. All too often, therapy arms developed in a collaborative effort suffer from too much arbitration and result in a trial where the therapeutic regimens are quite similar. Scientific progress from such trials is minimal.

Many patients are not suitable for answering a particular question efficiently, and thereby may dilute the trial. Selection of the appropriate category of patients is dependent upon the question raised and is further complicated by the necessity of including sufficient numbers of patients in the sub-group for the results to be conclusive. The earlier published trials on ovariectomy and breast cancer and the interpretation of these trials may stand as examples of this phenomenon. Ovariectomy is said not to affect survival, perhaps "only" to give a prolongation of the disease-free interval following surgery. There may be a sub-group of patients in whom hormone therapy actually prolongs survival, but who are diluted by non-responders and cannot be identified. From our current knowledge, it can be estimated that of

100 patients, 40% would be premenopausal and 60% postmenopausal. Thirty percent of premenopausal and 60% of postmenopausal patients have tumours that are positive for oestrogen receptors (ER^+). In each category, approximately 50% of ER^+ tumours will respond to hormone therapy. This gives 6 and 18 patients in each group, respectively, who will respond. The responders may well not be identified in a large clinical study unless the important factors are taken into account.

Results from controlled studies have shown that both adjuvant hormone therapy (Cole, 1968; Nissen-Meyer, 1967; Ravdin et al., 1970; Meakin et al., 1977) and single-agent or multiple-drug chemotherapy (Nissen-Meyer et al., 1978; Fisher et al., 1975; Fisher et al., 1977; Bonadonna et al., 1977) may significantly decrease the early disease relapse rate overall or in sub-groups of patients with operable breast cancer and histologically positive lymph nodes. In two studies, the long-term survival rate was improved by chemotherapy (Nissen-Meyer et al., 1978) or by hormone therapy in a sub-group of premenopausal women over 45 years of age (Meakin et al., 1977).

Results demonstrate that the same adjuvant chemotherapy is more efficient in premenopausal patients than in those who are postmenopausal (Fisher et al., 1977; Bonadonna et al., 1977). CMF medication produced amenorrhoea in 78% of premenopausal patients (Bonadonna et al., 1977). The relapse rate was lower in premenopausal women with CMF-induced amenorrhoea (10%) than in premenopausal CMF-treated patients without amenorrhoea (27%).

A synergistic effect of simultaneous cytotoxic chemotherapy and hormone therapy has been demonstrated in advanced breast cancer (Brunner et al., 1977; Ahmann et al., 1977). A tendency to better results in premenopausal patients was found when chemotherapy was combined with ovariectomy. The combined-modality treatment was associated with longer remission and survival. It is thus possible that combined hormone and chemotherapy may be biologically superior to either treatment modality alone.

Several options, such as alternative non-cross-resistant drug combinations, prolongation of adjuvant therapy, intensified chemotherapy, radiotherapy (Stjernswärd, 1977), and immunotherapy, were considered at the group meeting. However, it was decided to explore the role of hormone therapy in combination with chemotherapy, which can potentially bring about a therapeutic improvement with a relatively small increase in morbidity. Patients would be treated according to hormonal age, pooling premenopausal and perimenopausal patients. Furthermore, premenopausal and perimenopausal women would be divided into two groups according to nodal status: those with one to three positive nodes, in whom CMF is apparently effective, and those with four or more positive nodes, for whom a more efficient therapy than CMF must be sought.

The schema of the four studies activated by this group is presented in Fig. 1. No data are available to show any benefit of adjuvant therapy in the postmenopausal patients. Therefore, a control group is essential. Further, it was decided that cytotoxic therapy was not justified for patients between 66 and 80 years of age, but that the effect of tamoxifen should be evaluated.

The Study Group is one of the few groups, if not the only one at the moment, that – thanks to the accrual – can not only stratify breast cancer patients with positive operable lymph nodes according to some known prognostic factors, such as age, menstrual status, and number of tumour-involved lymph nodes, but also treat them specifically. This is a first step towards the future, when probably further factors, such as hormone-receptor status of the primary tumour, will also be used for the design of selective therapy for identifiable sub-groups of patients with varying prognosis, so as not to over- or undertreat our patients.

Project Title: Search for optimal adjuvant therapies, combining hormone and chemotherapy, in operable breast cancer.

Patient Population: Patients with histologically proven breast cancer who undergo surgical treatment, total mastectomy plus axillary clearance or modified radical mastectomy, and are classified post-surgically as $T1_A$ or $_B$, $T2_A$ or $_B$, $T3_A$ N(+)$M_{\text{"0"}}$.

Patient Entry: Patients are entered into the study following surgery but before the end of the 6-week postoperative period.

	After Surgery	Randomization
Scheme I:	Pre- and perimenopausal, 1–3 nodes positive	→ CMF → CMF P
Scheme II:	Pre- and perimenopausal, 4 or more nodes positive	→ CMF P → Ovariectomy + CMF P
Scheme III:	Postmenopausal, at least 1 node positive, 65 years or younger	→ Observation → CMF P + TAM → P + TAM
Scheme IV:	Postmenopausal, at least 1 node positive, 66 to 80 years	→ Observation → P + TAM

C, cyclophosphamide	100 mg/m² p.o. days 1 through 14 of each cycle
M, methotrexate	40 mg/m² i.v. on days 1 and 8 of each cycle
F, 5-fluorouracil	600 mg/m² i.v. on days 1 and 8 of each cycle
P, prednisone	7.5 mg/day p.o. (5 mg a.m., 2.5 mg p.m.)
TAM, tamoxifen	20 mg p.o. once daily

Fig. 1. Ludwig breast cancer studies I, II, III and IV, activated 1 July 1978.

The Statistical Plan

Small trials may create situations in which poor therapies are accepted for further study or promising therapies are dropped. The first type of error is of significant concern but it is probable that the true situation will be realised during the prolonged use of the therapy. The latter error, however, is of crucial importance. A promising therapy may not be adequately tested

Table 2. Entry of patients in multinational trial conducted by LUDWIG BREAST CANCER STUDY GROUP

	Estimated number of patients per year	Estimated number of patients per treatment arm per year
Premenopausal, 1–3 (+) nodes	156	78
Premenopausal, 4 or more (+) nodes	84	42
Postmenopausal	360	120

Table 3. Median time to recurrence (in years)

	Premenopausal	Postmenopausal
1–3 (+) nodes	2.9	6.9
4 or more (+) nodes	1.3	2.0
Overall	2.3	4.4

and may subsequently be shelved. It may be years before it is brought back for a retest and the situation corrected.

The entry of patients should not continue for more than $2\frac{1}{2}$–3 years, at the most. If studies drag on, the results of other trials may lead to strong pressure to change the on-going study or even make it unethical to continue. Furthermore, new findings, such as hormone receptor status, make it logically desirable to use these parameters as soon as possible, not only for stratification but also for selection of therapy, to avoid overtreatment or undertreatment of the patients.

The objective of our breast cancer study was to compare the various therapy regimens with regard to the disease-free interval. It is assumed that an increase of 50% or more in the median time to recurrence would be a medically significant finding, and that any less pronounced change would not be of sufficient interest to warrant the large number of patients necessary for the evaluation. This trial is designed to give a high likelihood (probably of at least 0.90) that an increase of 50% in the median time to recurrence will be detected, if such a difference really exists. What this means to the investigator is that whether positive or negative, the trial results will be conclusive.

It is estimated that 600 suitable patients will be assigned to the studies per year. Roughly speaking, the entry of the patients shown in Table 3.

The following data (FISHER et al., 1977) and the assumption of an exponential recurrence rate were utilised in the determination of the necessary sample size.

The sensitivity of a clinical trial to detect differences depends on two factors: the number of patients and the length of follow-up. With more patients entered, a shorter follow-up is needed, and when fewer patients are entered a longer follow-up is necessary.

Table 4. Probability of detecting a 50% increase in median time to recurrence

Years of follow-up	Years of patients entry		
	$1\frac{1}{2}$	2	$2\frac{1}{2}$
0	0.30	0.44	0.57
1	0.50	0.65	0.76
2	0.59	0.76	0.86
3	0.72	0.84	0.91

For the premenopausal patients with one to three positive nodes the probability of detecting a 50% increase in the median time to recurrence (based upon a one-tailed statistical test with $P = 0.05$), assuming an accrual of 78 patients per arm per year is given in Table 4.
It is evident that $2\frac{1}{2}$ years of accrual (a total of 195 patients per arm) succeeded by 2–3 years follow-up will be necessary.
Similar calculations for the remaining studies indicate that they will each require 2–3 years of accrual succeeded by 2–3 years of follow-up to achieve the desired precision.

Data Network

Timely collection of the required data is an essential element of a clinical trial that is often neglected. The establishment of an effective data-flow network should be part of the protocol style document. The role of the computer as an integral part of the conduct of a large modern clinical trial includes both the monitoring of the trial and the analysis of the results. Computer-generated data requests and status lists help to maintain a continuous data flow.
In the past few years the science of conducting clinical trials has advanced to the age of specialisation. Each participant in the Ludwig Breast Cancer Study Group has an identified "data manager" – a new concept to many investigators. This individual is responsible for ensuring that all forms are submitted punctually, and also responds to data or clarification requests from the group data manager at the Statistical Centre. Much of the data collection and processing does not require physician handling. An individual with a medical background and an aggressive attitude towards accurate data collection is a valuable component in the conduct of a clinical trial.

Discussion

The international resources pooled by the Ludwig Breast Cancer Study Group create a structure with the potential for significant contribution in the search for the role of adjuvant therapy in operable breast cancer. A view of the entire clinical trial process, with primary consideration given to the eventual analysis of results and subsequent impact on therapy, allows evaluation and permits a proper perspective to be given to aspects of the medical and statistical plan. The formulation of an efficient mechanism to perform these trials requires an exchange of ideas between the physician and biostatistician, and also demands specialisation and delineation of areas of responsibility.

Summary

Consideration of a set of principles is a necessary background to the correct design and conduct of a clinical trial. This involves planning of the collaborative effort, setting up of both a medical and a statistical plan, and the development of a data network. The Ludwig Breast Cancer Study Group has been formed on an international basis according to these principles. This approach to clinical trials is designed to maximise the scientific pay-off.

References

Ahmann, D. L., O'Connell, M. J., Hahn, R. G., Bisel, H. F., Lee, R. A., Edmonson, J. H.: An evaluation of early or delayed adjuvant chemotherapy in premenopausal patients with advanced breast cancer undergoing oophorectomy. N. Engl. J. Med. *297,* 356–360 (1977)

Bonadonna, G., Rossi, A., Valagussa, P., Banfi, A., Veronesi, U.: The CMF program for operable breast cancer with positive axillary nodes. Cancer *39,* 2904–2915 (1977)

Brunner, K. W., Sonntag, R. W., Alberto, P., Senn, H. J., Martz, G., Obrecht, P., Maurice, P.: Combined chemo- and hormonal therapy in advanced breast cancer. Cancer *39,* 2923–2933 (1977)

Cole, M. P.: Suppression of ovarian function in primary breast cancer. In: Prognostic factors in breast cancer. Forrest, A. P. M., Kunkler, E. S. (eds.), pp. 146–156. Edinburgh, London: Livingston 1968

Fisher, B., Slack, N., Katrych, D. L., Wolmar, K. N.: Ten year follow-up of breast cancer patients in a cooperative clinical trial evaluating surgical adjuvant chemotherapy. Surg. Gynecol. Obstet. *140,* 528–534 (1975)

Fisher, B., Glass, A., Redmond, C., Fisher, E. R., Barton, B., Such, E., Carbone, P., Economou, S., Foster, R., Frelick, R., Lerner, H., Levitt, M., Margolese, R., MacFarlane, J., Plotkin, D., Shibata, H., Volk, H. (and other cooperating investigators): L-Phenylalanine Mustard (L-PAM) in the management of primary breast cancer. Cancer *39,* 2883–2903 (1977)

Freiman, J. A., Chalmers, T. C., Smith, H., Jr., Kubler, R.: Importance of beta type error and sample size in the randomized control trial. N. Engl. J. Med. *299,* 690–694 (1978)

Meakin, J. W., Allt, W. E. C., Beale, F. A., Brown, T. C., Bush, R. S., Clark, P. M., Fitzpatrick, P. J., Hawkins, N. V., Jenkin, R. D. T., Pringle, J. F., Rider, W. D.: Ovarian irradiation and prednisone following surgery for carcinoma of the breast. In: Adjuvant therapy of cancer. Salmon, S. E., Jones, S. E. (eds.), pp. 95–99. Amsterdam: Elsevier/North Holland, Biomed. Press 1977

Nissen-Meyer, R.: The role of prophylactic castration in the therapy of human mammary carcinoma. Eur. J. Cancer *3,* 395–403 (1967)

Nissen-Meyer, R., Kjellgren, K., Malmio, K., Mansson, B., Norin, T.: Results with one short course with cyclophosphamide after mastectomy for breast cancer. Cancer *4,* 2088–2098 (1978)

Ravdin, R. G., Lewinson, E. F., Slack, N. H.: Results of a clinical trial concerning the worth of prophylactic oophorectomy for breast carcinoma. Surg. Gynecol. Obstet. *141,* 1055–1064 (1970)

Stjernswärd, J.: Adjuvant radiotherapy trials in breast cancer. Cancer *39,* 2846–2867 (1977)

29. *Establishment of Uniformity in Steroid Receptor Analyses Used in Cooperative Clinical Trials of Breast Cancer Treatment*

J. L. Wittliff, B. Fisher, and J. R. Durant

University of Louisville, School of Medicine and The Cancer Center, Department of Biochemistry, P.O. Box 35260, Louisville, KY 40232 (USA)

Introduction

It is well established that the hormonal milieu of the patient significantly influences the growth rates of certain breast tumors. Clinical observations since the turn of the century indicate that 25%–40% of breast cancers respond to the surgical removal of hormone-producing glands such as the ovaries in the premenopausal woman or the adrenals in the postmenopausal patient. Administration of pharmacologic doses of estrogens and androgens also may bring about breast tumor remissions.

An obvious problem for the surgeon or oncologist treating the breast cancer patient has been to identify the individual most likely to respond to endocrine manipulation. Until recently, clinical factors such as previous response to hormone therapy, disease-free interval, age and menopausal status, and location of the dominant metastatic lesion were the principal criteria for selecting therapeutic regimens for these women.

Investigations during the past decade have elucidated the mechanism by which steroid hormones influence the differentiation and development of target organs (e.g., Jensen et al., 1974; Wittliff, 1975; Buller and O'Malley, 1976). A prerequisite for responsiveness appears to be a cellular protein termed the steroid receptor or steroid binding protein. Receptor proteins are found in a variety of concentrations (500–20,000 binding sites) in target cells but are virtually absent in nontarget tissues. An important property is that the steroid hormones associate with their characteristic receptor protein in a manner exhibiting high affinity and ligand specificity. Since the original report of Folca and co-workers (1961) indicating a greater uptake of labeled hexestrol by breast tumors of patients showing a response to ablative therapy, numerous studies (e.g., Jensen et al., 1971; Wittliff, 1974; McGuire et al., 1975) have shown that approximately one-half of all biopsies of malignant breast tumors contained estrogen receptors. Furthermore, 55%–60% of the patients exhibiting estrogen receptors were responsive to hormone therapies of the additive or ablative types. The use of this single biochemical criterion by the physician has increased by two- or threefold the accuracy of selecting an endocrine manipulation likely to produce an objective remission in the patient with advanced breast cancer.

Mechanism of Interaction with Target Cells

Our current understanding of the sequence of events which follows the interaction of a steroid hormone with a target cell (Fig. 1) evolved from the original "two-step mechanism" suggested

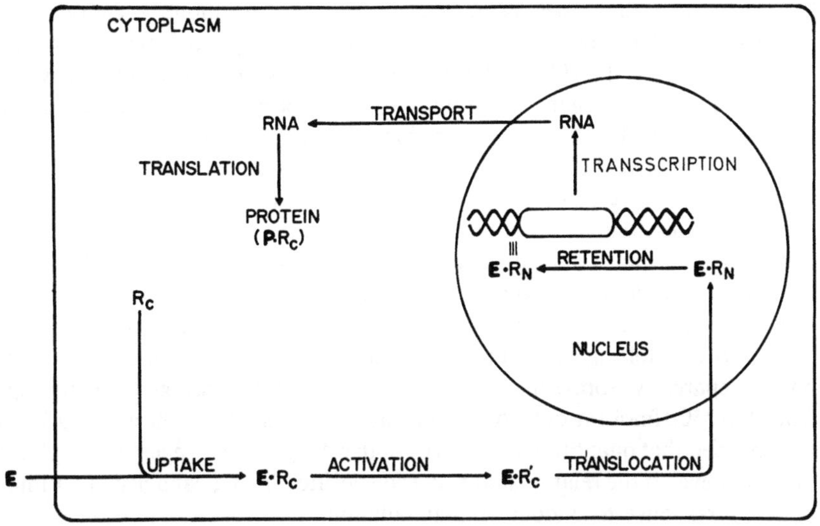

Fig. 1. Proposed interrelationship of estrogen and progestin receptors. The cytoplasmic form of the receptors is designated as ER_C, the nuclear form as ER_N, the progestin receptors as PR_C and the estrogenic hormone as E

independently by GORSKI and co-workers (1968) and by JENSEN and colleagues (1968). These workers utilized uterine tissues from rodents for these early studies. Investigations from the authors' laboratory suggest that similar cascade of events exists in normal and neoplastic mammary cells. Steroid hormones are transported in the plasma compartment by a number of proteins including albumin, testosterone-estradiol-binding globulin, each with a characteristic affinity and capacity. The unbound steroid enters the cell apparently by passive diffusion and combines with its specific receptor protein in a reaction termed uptake (Fig. 1). Prior to translocation into the nucleus, the steroid-receptor complex must undergo an activation step (PARK and WITTLIFF, 1977). After it enters the nucleus, the steroid hormone-receptor complex associates with the chromatin in an event called retention. This interaction stimulates RNA synthesis resulting in the formation of certain breast cell proteins. Thus the steroid receptor appears to be a prerequisite for responsiveness to hormonal perturbations; in its absence alterations in macromolecular synthesis do not occur at physiologic hormone concentrations. Normal breast cells contain specific binding proteins for estrogen, progestins, glucocorticoids and androgens of variable quantities depending upon the stage of mammary gland differentiation (WITTLIFF, 1975).

Properties of Estrogen Receptors in Human Breast Carcinoma and Their Clinical Significance

The concept underlying endocrine therapy is that certain tumors have retained the cellular mechanism to respond to the same hormonal stimuli as their normal progenitor cells. Only recently it was demonstrated that the presence of estrogen receptors provide a molecular basis for the distinction between human breast carcinomas that are responsive to hormonal therapy or to endocrine organ ablative surgery and those which are not (e.g., JENSEN et al., 1971; WITTLIFF, 1974; McGUIRE et al., 1975).

Steroid receptors have been estimated in a variety of hormone target organs using methods ranging from administration in vivo of labeled steroid to procedures in vitro (e.g., FOLCA et al., 1961; JENSEN et al., 1975; WITTLIFF, 1975). Two methods have proven useful for the determination of estrogen and progesterone receptors in human breast carcinomas by the clinical chemist. The titration procedure (Figs. 2 and 3), which utilizes dextran-coated charcoal to remove the unbound steroid from that associated with the intracellular receptor, provides a measure of the binding capacity and the affinity. Usually binding capacity is expressed as femtomoles of ^{3}H-labeled steroid bound per mg cytosol protein. It is generally accepted that less than 3 fmol/mg cytosol protein represents a quantity of estrogen binding sites usually correlated with the lack of response of a breast cancer patient given endocrine therapy (MCGUIRE et al., 1975; 1978). Although there appears to be a "borderline" range of values from 3 to 10 fmol/mg cytosol protein, estrogen binding capacities of >10 fmol of estrogen bound apparently represent a "receptor positive" tumor. Estrogen binding capacities ranging from 3 to 2500 fmol/mg cytosol protein have been observed in the authors' laboratory. It is recommended that quantitative values of both estrogen and progestin receptors be reported in order to develop the relationship between specific binding capacity of a tumor biopsy and a patient's response to endocrine manipulation.

Typical titration curves of estrogen and progestin binding sites are seen in Figs. 2 and 3. To determine specific binding the analyses must be performed in the presence of a competitive inhibitor of the association of ^{3}H-ligand with the receptor. We routinely use unlabeled

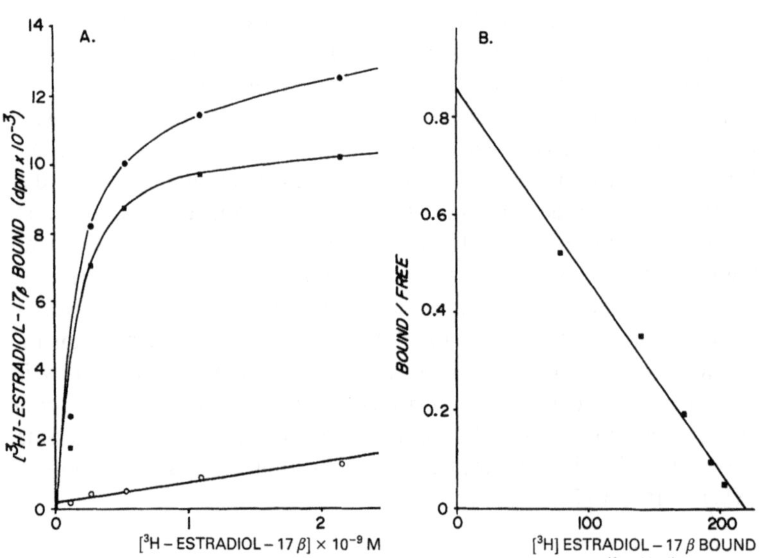

Fig. 2. Titration analysis of estrogen receptors in human breast carcinoma. **A** Aliquots (0.1 ml) of cytosol prepared from a frozen powder of human breast tumors were incubated in triplicate with 0.1 ml [^{3}H] estradiol-17β solutions in homogenization buffer containing increasing amounts of radioactive ligand either in the absence (●) or presence (○) of a 200-fold excess of diethylstilbestrol. Specific binding (■) was estimated as the difference between total binding and binding in the presence of the competitor. **B** The titration data from A were plotted according to the method of Scatchard. The dissociation constant (K_d) determined from the slope of the curve was 2.1×10^{-10} *M* for this preparation. The binding capacity of the estrogen receptor complexes was estimated from the intercept on the abscissa and gave a value of 198 fmol/mg cytosol protein

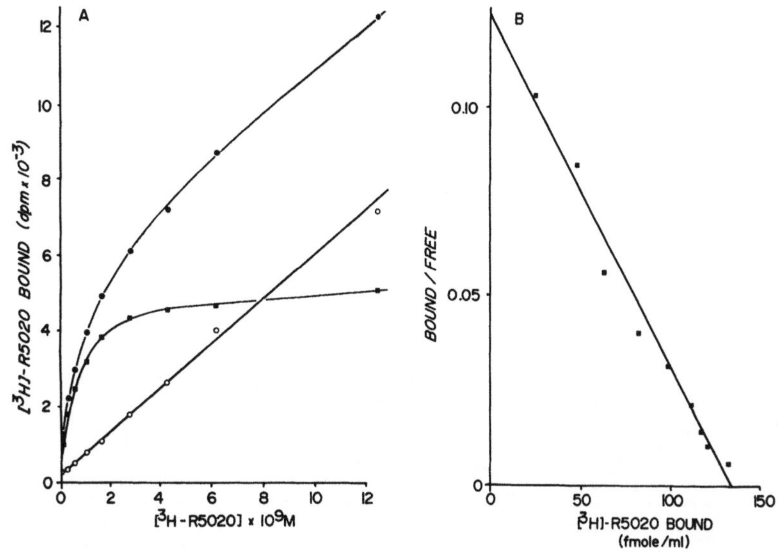

Fig. 3. Titration analysis of progestin receptors in human breast carcinoma. **A** Aliquots of cytosol were prepared and analyzed as described in Fig. 2 except that [³H]R5020 was used in the absence (●) or presence (○) of unlabeled R5020. Specific binding (■) was calculated similarly. **B** When the specific binding data from A were plotted according to the method of Scatchard, a K_d value of 1.1×10^{-9} *M* and a specific progestin binding capacity of 74 fmol/mg cytosol protein were estimated

diethylstilbestrol in a 200-fold excess since this competitor associates with the estrogen receptor with a $K_d \sim 10^{-9}$ *M*. Another important advantage of using this compound as an inhibitor is that it has a low affinity for sex-steroid binding proteins of plasma which may contaminate cytosol preparations binding proteins of plasma which may contaminate cytosol preparations from human breast tumors. Generally, the dissociation constant of estrogen-receptor complexes ranges from 10^{-10} to 10^{-11} *M*, indicating a high affinity. Our experience indicates the titration assay is equally useful for the clinical determination of receptors for progestins, glucocorticoids and androgens in human breast tumors as long as consideration of the [³H] ligand is given.

The sucrose gradient method which separates the various forms of the steroid receptors assesses certain molecular properties of those proteins in a tumor extract (Fig. 4). Using this method, it has been determined that the sedimentation profiles of both estrogen and progestin receptors in human breast carcinomas fall into four general categories (Jensen et al., 1971; Wittliff, 1974; Horwitz and McGuire, 1975; Wittliff et al., 1977). These are tumors which contain specific steroid binding components migrating at either 8-s, 4-s, or both 8-s and 4-s (Fig. 4) and those in which receptors are undetectable. A more accurate estimation of the sedimentation coefficients of these molecular forms has been made using a number of marker proteins. From these data the higher molecular weight species of the estrogen receptor sedimented at 7.6–8.1-s while the lower molecular weigth form sedimented at 4.0–4.6-s under conditions of low ionic strength. Occasionally we have observed specific estrogen binding components sedimenting at < 4-s under these same conditions. Some investigators have used the sucrose gradient method to quantitate the steroid binding capacity of human breast tumors (Wittliff et al., 1972; Jensen et al., 1975). When a saturating concentration of [³H] ligand as well as an excess of a competitor are used in this assay, the estimation of spe-

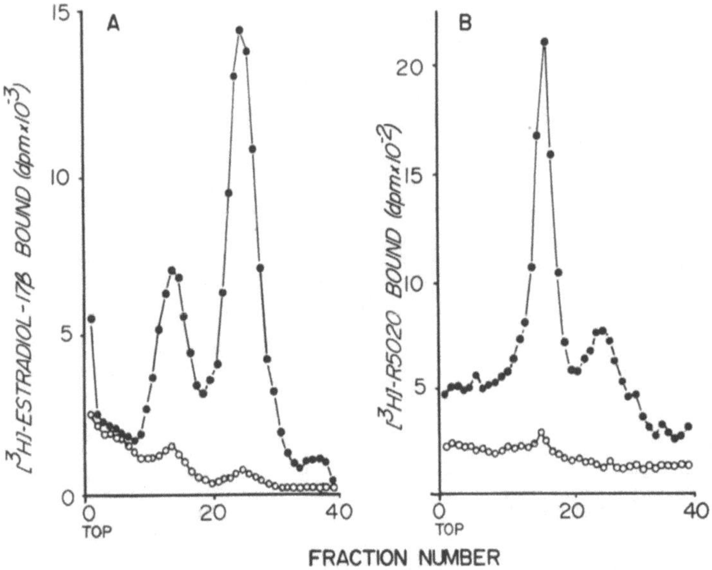

Fig. 4. Sucrose gradient separation of estrogen and progestin (R5020) receptors in human breast carcinoma. Tumor cytosol was reacted either with [^{3}H]estradiol (A) or with [^{3}H]R5020 (B) for 4 h at 3° C in the presence (○) or absence (●) of a 200-fold excess of unlabeled competitor. Note the presence of both 8-s and 4-s forms of these steroid receptors in the single breast carcinoma analyzed

cific binding capacity is in good agreement with that determined by the titration analyses (WITTLIFF and SAVLOV, 1975).

In 1969 the principal author and his co-workers began a longterm study to examine the original hypothesis set forth by JENSEN and colleagues (1967; 1971) that the presence of specific estrogen binding components in breast carcinomas was predictive of a patient's response to endocrine therapy. Using sucrose gradient separation of specific estrogen binding proteins in cytosol fractions of biopsies of primary and metastatic breast carcinomas, four types of receptor profiles have been demonstrated as discussed earlier. The majority of breast tumors containing estrogen receptors exhibited either the 8-s species alone or both the 8-s and 4-s forms (Fig. 4). From 10% to 15% of breast carcinomas contained only the 4-s type of estrogen receptor using sucrose gradients of low ionic strength (WITTLIFF, 1976). In spite of the differences in sedimentation properties, the ligand binding specificities and affinities of the 8-s and 4-s species of estrogen receptors were similar. The fourth category comprising approximately half of the infiltrating ductal carcinomas of the breast examined were those that did not contain any type of estrogen binding component.

A summary of our results relating a breast cancer patient's response to endocrine therapy with the presence of specific forms of the estrogen receptors in breast tumor biopsies is presented in Table 1. No objective remissions have been observed in patients with advanced breast carcinoma who had tumor biopsies which were estrogen receptor negative regardless of the type of hormone therapy administered (WITTLIFF et al., 1978). This correlation is far better than that reported for the collective results presented at the International Workshop (MCGUIRE et al., 1975). Approximately 75% of the patients administered various types of hormone therapy in which the biopsies contained either the 8-s species alone or both the 8-s and 4-s forms of estrogen receptors exhibited objective remissions. As indicated by the foot-

Table 1. Relationship between response to endocrine therapy and the presence of estrogen receptors in tumor biopsy

	Objective remissions according to estrogen receptor species in tumor		
Endocrine therapy[a]	8–9 s 8–9 s and 4–5 s	4–5 s	Undetectable
Ablative	17/21	1/8	0/11
Additive	16/23	3/15	0/33
Total	33/44	4/23	0/44

[a] Nine additional patients exhibited remissions but had unclassified estrogen receptor-positive tumors; 5 responded to estrogen, 3 responded to androgen therapy, and one responded to oophorectomy (Adapted from WITTLIFF et al., 1978).

note to Table 1, nine additional patients exhibited remissions to endocrine therapy whose tumors were examined only by titration analysis, the molecular forms of estrogen receptors in these specimens were not distinguished. Of 23 patients whose tumors contained exclusively or predominantly the 4–5-s forms of estrogen receptors and who were administered hormone therapy only four responded objectively. These data suggest that these molecular forms of estrogen receptors in human breast cancer have clinical significance.

Our earlier results clearly showed that the 8-s estrogen receptor of lactating mammary gland was composed of at least two components each with different ionic properties as measured by DEAE-cellulose chromatography (WITTLIFF et al., 1978). Unlike normal mammary cells, the 8-s estrogen receptor of human breast tumors separated into a variable number of components each with different ionic properties (KUTE et al., 1978). Furthermore, the 4-s estrogen receptor of human breast tumors also separated into at least two components each with different ionic properties. These data indicate the estrogen receptors of human breast cancers exhibit molecular heterogeneity. They also suggest that the molecular properties of estrogen receptors in human breast biopsies may be related to clinical responsiveness of patients given hormonal manipulations. In contrast to endocrine responsive tumors, ALLEGRA et al. (1978) suggested that breast cancer patients with estrogen receptor negative tumors showed an increased response rate to cytotoxic chemotherapy. Thus both the quality (integrity) and quantity (number of binding sites) of estrogen receptors appear to be important as predictive indices when the oncologist is faced with the selection of a therapy likely to produce an objective remission. These latter considerations clearly impose a requirement for rigid quality control of steroid receptor analyses in the clinical laboratory.

Establishment of Uniformity of Steroid Receptor Analyses

An extensive problem for the clinical chemist has been the lack of uniformity in the methods of receptor analyses in the clinical laboratory and in the expression of specific steroid binding data. Certain clinical cooperative groups, namely the National Surgical Adjuvant Breast Project (NSABP) with headquarters at the University of Pittsburgh and the Southeastern Cancer Study Group (SECSG) with headquarters at the University of Alabama have initiated experimental therapeutic protocols requiring analyses of estrogen and progestin receptors of breast tumors. Thus the establishment of assay uniformity and quality control is imperative to insure meaningful correlations between laboratory results and clinical response.

Firstly, we have generated a number of tissue reference powders composed of various quantities of frozen, pulverized organs such as uterus, breast, muscle, and liver as well as certain types of sera (e.g., of pregnancy). Breast tumors also were added to certain powders. Each of these reference powders is formulated in such a manner to contain different combinations of estrogen and progestin receptors, i.e., estrogen receptor positive, progestin receptor negative; estrogen receptor positive, progestin receptor positive, etc. Routinely, a laboratory from an institution participating in the cooperative trial is sent a set of four tissue powders frozen in dry ice. The laboratory analyzes these using "in house" methodology and returns the results to the headquarters of the NSABP or of the SECSG for comparison with data generated by other laboratories in the Cooperative Group and by the Reference Laboratory. Presently, we have developed 95% confidence intervals of the specific steroid binding capacities of each powder using the titration analysis and dextran-coated charcoal. These data provide preliminary guidelines regarding the determination of agreement of assay results among the laboratories of the Cooperative Groups (see Table 2). As our program improves, we plan to develop tolerance limits which appear to more accurately express agreement in statistical terms. The dextran-coated charcoal procedure appears to be the most widely utilized for estimating estrogen and progestin receptors of human breast tumors by clinical laboratories in the United States and Canada.

Furthermore, if a laboratory used by a member of the NSABP or of the SECSG needs assistance with the development of a receptor procedure or with the modification of an established method, our laboratory also accomodates them either at the University of Louisville or at their institution. Thus far, we have participated in the establishment of uniformity in steroid receptor analyses in more than one hundred laboratories in North America [55 laboratories used by NSABP institutions; 15 laboratories used by SECSG institutions; 36 laboratories not participating directly in clinical trials (including commercial institutions)] and in the development of steroid receptor reference facilities at the University of Düsseldorf in West Germany and at the University of Innsbruck in Austria.

An important consideration every laboratory contributing data to a cooperative treatment trial must evaluate is the extent of variability expected in steroid receptor analyses. To determine the amount of variation we suggest that each person measuring steroid receptors in

Table 2. Criteria for agreement of results from steroid receptor analyses of reference powders by institutions of the NSABP and the SECSG

1.	All (+)
2.	3 (+), 1 (±)
3.	2 (+), 2 (±)
4.	1 (+), 3 (±)
5.	All (±)

(+), within 95% confidence interval;
(±), outside 95% confidence interval but agreement on receptor status;
(–), nonagreement.

Table 3. Analyses of estrogen receptors in reference powders used to establish uniformity of these assays in clinical trials

	Reference powder[a]		
Technician	No. 1	No. 2	No. 3
1	262 ± 15[a]	189 ± 48	59 ± 6
2	208 ± 11	149 ± 9	70 ± 9
3	227 ± 18	138 ± 3	63 ± 5
4	234 ± 18	181 ± 8	74 ± 5
5	190 ± 31	153 ± 6	65 ± 3

[a] Mean ± standard error of three determinations expressed as fmol/mg cytosol protein. Specific estrogen binding capacity was determined by titration analyses using the dextran coated charcoal procedure.

a clinical laboratory estimate the receptor content on a series of tissue reference powders using at least three titration analyses.

The results of such an experiment whereby five different individuals performed three separate estrogen receptor analyses on three different tissue reference powders is shown in Table 3. The random variation within the powders determined from the data in Table 4 was 30.4 fmol/mg cytosol protein for this particular experiment. Surprisingly the amount of variation in the results estimated between the five individuals participating in this experiment was *less* than the amount of random variation expected, i.e., 10.7 fmol/mg (the other source of variance came from within the powders, 30.4 fmol/mg) cytosol protein. These types of data are useful in bringing about quality control within a laboratory. We recommend that each facility analyzing steroid receptors in clinical material develop a tissue reference powder for daily monitoring of procedures. Because of the lability of these intracellular proteins, the selection of a tissue for preparation of the reference powder is critical. We have had good experience with calf uterus frozen in liquid nitrogen shortly after removal and pulverized while in the frozen state. The advantage of a tissue powder over a reference cytosol or a lyophilyzed tissue is that it permits evaluation of the homogenizing procedure, clearly a critical step in the quantification of steroid receptor analyses.

In summary, it is generally accepted that estrogen and progestin binding capacities of tumor biopsies be included with other criteria used in the selection of endocrine therapies for the patient with advanced breast cancer. Data from the authors' laboratory and those of other investigators suggest that a new generation of clinical tests performed directly on the tumor specimen will not only provide information on the response potential (binding site levels) of a carcinoma but will access the quality and possibly the duration of the remission.

Acknowledgements

The authors acknowledge the important contributions of Mr. Dewitt T. Baker, Jr., and Ms. Sandra A. Wiehle of the Reference Laboratory, Ms. Leslie N. Kane and Mr. Miles Hall of the Clinical Laboratory and Dr. Pamela Wheeler Feldhoff. The authors express their appreciation to Mr. John Sandoz for his assistance with the entry of data into the computer bank and to Diane S. Mason for her assistance with the typescript. Portions of these studies were supported in part by a developmental grant from the American Cancer Society and by funds from USPHS grants to the National Surgical Adjuvant Breast Project and to the Southeastern Cancer Study Group (CA-19657) awarded by the National Cancer Institute.

References

Allegra, J. C., Lippman, M. E., Thompson, E. B., Simon, R.: An association between steroid hormone receptors and response to cytotoxic chemotherapy in patients with metastatic breast cancer. Cancer Res. *38,* 4299–4307 (1978)

Buller, R. E., O'Malley, B. W.: The biology and mechanism of steroid hormone receptor interaction with eukaryotic nucleus. Biochem. Pharmacol. *25,* 1–12 (1976)

Folca, P. J., Glascock, R. F., Irvine, W. T.: Studies with tritiumlabeled hexoestrol in advanced breast cancer. Lancet *1961 II,* 789

Gorski, J., Toft, D., Shyamala, G., Smith, D., Notides, A.: Hormone receptors: studies on the interaction of estrogen with the uterus. Recent Prog. Horm. Res. *24,* 45–80 (1968)

Horwitz, K. B., McGuire, W. L.: Specific progesterone receptors in human breast cancer. Steroids *25,* 497–505 (1975)

Jensen, E. V., Block, G. E., Smith, S., Kyser, K., DeSombre, E. R.: Estrogen receptors and breast cancer response to adrenalectomy. Natl. Cancer Inst. Monogr. *34,* 55–79 (1971)

Jensen, E. V., Mohla, S., Gorell, T. A., DeSombre, E. R.: The role of estrophilin in estrogen action. Vitam. Horm. *32,* 89–127 (1974)

Jensen, E. V., Polley, T. Z., Smith, S., Block, G. E., Ferguson, D. J., DeSombre, E. R.: Prediction of hormone dependency in human breast cancer. In: Estrogen receptors in human breast cancer. McGuire, W. L., Carbone, P. P., Vollmer, E. P. (eds.), pp. 37–56. New York: Raven Press 1975

Jensen, E. V., Suzuku, T., Kawashima, T., Stumpf, W. E., Jungblut, P. W., DeSombre, E. R.: A two-step mechanism for the interaction of estradiol with rat uterus. Proc. Natl. Acad. Sci. *59,* 632–639 (1968)

Kute, T. E., Heidemann, P., Wittliff, J. L.: Molecular heterogeneity of cytosolic forms of estrogen receptors from human breast tumors. Cancer Res. *38,* 4307–4313 (1978)

McGuire, W. L. (ed.): Hormones, receptors and breast cancer. New York: Raven Press 1978

McGuire, W. L., Carbone, P. O., Vollmer, E. P. (eds.): Estrogen receptors in human breast cancer. New York: Raven Press 1975

Park, D. C., Wittliff, J. L.: Assessment of "activation" of estrogen receptors in lactating mammary gland using DNA-cellulose binding. Biochem. Biophys. Res. Commun. *78,* 251–257 (1977)

Wittliff, J. L.: Specific receptors of the steroid hormones in breast cancer. Semin. Oncol. *1,* 109–119 (1974)

Wittliff, J. L.: Steroid-binding proteins in normal and neoplastic mammary cells. In: Methods in cancer research. Vol. XI. Busch, H. (ed.), pp. 298–354. New York: Academic Press 1975

Wittliff, J. L., Beatty, B. W., Savlov, E. D., Patterson, W. B., Cooper, R. A., Jr.: Estrogen receptors and hormone dependency in human breast cancer. In: Breast cancer: a multidisciplinary approach. St. Arneault, G., Band, P., Israël, L. (eds.), pp. 59–77. Berlin, Heidelberg, New York: Springer 1976

Wittliff, J. L., Hilf, R., Brooks, W. F., Jr., Savlov, E. D., Hall, T. C., Orlando, R. A.: Specific estrogen-binding capacity of the cytoplasmic receptor in normal and neoplastic tissues of humans. Cancer Res. *32,* 1983–1992 (1972)

Wittliff, J. L., Lewko, W. M., Park, D. C., Kute, T. E., Baker, D. T., Jr., Kane, L. N.: Steroid binding proteins of mammary tissues and their clinical significance in breast cancer. In: Hormones, receptors and breast cancer. McGuire, W. L. (ed.), pp. 325–359. New York: Raven Press 1978

Wittliff, J. L., Mehta, R. G., Kute, T. E.: Interaction of R5020 with binding sites in normal and neoplastic mammary tissues. In: Progesterone receptors in normal and neoplastic tissues. McGuire, W. L., Raynaud, J. P., Baulieu, E. E. (eds.), pp. 39–57. New York: Raven Press 1977

VIII. Anti-Oestrogen Treatment in Breast Cancer – A Comprehensive Review

30. Clinical Experience with Tamoxifen in Advanced Breast Cancer

B. A. Stoll

St. Thomas' Hospital, Department Oncology, London SE1 7EH (U.K.)

The discussion on clinical experience with tamoxifen concentrated on 18 questions answered by a panel, which reached the following conclusions:

1) What is the Response Rate to Tamoxifen and the Duration of Response?

When tamoxifen is used as the first method of systemic therapy in advanced breast cancer, objective evidence of tumour regression (over 50% decrease in size) occurs in about 30%–35% of cases overall, and complete regression occurs in about one-third of these cases. When it is used as secondary therapy, the objective response rate is lower – only about 20%–25%. The mean duration of response reported is 9–15 months in large series, and many of the patients on whose experience this is based were still alive at the time of the reports. Remissions of 3–4 years are not uncommon. In addition to objective regression of the tumour, a subjective response occurs in about 60% of patients treated. It includes a general feeling of well-being, increased appetite and weight, and relief of bone pain even without recalcification of bone metastases. The cause of the last observation is not known.

2) What is the Optimum Dosage Level for Tamoxifen in Breast Cancer?

Pharmacokinetic mechanisms of tamoxifen in man need further investigation. Early reports suggested that 40 mg tamoxifen daily yielded a higher response rate than did 20 mg daily, but this was not confirmed in later reports. The avoidance of unnecessarily high dosage of tamoxifen – as used by some trialists – may be particularly important when it is used for long-term adjuvant therapy, and it might be advisable to adjust the dosage according to the body surface. Further clinical trials are necessary to clarify this point, and also to correlate oral intake of the drug with circulating levels in the blood. Furthermore, we need more information on how to fractionate drug dosage over the 24 h, because it appears that tamoxifen has a fairly long half-life in the blood.

3) What is the Correlation Between Response to Tamoxifen and Previous Treatment?

It is not certain whether response to tamoxifen is more likely after previous failure of hormonal therapy or after failed cytotoxic therapy, but both occur in a small proportion of cases. A degree of case selection obviously accounts for the divergent results published.

However, most reports agree that there is about a 60% likelihood of response to secondary tamoxifen therapy after objective response to another form of hormonal therapy has been lost. Response to tamoxifen therapy may occur even when high-dosage oestrogen therapy or hypophyseal ablation no longer control the disease, but it is better given *before* these methods, because it is just as effective and its morbidity and side effects are less. The few available reports suggest that response to oestrogen therapy is unlikely after loss of response to tamoxifen therapy.

4) What is the Correlation Between Response to Tamoxifen and Age Group?

Age is also an important factor in the prediction of response to tamoxifen therapy. The response rate rises with increasing age, being less than 30% up to the age of 55 but about 50% after the age of 70. When the response rate is assessed in relation to the menopause, it is about 20% in the first 5 years after the menopause, 30% between 5 and 10 years after the menopause, and over 40% in patients in whom the menopause has occurred more than 10 years previously. Like high-dosage oestrogen therapy, tamoxifen shows its best results in the elderly patient with slow-growing soft-tissue involvement from breast cancer.

5) What is the Correlation Between Response to Tamoxifen and Site of Metastasis?

There is universal agreement that tamoxifen therapy shows its highest response rate in the case of soft-tissue involvement – advanced primary breast cancer, infiltrating skin nodules, and regional metastatic nodes. The response rate in such cases is approximately 40% overall for all age groups. There is less agreement over the response rate of bone metastases, and reported rates vary with the criteria of response. Overall figures suggest a 10%–20% likelihood of response to tamoxifen in the case of bone metastases, and this is similar to the response rate to high-dosage oestrogen. For visceral metastases the overall response rate is about 20%–30%, but it varies in each series according to selection of cases. The best responses are in lung and peritoneal deposits, although occasional responses of liver metastases may occur in oestrogen receptor-positive (ER) cases.

6) What is the Relationship of Oestrogen Receptor Assay to Response Rate?

Accumulated data now make it clear that tumour regression after tamoxifen therapy occurs in 50%–60% of ER+ cases but in only 5%–10% of ER– cases. The correlation is almost identical with that seen with other endocrine treatments. There was some confusion when early reports failed to show a clear correlation between ER assay of the tumour and the likelihood of response to tamoxifen therapy. This may have been because the majority of cases reported in the early series had previously failed to respond to cytotoxic therapy or other forms of hormonal treatment, resulting in a type of case selection. Although ER+ cases tend to show longer recurrence-free intervals, there is no clear evidence so far that the response rate to tamoxifen increases with increasing length of the recurrence-free interval.

7) What is the Role of Tamoxifen in Premenopausal Breast Cancer?

To date there are reports of about 120 premenopausal patients with advanced breast cancer treated with tamoxifen. They represent the cumulative experience of about 10 different centres. About 30% of cases have shown evidence of tumour regression (over 50% decrease in size of the tumor), and the figure is almost identical with the response rate in postmenopausal patients. Surprisingly, oestradiol levels in the serum have been found to be raised in tamoxifen-treated patients, even in those showing tumour regression on therapy. After loss of response to tamoxifen therapy a second response has been occasionally obtained by castration.

8) What is the Role of Tamoxifen in the Adjuvant Treatment of Operable Breast Cancer?

Interest in the use of tamoxifen for adjuvant treatment of operable breast cancer has increased for two major reasons. Firstly, it has recently become clear that current trials of cytotoxic adjuvant therapy in breast cancer are showing significant delay in recurrence only in premenopausal and not in postmenopausal Stage II cases, which suggests that at least part of the benefit must be achieved through endocrine mechanisms. Secondly, recent reports of a randomised trial show that a combination of X-ray castration and prednisone given after surgery not only delays recurrence but actually increases 10-year survival in premenopausal women over the age of 45 with operable breast cancer.
A number of randomised clinical trials have been set up with tamoxifen used as adjuvant therapy in either Stage I or Stage II breast cancer. It will be several years before we can assess its long-term effect on recurrence and survival and compare it with that of cytotoxic therapy alone and that of a combination of tamoxifen and cytotoxic treatment.

9) What is the Role of Tamoxifen in Male Breast Cancer?

Because breast cancer is rare in the male, it is difficult to establish the best forms of treatment. Different authors have reported occasional cases of the advanced disease treated with tamoxifen, either alone or in combination with some other therapy. Partial or complete regression of tumour has been noted occasionally with tamoxifen therapy alone, and in some patients the response has lasted a year or longer. Tamoxifen appears to be well tolerated by males and it is worth a trial as the first treatment in advanced breast cancer, especially as an alternative to the psychologically distressing operation of castration and the feminising effects of oestrogen therapy.

10) What is the Effect of Tamoxifen on the Serum Prolactin Level?

According to one report, administration of tamoxifen reduced the circulating prolactin level and also the TRH-stimulable prolactin level in the serum, but this was not confirmed in another report. Such information may be important for the assessment of the role of prolactin in the growth of human breast cancer, because high-dosage oestrogen therapy has a similar effect to tamoxifen on the growth of advanced breast cancer, yet the former undoubtedly stimulates the release of prolactin from the pituitary gland.

11) What is the Effect of Tamoxifen on Pregnancy?

There is no evidence that tamoxifen is mitogenic or teratogenic in animals. We have little information on the effect of its continuous administration during human pregnancy. However, it has been used in the induction of ovulation in infertile women, and in the case of one woman who received three courses of the agent during the first trimester of pregnancy a normal baby was subsequently born.

12) What is the Tolerance to Tamoxifen and the Incidence of Side Effects?

In considering tolerance and side effects we must distinguish between mild side effects not interfering with the continuation of treatment and those that necessitate stopping or interrupting treatment. Mild side effects include moderate increase in weight, hot flushes, headache, pruritus vulvae, depression, slight nausea, and transient thrombocytopenia. These are generally reported in about 25% of patients in each series. On the other hand, in a recent survey of 1000 treated patients collected from several series, complications causing cessation of treatment occurred in less than 3% of all cases, and this compares with a 15%–20% withdrawal from therapy in the case of high-dosage oestrogen therapy.

The symptoms leading to interruption or cessation of tamoxifen treatment are mainly severe gastrointestinal symptoms, dizziness, skin rash, hypercalcaemia, and increase in tumour pain. Tamoxifen therapy is well tolerated even in patients with congestive cardiac failure. Many patients have now been on treatment for 5 years or longer without significant problems.

13) What is the Way to Manage Hypercalcaemia Following Tamoxifen Treatment?

It is important to define our terms. A rise in the serum calcium level within 14 days of the initiation of any type of hormonal therapy is usually ascribed to such therapy. Hypercalcaemia is thought to result from excessive calcium mobilisation in the presence of lytic metastases in bone, and may occur occasionally following tamoxifen therapy. It is sometimes associated with an increase in pain at the site of bone metastases. The incidence of hypercalcaemia during tamoxifen therapy varies in different reports, and it is possible that in some reported cases the calcium level may have been raised *before* hormonal therapy was instituted.

If serum calcium levels are not unduly high it is generally agreed that it is necessary only to stop tamoxifen therapy for about a week for the levels to return to normal in most cases. High levels of serum calcium are life-threatening, however, and it is therefore essential also to institute corticosteroid therapy and other forms of systemic therapy designed to reduce serum calcium levels, e.g., enhanced diuresis. When the hypercalcaemia settles, the corticosteroid can usually be safely discontinued and tamoxifen restored.

14) What is the Relationship of Oestrogen Receptor Assay to the Likelihood of Hypercalcaemia Developing During Anti-Oestrogen Therapy?

Two different observers have commented that the majority of patients showing evidence of hypercalcaemia soon after the initiation of anti-oestrogen therapy have tumours in which the results of ER assay are positive. A similar observation has also been made in the case of oestrogen-induced hypercalcaemia. Hormonally induced hypercalcaemia seems therefore to indicate the likelihood of a hormone-sensitive tumour, and this may explain why recalcification of bone metastases often occurs when hormone therapy is continued subsequently.

15) What is the Significance of Thrombocytopenia Complicating Tamoxifen Therapy?

Reports on the appearance of thrombocytopenia following tamoxifen therapy show widely divergent incidence rates, but overall the rate of occurrence is certainly less than 10%. In the vast majority of cases the depression in the count is slight and transient, but occasionally the platelet level has been noted to fall below 50000 mm^3. In such a case, interruption of the treatment for 1–2 weeks allows the blood count to recover. It is suspected by some that the fall in platelet count may indicate a previously undetected replacement of the bone marrow by tumour.

16) How do the Clinical Effects Compare with Those of Clomiphene and Nafoxidine?

Two other anti-oestrogens – clomiphene citrate and nafoxidine – have both been claimed to yield an overall 30% response rate in advanced breast cancer. Not only do they show a similar overall response rate to tamoxifen therapy, but there is a similar variation of their effectiveness with age group and site of metastases. Severe side effects of clomiphene at the therapeutic dose include nausea and vomiting, hot flushes, blurred vision, and a danger of cataract, while those of nafoxidine include gastrointestinal symptoms, the development of skin hypersensitivity to sunlight, and a predisposition to cataract. All agree that the side effects of tamoxifen are minimal in comparison, although the spectrum of activity of all three agents appears to be similar in the treatment of breast cancer.

17) What is the Significance of a Flare Following Tamoxifen Therapy?

A flare in breast cancer following the initiation of hormonal therapy of any type usually involves an increase in pain, redness or swelling over soft tissue metastases, or a sudden increase in pain at the site of presumed tumour deposits. This is reported in 1%–2% of cases treated with tamoxifen, and usually appears within 7 days of the initiation of treatment. Whatever its cause, it seems to indicate hormone sensitivity, because there is evidence of tumour regression in a high proportion of cases if tamoxifen therapy is continued.

18) What is the Evidence for Tumour Acceleration by Tamoxifen?

This question is related to the previous one. It has often been suggested that a local flare indicates an increase in the growth rate of breast cancer as a result of growth stimulation by tamoxifen. However, in cases where several measurements of the tumour size have been plotted carefully *before* the initiation of therapy, there is no evidence of an increase in the slope of the growth curve during the period of the flare. It was suggested that the local reaction might be due to the release of some prostaglandin-like agent and that it is safe to continue tamoxifen therapy in these cases, perhaps with the addition of antiphlogistic agents or corticosteroids to control the local reaction.

31. The Place of Tamoxifen in the Treatment of Breast Cancer

P. S. Schein

Vincent-T.-Lombardi Cancer Research Center, Georgetown University, School of Medicine, Section of Medical Oncology, 3800 Reservoir Road, Washington D.C. (USA)

The aim of a round-table discussion was to place the current clinical data into a more complete prospective, and to identify the issues that remain to be resolved. There is general agreement that, with proper case selection, tamoxifen is both effective and relatively nontoxic.
One of the main questions is the problem of patient selection, and specifically the role of receptor measurements.
What criteria exist for the designation "estrogen receptor-rich (ER-rich) tumor"? Cut-off values ranging from 10—20 fmol/mg cytosol protein have been reported. In the experience of JENSEN there was very little prospect of response if there were no detectable receptors in the tumor. The number of receptors he considered necessary for an objective remission was arrived at empirically, based upon a retrospective analysis of clinical and laboratory data from his own institution. The threshold level for ER-rich differed between the pre- and postmenopausal patients. Two levels of prediction should be used, unless one determines the nucleus-occupied as well as the cytoplasmic receptor in the premenopausal group. JENSEN described his method of nuclear exchange for tumors removed from patients exposed to endogenous or exogenous estrogens; it employs silver nitrate as a means of dissociating the hormone from the receptor, the reaction being carried out at 0° C so as to avoid decomposition of the receptor. While the majority of investigators have reported their receptor data in terms of femtomoles per milligram of protein, JENSEN recommended the data be expressed in terms of grams of tumor or micrograms of DNA. The use of cytosol protein, unless it is corrected for contaminating serum protein, can result in a false estimate of receptor concentration. Patients with the highest concentrations of ERs have a greater probability of achieving an objective response with hormonal therapy. Similarly, the rate of remission is significantly higher in tumors containing both ERs and progesterone receptors (PgRs) than in tumors that have only ERs. Nevertheless, patients with only ERs should not be denied endocrine therapy, since an estimated 30% will respond. In terms of practical utility, the PgR currently has limited value. There is also some question as to whether the PgR functions as an independent prognostic variable, since positive cases also have the higher levels of estrogen receptors.
MAASS and JENSEN both agreed that correlations between receptor-rich tumors and clinical response have been most favorable with ablative therapy. While it is accepted that patients with receptor-rich tumors are the most likely to benefit from tamoxifen, there are examples of response in receptor-poor cases. This was most notable in the studies presented by ENGELSMAN and in the series of MAASS. These authors emphasized that additional studies in

"borderline" receptor cases are needed to clarify these initial results. It was generally agreed that, given the variability in methodology and patient populations, each institution must decide empirically what level of ER concentration constitutes a positive value; this determination should be based upon the retrospective correlation with clinical response.

The principal application for tamoxifen in the management of breast cancer has been in the treatment of postmenopausal patients with advanced stages of the disease. Additional aspects of the central question of patient selection are raised in the discussions on the position of tamoxifen in relation to other therapeutic options, endocrine and nonendocrine, already available for this group of patients.

HENNINGSEN stated his preference for endocrine therapy, and specifically tamoxifen, as the initial treatment. He emphasized the general clinical features of the postmenopausal patient, including a high incidence of ER-rich neoplasms, relatively slow tumor growth, high remission rates, and long durations of response, averaging 27 months in his series. The low frequency of serious toxic reactions stands in contrast to the effects of cytotoxic chemotherapy. This basic position was confirmed by several others.

CAVALLIS' experience with tamoxifen has not been as optimistic, and he reports only a 23% remission rate and 12 months median duration of response for previously untreated postmenopausal patients. This compared with a 50% response rate with chemotherapy. Chemotherapy is his preferred initial treatment for patients with extensive hepatic metastases or large tumor mass. MOURIDSEN advocated the use of chemotherapy for younger postmenopausal patients (less than 65 years) for whom there is no information on ER status.

It was stressed that the ER status of the patient is only one variable in the decision-making process. MAASS takes into account the age of the patient, the disease-free interval, and the localization of metastases. Hepatic and cerebral metastases have represented very poor contraindications for endocrine therapy based upon past experience with other hormonal therapies. SCHEIN suggested that our concepts regarding the responsiveness of hepatic metastases may be subject to revision; several series with tamoxifen have yielded response rates of 40%–60% for ER+ liver-dominant disease.

ENGELSMAN regards the rate of tumor proliferation as an essential factor in patient selection. With slow-growing neoplasms he would use tamoxifen as the sole therapy. However, with a history of rapid tumor growth, chemotherapy is indicated even if the neoplasm is ER-rich. This author raised the question of combined endocrine and chemotherapy in such cases.

There is at present no basis upon which to choose between tamoxifen and estrogen as the initial endocrine therapy for the postmenopausal patient. Several reports state a preference for tamoxifen because of its reduced toxicity.

It has been assumed that the principal role of the available ablative procedures, adrenalectomy and hypophysectomy, is the removal of a secondary source of estrogenic hormones. Can tamoxifen replace the past use of ablative therapies?

HENNINGSEN reported that in Heidelberg adrenalectomies are no longer performed and tamoxifen has been substituted. MOURIDSEN held that many breast cancer patients in Europe do not live near facilities where ablative procedures are readily available, and tamoxifen represents a worthwhile alternative for such cases. SCHEIN described the early results of PEARSON, who reported that 26% of patients who had obtained objective remission following hypophysectomy responded to tamoxifen. Similarly, a significant proportion of patients responding to tamoxifen achieved a secondary remission with the ablative procedure. These data raise serious questions as to whether tamoxifen can strictly be considered a substitute for ablative therapy. An additional consideration relates to the mechanism of action of tamoxifen; does it act solely as an antiestrogen, or does it possess an additional element of independent cytotoxicity? These questions remain open, and controlled trials are needed to determine whether tamoxifen can serve a complementary or additive role in conjunction with hypophysectomy and adrenalectomy.

The position of tamoxifen in the management of premenopausal women with advanced stages of disease has not yet been determined. This will require the completion of ongoing controlled trials comparing the response to tamoxifen in conjunction with, or as a substitute for, oophorectomy.

SCHEIN expressed his concern about the current trend of combining tamoxifen and cytotoxic chemotherapy, which he feels should be done with caution until data that unequivocally support this approach are available. Only a limited number of palliative treatment options are available for the patient with advanced breast cancer. The initial use of combined therapy imposes significant limitations on the management of the eventual relapse. Do the results of current trials support the use of combined therapy? There are no definitive data to indicate that combined therapy is superior to the sequential use of endocrine and cytotoxic regimens. The completed studies on the basis of which positive results are reported have design flaws. MOURIDSEN emphasized the need for continued clinical trials so that a maximally effective therapy can be developed and brought to the adjuvant situation, where treatment is not palliative but curative in intent.

The role of tamoxifen as an adjuvant therapy, when used alone or with chemotherapy, has still to be determined. Controlled trials for pre- and postmenopausal women, correlated with receptor status, are now in progress in several centers and cooperative groups.

In summary, tamoxifen represents a valuable addition to the theurapeutic armamentarium for breast cancer, and in particular for the postmenopausal patient with a metastatic receptor-rich tumor. A more complete understanding of this antiestrogen's role for premenopausal women and in adjuvant therapy awaits the results of current controlled trials.

Final Remarks

Final Remarks

As a final remark, it seems appropriate to update a pentalinear expression first recorded by PINCUS and VOLLMER[2] nearly twenty years ago at a time when a truly effective medical approach to the endocrine therapy of breast cancer was still only a pious hope.

A lady, with growth neoplastic,
Thought ablation to be a bit drastic.
She preferred that her ill
Might be cured with a pill
Which today is no longer fantastic.

That hope has become reality for metastasising breast cancer. And what once was fantasy may now be fact for many patients.

E. V. Jensen[1]

---

1 The University of Chicago, Ben May Laboratory for Cancer Research, 950 East 59th Street, Chikago, IL 60637 (USA).

2 G. PINCUS and E. P. VOLLMER, eds. *Biological Activities of Steroids in Relation to Cancer.* Proceedings. New York, Academic Press, 1960. p. 381.

Subject Index

Recent Results in Cancer Research

Sponsored by the Swiss League against Cancer. Editor in Chief: P. Rentchnick, Genève

For information about Vols. 1–9, please contact your bookseller or Springer-Verlag

10 Nelson, R. S.: Radioactive Phosphorus in the Diagnosis of Gastrointestinal Cancer.
11 Freeman, R. G. and J. M. Knox: Treatment of Skin Cancer.
12 Lynch, H. T.: Hereditary Factors in Carcinoma.
13 Tumours in Children, 2nd Edition. Edited by H. B. Marsden and J. K. Steward.
14 Odartchenko, N.: Production Cellulaire Erythropoïétique.
15 Sokoloff, B.: Carcinoid and Serotonin.
16 Jacobs, M. L.: Malignant Lymphomas and Their Management.
17 Normal and Malignant Cell Growth. Edited by R. J. M. Fry, M. L. Griem, and W. H. Kirsten (Symposium).
18 Anglesio, E.: The Treatment of Hodgkin's Disease.
19 Bannasch, P.: The Cytoplasm of Hepatocytes during Carcinogenesis. Electron- and Lightmicroscopical Investigations of the Nitrosomorpholineintoxicated Rat Liver.
20 Rubidomycin. A new Agent against Cancer. Edited by J. Bernard, R. Paul, M. Boiron, C. Jacquillat, and R. Maral.
21 Scientific Basis of Cancer Chemotherapy. Edited by G. Mathé (Symposium).
22 Koldovský, P.: Tumor Specific Transplantation Antigen.
23 Fuchs, W. A., J. W. Davidson, and H. W. Fischer: Lymphography in Cancer. With contributions by G. Jantet and H. Rösler.
24 Hayward, J.: Hormones und Human Breast Cancer. An Account of 15 Years Study.
25 Roy-Burman, P.: Analogues of Nucleic Acid Components. Mechanisms of Action.
26 Tumors of the Liver. Edited by G. T. Pack and A. H. Islami.
27 Szymendera, J.: Bone Mineral Metabolism in Cancer.
28 Meek, E. S.: Antitumour and Antiviral Substances of Natural Origin.
29 Aseptic Environments and Cancer Treatment. Edited by G. Mathé (Symposium).
30 Advances in the Treatment of Acute (Blastic) Leukemias. Edited by G. Mathé (Symposium).
31 Denoix, P.: Treatment of Malignant Breast Tumors. Indications and Results.
32 Nelson, R. S.: Endoscopy in Gastric Cancer.
33 Experimental and Clinical Effects of L-Asparaginase. Edited by E. Grundmann and H. F. Oettgen (Symposium).
34 Chemistry and Biological Actions of 4-Nitroquinolin 1-Oxide. Edited by H. Endo, T. Ono, and T. Sugimura.
35 Penn, I.: Malignant Tumors in Organ Transplant Recipients.
36 Current Concepts in the Management of Lymphoma and Leukemia. Edited by J. E. Ultmann, M. L. Griem, W. H. Kirsten, and R. W. Wissler (Symposium).
37 Chiappa, S., R. Musumeci, and C. Uslenghi: Endolymphatic Radiotherapy in Malignant Lymphomas. With contributions by G. Bonadonna, B. Damascelli, G. Fava, F. Pizzetti, U. Veronesi.
38 Koller, P. C.: The Role of Chromosomes in Cancer Biology.
39 Current Problems in the Epidemiology of Cancer and Lymphomas. Edited by E. Grundmann and H. Tulinius (Symposium).
40 Langley, F. A. and A. C. Crompton: Epithelial Abnormalities of the Cervix Uteri.
41 Tumours in a Tropical Country. A Survey of Uganda (1964–1968). Edited by A. C. Templeton.
42 Breast Cancer: A Challenging Problem. Edited by M. L. Griem, E. V. Jensen, J. E. Ultmann, and R. W. Wissler (Symposium).
43 Nomenclature, Methodology and Results of Clinical Trials in Acute Leukemias. Edited by G. Mathé, P. Pouillart, L. Schwarzenberg (Symposium).
44 Special Topics in Carcinogenesis. Edited by E. Grundmann (Symposium).
45 Koldovský, P.: Carcinoembryonic Antigens.
46 Diagnosis and Therapy of Malignant Lymphoma. Edited by K. Musshoff (Symposium).
47 Investigation and Stimulation of Immunity in Cancer Patients. Edited by G. Mathé and R. Weiner (Symposium).
48 Platinum Coordination Complexes in Cancer Chemotherapy. Edited by T. A. Connors and J. J. Roberts (Symposium).
49 Complications of Cancer Chemotherapy. Edited by G. Mathé and R. K. Oldham (Symposium).
50 Cancer Registry, Edited by E. Grundmann and E. Pedersen (Symposium).

51 Gliomas. Current Concepts in Biology, Diagnosis and Therapy. Edited by J. HEKMATPANAH (Symposium).

52 The Ambivalence of Cytostatic Therapy. Edited by E. GRUNDMANN and R. GROSS (Symposium).

53 A. CLARYSSE, Y. KENIS, and G. MATHÉ: Cancer Chemotherapy.

54 Malignant Bone Tumors. Edited by E. GRUNDMANN.

55 MATHÉ, G.: Cancer Active Immunotherapy, Immunoprophylaxis, and Immunorestoration.

56 Lymphocytes, Macrophages, and Cancer. Edited by G. MATHÉ, I. FLORENTIN, and M.-C. SIMMLER (Symposium).

57 Breast Cancer: A Multidisciplinary Approach. Edited by G. ST. ARNEAULT, P. BAND, and L. ISRAËL (Symposium).

58 B. S. SCHOENBERG: Multiple Primary Malignant Neoplasms.

59 Selective Heat Sensitivity of Cancer Cells. Edited by A. ROSSI-FANELLI, R. CAVALIERE, B. MONDOVI, and G. MORICCA.

60 Tumors of the Male Genital System. Edited by E. GRUNDMANN and W. VAHLENSIECK (Symposium).

61 D. METCALF: Hemopoietic Colonies.

62 Tactics and Strategy in Cancer Treatment. Edited by G. MATHÉ (Symposium).

63 Antitumor Antibiotics. Edited by S. K. CARTER, H. UMEZAWA, J. DOUROS, and Y. SAKURAI (Symposium).

64 Lymphoid Neoplasias I: Classification, Categorization, Natural History.

65 Lymphoid Neoplasias II: Clinical and Therapeutic Aspects.
Lymphoid Neoplasias I & II. Proceedings of the 1977 CNRS-EORTC International Colloquium. Editors: G. MATHÉ, M. SELIGMANN, M. TUBIANA. Devided into two volumes.

66 Carcinogenic Hormones. Edited by C. H. LINGEMAN.

67/68 Adjuvant Therapies and Markers of Post-Surgical Minimal Residual Disease I & II. Proceedings of the 1978 Annual Plenary Meeting of the EORTC. Editors: G. BONADONNA, G. MATHÉ, S. E. SALMON. Divided into two volumes:

67 Markers and General Problems of Cancer Adjuvant Therapies.

68 Adjuvant Therapies of the Various Primary Tumors.

69 Strategies in Clinical Hematology. Edited by R. GROSS and K.-P. HELLRIEGEL.

70 New Anticancer Drugs. Edited by S. K. CARTER

71 Endocrine Treatment of Breast Cancer. Edited by B. HENNINGSEN, F. LINDER, C. STREICHELE.

MIX
Papier aus verantwortungsvollen Quellen
Paper from responsible sources
FSC® C105338

If you have any concerns about our products,
you can contact us on
ProductSafety@springernature.com

In case Publisher is established outside the EU,
the EU authorized representative is:
Springer Nature Customer Service Center GmbH
Europaplatz 3, 69115 Heidelberg, Germany

Printed by Libri Plureos GmbH
in Hamburg, Germany